# WESTERN CIVILIZATION FROM 1500

*4th Edition*

**Ahmed H. Ibrahim, Ph.D.**
Missouri State University
Springfield, MO

Walther Kirchner, Ph.D.

**Contributing Editor**
Chad Ross, Ph.D.
University of Missouri
Columbia, MO

# Collins

*An Imprint of HarperCollinsPublishers*

**WESTERN CIVILIZATION FROM 1500.** (Fourth edition.) Copyright © 1958, 1966 by Harper & Row, Publishers, Inc. Copyright © 1975 by Walther Kirchner. Copyright © 1991, 2007 by HarperCollins Publishers. All rights reserved. Printed in the United States. No part of this book may be used or reproduced in any manner whatsoever without written permission except in the case of brief quotations embodied in critical articles and reviews. For information address HarperCollins Publishers, 10 East 53rd Street, New York, NY 10022.

**An American BookWorks Corporation Production**

HarperCollins books may be purchased for educational, business, or sales promotional use. For information please write: Special Markets Department, HarperCollins Publishers, 10 East 53rd Street, New York, NY 10022.

---

Library of Congress Cataloging-in-Publication Data

Ibrahim, Ahmed H. (Ahmed Hassan), 1957-
Western civilization from 1500 / Ahmed H. Ibrahim, Walter Kirchner ; contributing editor, Chad Ross. – 4th ed.
    p. cm. – (Collins college outlines series)
  Includes bibliographical references and index.
  ISBN: 978-0-06-088160-3
  ISBN-10: 0-06-088160-7
  1. Civilization, Western—History. I. Kirchner, Walter. II. Ross, Chad. III. Title.

CB245.I27 2007
909′.09821—dc22                                                 2007060877

---

07 08 09 10 11 CW 10 9 8 7 6 5 4 3 2 1

# Contents

Preface .... v
Chapter 1: The Ancient World: Foundation of the West .... 1
Chapter 2: The Medieval Heritage .... 12
Chapter 3: The Beginning of "The Modern Age" (1492-1517) .... 23
Chapter 4: The New Monarchies (1455-1519) .... 36
Chapter 5: The Age of the Reformation (1517-1555) .... 43
Chapter 6: The Aftermath of Renaissance and Reformation (1555-1603) .... 58
Chapter 7: The Emergence of the Modern State System (1603-1648) .... 74
Chapter 8: The Age of Louis XIV (1643-1715) .... 91
Chapter 9: The Age of Enlightenment (1715-1774) .... 109
Chapter 10: The Age of Revolution (1775-1795) .... 130
Chapter 11: The Napoleonic Era (1795-1815) .... 140
Chapter 12: Nationalism, Liberalism, Industrialism (1815-1830) .... 155
Chapter 13: Society, Arts, and Sciences (1815-1848) .... 167
Chapter 14: The Bourgeois Era and Revolution (1830-1848) .... 179
Chapter 15: Political Reorganization (1848-1870) .... 192
Chapter 16: Revaluation of Values (1848-1870) .... 207
Chapter 17: The Era of Bismarck (1870-1890) .... 217
Chapter 18: Economic and Cultural Trends (1870-1914) .... 232
Chapter 19: The Road to World War I (1890-1914) .... 247
Chapter 20: War, Peace, and Revolution (1914-1919) .... 264
Chapter 21: The Twilight of Liberalism (1921-1929) .... 279
Chapter 22: Depression, Fascism, and War (1929-1945) .... 298
Chapter 23: The Postwar Era (1947-1967) .... 318
Chapter 24: A World in Transition (1968-1984) .... 336
Chapter 25: The End of the Cold War and the New Challenges (1985-Present) .... 348

Index .... 361

# Preface

Walther Kirchner's *Western Civilization from 1500* has been, for many years, among the most important supplemental works in the study of Western civilization. Since it first appeared in 1958, it has gone through three editions, which were published in 1966, 1975 and 1991. After Professor Kirchner's death in June 2004, I completed work on this fourth edition.

For the fourth edition, I have made many changes affecting almost every chapter. Many significant events have taken place in many Western societies since the early 1990s, and coverage of these affairs has been added. Further, new research regarding earlier times has been incorporated into each chapter. Since a variety of high-quality materials addressing the history of Western civilization since 1500 continue to appear in great abundance, I have expanded the bibliographic references found at the end of each chapter to accommodate the most recent general studies and monographs dealing with this topic. Despite the additions and changes, the total length of the work, 25 chapters, is about the same as the previous edition. Each chapter includes a brief introduction, a general perspective, and a "test-yourself" question-and-answer section. In addition, this fourth edition makes maps of previous editions clearer and more effective and adds numerous new ones.

To better understand key developments in the past five centuries, I have been careful to avoid superficial generalizations that oversimplify historical periods and transitions. I have attempted to state and interpret as many facts as possible, given the space, in order to provide students with a frame of reference within which to comprehend the principal events and eras in Western history.

I am very grateful to the many friends and family members who have provided encouragement and support during the time needed to complete this project. In particular, my thanks go to Marina G. Ibrahim, John Chuchiak, and Dale Streeter. I also would like to thank Fred Grayson of the American BookWorks Corporation. for inviting me to undertake this project.

I hope that this fourth edition will be as useful to students and general readers as earlier editions have been. In this way, the memory of Walther Kirchner will be commemorated.

**Ahmed H. Ibrahim**
**Springfield, Missouri**
**Summer 2006**

**CHAPTER 1**

# The Ancient World: Foundation of the West

**ca. 720 B.C.E.** Homer, *Iliad*
**ca. 680 B.C.E.** Homer, *Odyssey*
**ca. 470-399 B.C.E** Socrates
**ca. 450-420 B.C.E** Herodotus, *Histories*
**ca. 428-347 B.C.E** Plato
**ca. 420-400 B.C.E.** Thucydides, *History of the Peloponnesian War*
**ca. 384-322 B.C.E.** Aristotle
**264 B.C.E.** All of Italy under Roman control
**ca. 106-43 B.C.E.** Cicero, the greatest Latin orator
**27 B.C.E.-14 C.E.** Cesar Augustus's rule
**121 C.E.-180 C.E.** Marcus Aurelius's rule
**476 C.E.** Fall of Western Roman Empire

*The Modern Age begins around 1500 C.E. Historians generally date it from the year 1492 C.E. By then, Western civilization had undergone an evolution of more than five thousand years. Great empires and civilizations had arisen—and disappeared. Egyptians, Babylonians, Hittites, Assyrians, Persians, Hebrews, Phoenicians, Etruscans, Greeks, and Romans had acted on the stage of Western history. All of them had flourished in the same comparatively small area, restricted to lands that surrounded the eastern Mediterranean basin and extended eastward to India and the valley of the Tigris and Euphrates rivers. Geographic links connected the various peoples; their commercial enterprises, religious beliefs, artistic creations, and political fates were interwoven. The inventions and achievements of each civilization nourished the thought and the work of civilizations that came after it.*

*Time has annihilated most of what they produced. Our knowledge of the oldest precursors of Western civilization has increased, however, owing to the recent work of archaeologists. Yet any direct impact of the Egyptians and Babylonians, Persians and Phoenicians, or Hittites and Etruscans is hard to find because there are few surviving monuments. Only indirectly has their legacy been preserved. These older cultures affected the Greeks and Romans and, through them, modern Western civilization. Even the influence of the Hebrews can be seen only indirectly, chiefly in the ethical principles that have come down to us through Christianity.*

*Figure 1-1 The major Greek City States during the Peloponnesian Wars*

## ■ GREEK CONTRIBUTIONS TO MODERN WESTERN CIVILIZATION

*The influence of the ancient Greeks can be felt directly in almost all facets of modern life. Greek culture has had a major impact on Western civilization.*

### Language

The first indication of Greece's significance is shown in the treasure trove of words that the modern world has embraced. Examples include such English words as philosophy, history, mathematics, aesthetics, mysticism, architecture, poetry, choir, monarchy, democracy, barbarism, theory, paper, and atom. Such words are not important simply for having entered our vocabulary. Rather, their importance lies in the fact that the concepts for which they stand have retained meaning for modern people. The thoughts behind them have enriched our thinking, and the ideas they represent have remained valid through the ages.

### Philosophy

Greek thought ranged widely and freely, restrained by clear and logical minds, but unimpeded by a written set of values, an enforced creed, or a dogma. This was perhaps the most important factor that helped to make the concepts of ancient Greece permanent and usable tools. The Greeks loved wisdom and sought a path to wise living. They studied the reality that surrounded them and tried first to understand it, then to master it. To achieve such mastery, they looked to noble qualities in human nature, to self-control, fortitude, and temperance. They studied themselves, both as individuals with individual aspirations and as members of a community with a common destiny. They searched for a compromise between the ideal state of human beings and the limited status imposed upon them by nature. The Greeks initiated various philosophical schools, including the Sophists, the Epicureans, the Stoics, and the Cynics. Socrates, Plato, and Aristotle (4th century B.C.E.) created systems of logic and concepts of ethics that still act as guides. They considered and developed various ways to direct people in their search for knowledge and drive to action. They recognized that the human mind cannot comprehend everything and that there are limits. Within these limits, philosophical investigations moved throughout the history of Western civilization.

## Science

With their rational procedures and their reliance upon logical deduction, the Greeks achieved remarkable insights into the works of nature. They arrived at these insights through speculation rather than observation and experimentation. This, to be sure, limited their achievement. Since they failed to evolve physical instruments that could have supplemented their methods and measured their results, they reached numerous erroneous conclusions. These, too, contributed to a lasting heritage: as the errors played an important role in the Greek view of the universe, so too, to a large extent, did they dominate Western thought well into the 19th century.

Simultaneously, however, the Greeks developed views that modern investigations have proved to be correct to an astounding degree. By means of logical deduction, they anticipated many findings acceptable to the modern world, and they prepared the way for fundamental procedures and discoveries. Among such significant achievements were those of Pythagoras, Archimedes, and Euclid in mathematics; of Democritus, who postulated an atomic theory; and of Thales, who taught that the Earth is a sphere.

In medicine, the works of Asclepiades, Hippocrates, and Galen have guided the medical profession into the present. They set forth fundamental concepts about the duties of a doctor (the Hippocratic Oath), and they recognized the value of sanitariums and healing springs, of hygiene and physical exercise. Moreover, recent psychological trends were anticipated by philosophers like Plato, who insisted on the interconnection of mind and body.

In zoology, data on the animal world were compiled by Aristotle. In geography, on the basis of philosophical speculation and travel accounts, a picture of the globe was drawn which, notwithstanding all its faults, determined the views of geographers well into the Modern Age and has given direction to almost 2,000 years of mapmaking. A special contribution was made by Greek philosophers in the field of education. The Socratic method of teaching by asking questions and demanding logical answers has become an integral part of modern pedagogy. Invariably, the modern world has gone back to Greek models in its search for a satisfactory path to learning.

Greek principles have survived even in military tactics. Though weapons have changed, wedge-like formations for attack and the oblique arrangement of battle forces, as used and described by the Greeks, have retained their usefulness.

## Art

Marked by its devotion to beauty, Greek civilization's sense of harmony induced its people not only to seek a comprehensible picture of human beings and the universe, but also to express their thoughts and feelings in a form that would inspire generations to come.

Nowhere is this striving for harmony of form and content more vividly expressed than in their architecture. The Greek temple has remained the best example of serene "classical" beauty. Hardly a town exists in the entire modern Western world where the Greek temple has not been copied outright or has not, at least, affected the style of public and private buildings. The simplicity and vigor of the Doric column, the grace of the Ionian, and the restrained exuberance of the Corinthian have never ceased to charm and inspire builders and architects. They have imitated Greek friezes, gables, and porticoes, seeking to achieve a similar clarity of line and simplicity of concept. The use of mathematical forms may explain the marvelous proportions of Greek architecture to some degree, but it is the meaningful ideas created by the great masters that have given their work its overwhelming appeal throughout the ages.

As in architecture, Greek sculpture has often been praised for its true-to-life quality. This is illustrated in the statues of Phidias, Praxiteles, and others. However, it was not merely the sculptures that are of lasting value; rather, it is the fact that an abstract concept of beauty and a thoughtful approach to life were combined and expressed in such realistic form.

Unfortunately, we know too little to about Greek painting, music, and dance to make similar assertions. There are many indications, however, that in these arts, too, the Greeks created works of unsurpassed beauty. Some of their instruments, such as the flute and lyre, were inherited by later cultures. Being more perishable than stone and marble, painting and music could not be passed on to future generations in the same way as buildings and sculpture.

## Literature

Time has taken a similar toll upon the written works of Greece. Only a small fraction of what the Greeks composed has come down to the Modern Age. It is surprising, therefore, that Greek literature has had such an unparalleled influence on later cultures. The very words for different poetic forms—tragedy, comedy, lyric, epic—or for different verse meters—iamb, dactyl, hexameter—bear witness to the historical importance of their literature. The epics of Homer, the *Iliad* and the *Odyssey*, are cherished to this day, and many children have dreamed of the mighty deeds of his heroes. What modern reader would not be awed by the breadth of Homer's vision of the human race, his insight into human emotions, the charm and meaningfulness of his parables? What poet or lover of poetry would not be captured by the infinite warmth and tenderness of the lyrics of Sappho, Pindar, or Anacreon? Their names may be less familiar than Homer's, but their influence has been felt, both consciously and unconsciously. Their poetry has given direction to the form and content of songs and poems in all subsequent ages.

Equally potent has been the influence of the great Greek dramatists, Sophocles, Aeschylus, and Aristophanes. Their individual topics, whether mythological or political, may have lost their relevance, but the general significance of their work has remained undiminished. Antigone's appeal to unwritten laws that may be higher than any man-made rules, Oedipus's tragic involvement in predestined guilt, and Orestes's battle against the Furies who are persecuting him for a crime that was necessary and preordained—never have these problems lost their hold upon our imagination. Our relationship to necessity, to a fate buried within our own nature as well as imposed by external forces, is an issue that not only engaged the attention of Greek thinkers and dramatists continuously, but it has also captured, puzzled, shaken, and inspired the modern mind.

## History

Greek civilization has often been described as unconcerned with history or as hostile to it, yet it produced some of the greatest historians. Among them were Herodotus, Xenophon, and, especially, Thucydides. Thucydides was perhaps more conscious of the permanent significance of his work than were the poets (who, while giving expression to lasting thought, addressed themselves to contemporary audiences). As he himself states, Thucydides set out to write a history that was to be a treasure for all time. His method of presenting historical events did not establish standards. A science of history did not evolve in Greece. But, through his artistic genius, the perfection of his treatment, the range of his presentation, the scope of his insight into the human drama, and his awareness of the limitations of human understanding, Thucydides left a work that has proved to be the very treasure he aspired to create.

## Statecraft

The political problems of a country as small as Greece were, in many ways, very different from those facing modern, industrialized, large nation-states. The basic unit of the Greek society was the city-state, called the *polis*. What has made the political achievements of Athens, Sparta, Thebes, and others so imposing is that the people did not merely adjust themselves pragmatically to a given political form, but rather gave thoughtful consideration to the fundamental issues that confront any human community. They did not, like others, unrealistically take on the despotic models or priest-dominated systems of neighboring societies. Instead, they experimented with monarchy, aristocracy, oligarchy, democracy, and tyranny. Seeking independence, law, and order, and—at least in Athens—the free development of the citizen, they worked out constitutions of the most varied types.

Although they experienced, like others, the weaknesses of these respective forms of government, the Greek philosophers and writers set themselves to the task of investigating various aspects of these forms, evaluating their relative merits and dangers. In poems, tragedies, and comedies, or in philosophical treatises, they set forth the conflicts that exist between civic duties and personal aspirations, between society and individual. Thus, a body of political writings emerged that dealt not only with the realities of life in ancient Greece and the problems of government and citizenship there, but also with the ideal of a utopian state where conflicting forces might ultimately be reconciled.

## Sports

The same sense of harmony that inspired Greek art and the Greek search for political order caused the Greeks to strive for the development of the individual, not only as a vehicle of spiritual aspirations, but with pride in the physical side of life as well. The beauty of the human body was a cherished ideal, and valor was expected of all, along with strength, fleetness, and grace. It was to further such ideals that the Greeks favored sports and instituted sporting competitions. Regularly, they held great festivals at Olympia, Corinth, and Delphi. True to the tradition of harmonious development of spirit, mind, and body, they generally started these events with religious rites and a dedication to the gods. Then, over a period of several days, they held sports competitions, wherein racing, discus throwing, and wrestling played prominent roles. They concluded the celebrations with musical and literary performances in which composers, writers, and artists vied for laurels. Separate festivals with similar programs were held for women. These occasions played such a vital role in Greek life that the very calendar of Greece was constructed with reference to the Olympic Games.

## Survival of Greek Civilization

Enthusiasm for Greek life has induced many historians to idealize Greek institutions, Greek thought, and Greek habits to such an extent that they have neglected the darker aspects and conditions in Greece. Little has been said about some of the attitudes that lay behind the Greek artistic and philosophical achievements. Some have forgotten that the Greeks were vain and arrogant people, who considered the entire world outside their borders "barbaric." They were, to an extent, quarrelsome, greedy, brutal, and oppressive. Slavery was an integral part of their social institutions. On a number of occasions, politicians and demagogues sacrificed the welfare of the state to personal ambitions. Regardless, what has survived are the immortal works of the few: the depth of thought of the greatest minds, the longing for freedom and free development of nation and individual as expressed in deeds, the artistic creations that Grecian sensitivity to beauty made possible, the penetration of nature's secrets, and the understanding of human life and ways—these guide all Western civilization.

## ■ THE ROMAN CONTRIBUTIONS TO MODERN WESTERN CIVILIZATION

If the Greek heritage has been praised for its legacy of rationality, truth, and beauty, the Roman heritage has been extolled for its practicality. Scant justice, however, has thus been done to Rome, for Rome, too, left a large spiritual heritage to future generations in its innumerable monuments, one that can well challenge that of Greece.

### Language

Like the Greek language, Latin too has made inestimable contributions to the civilization of the modern world. Just as with Greek, numerous Latin terms are part of modern vocabularies as are the concepts and institutions they represent. Among Latin-English words are citizen, family, census, senate, monument, and arch. Other words, which originally were Greek, entered the Latin and were preserved by the Romans. The Western world thus owes to Rome a debt of thanks for a vast store of experience, embodied in language, that otherwise would have had to be painfully worked out independently and anew.

### History

Most important among the legacies of Rome are those contributions that have taught the modern world a rational, reasonable approach to political conduct and nation-building. The political genius of

Figure 1-2 *The Roman Empire at its Greatest Extent, ca. 117 C.E.*

Rome, its ability to rule itself and others, to adapt itself to changing conditions, to invent checks and balances in order to avoid excesses, to overcome the threats of social challenges, to regulate "the relationship of man to man," altogether constitute an unequaled lesson for Western civilizations.

Preserved and evaluated by Livius, Tacitus, and others, the history of Rome furnishes insight into the evolution not only of Rome, but also of any great people. Its history is embodied in the traditions of every Mediterranean nation, in monuments erected in the most diverse countries, in their languages, law codes, and institutions. These Roman achievements, unlike those of Greece in its time of glory, were less the work of a few individuals of outstanding genius than, as the German historian Theodor Mommsen once wrote, the result of "extraordinary deeds" by "ordinary men."

## Law

Underlying the structure of the mighty empire that was eventually built by the Romans was a concept of law which, though it had many roots in Greek philosophical thought and derived as well from the many examples provided by the political systems of other Mediterranean nations, was nonetheless unique in the ancient world. A living procedure, Roman law could adapt to constantly changing situations. Only toward the very end of the empire, when the decay of the state had progressed to a great degree, did the law become codified in its various aspects.

Roman law embraced relationships between individuals. It progressively defined civic rights and the role of the citizen within the common republic. Its vocabulary is still in use, and its procedures serve as models even today. Its stipulations in regard to property, the conduct of business, matters of inheritance, marriage, and divorce, and numerous other fields have influenced codes of justice in all Western nations. Moreover, the international rules devised by Rome represent the beginning of a long path toward the development of a universal organization that would do justice to all members of the society of nations.

## Architecture and Public Construction

In architecture, the Romans are known less for their originality than for their genius at adaptation. To a large extent, they adopted the artistic concepts that the Greeks had evolved. They built temples following the styles of Greece, which still inspire us through their harmony of form and elegance of structure.

What the Romans took over they also applied to other types of architectural projects and construction that reflect an enterprising spirit and an inventive genius not shown by the Greeks. To these projects, Rome lent much of that same kind of beauty that had flourished in Greece. Mighty waterworks were completed, aqueducts were installed, bridges with noble spans were constructed across rivers and canals, viaducts were laid across valleys, and a *Cloaca Maxima* (sewer system) was built that continues to astound modern engineers. The most distant parts of the empire were connected by a remarkable system of roads, many of them still in use. For hundreds of miles, walls and forts were erected along endangered borders.

Beyond such necessities—witnesses of the practical inclinations of an empire-building society—the Romans also created remarkable public monuments for the beautification and glory of their state. Such projects simultaneously helped to solve social problems by furnishing work for the unemployed and providing entertainment for the discontented classes. The Romans erected triumphal arches, constructed columns celebrating victories, and adorned these structures with inscriptions and representations of Rome's deeds of glory. They built public baths, the Colosseum and, in many cities, large arenas. The private houses of the rich, such as those found in long-buried Pompeii, were embellished with beautiful frescoes, sculptures, mosaics, and fountains.

## Literature

As was the case in architecture, Rome did not initiate many new styles in the field of literature. The Romans did not take many new literary approaches and did not show much originality. For its epic poetry,

Rome borrowed the hexameter from Greece. For its lyrics, Rome used and adapted the verse meters of Sappho, Alcaeus, and others. For its prose, it took the histories of Herodotus and Thucydides or the fables of Aesop as models. In the form and content of its drama, Rome reflected the tragedies and comedies of Greece. Virgil's *Aeneid*, one of Rome's most important literary masterpieces and a work of lasting grandeur, would have been impossible without the model of Homer's *Iliad* and *Odyssey*.

Nevertheless, at certain times, especially during the Renaissance, the literature of Rome has meant more to Western civilization than that of Greece. The writings of Cicero have been praised again and again as the embodiment of worldly wisdom, and they have exercised a profound influence. Stoic philosophy has become known chiefly through the writings of Seneca and Marcus Aurelius. Epicureanism found a home and tradition in the wealthy Roman Empire rather than in Greece. As for poets, Ovid and Horace are two of the better known to the modern world. For the stage, Rome produced the plays of Plautus, Terence, and Juvenal.

To these lasting contributions can be added the works of the great Roman historians—Livius, Caesar, Tacitus, and many others—who, by transmitting the deeds of compatriots through their writings, have helped to shape Western civilization. It is through their eyes that Rome's history is viewed, that Rome's glory is appraised, and that Rome's mistakes and vices are recognized. Roman moral judgment has permanently affected the attitude of the West, and Roman standards have become an inseparable part of the civilization within which modern people act.

## Survival of Rome

Like all great empires, Rome fell as corruption ran rampant within its bureaucracy. Greed motivated those who should have dispensed justice, and arbitrariness marked those who should have looked after the welfare of the state and its citizens.

The Romans extolled bravery, and in bloody conquests, they extended their empire. They exploited the lands and peoples they conquered. At home, disillusioned citizens longed for a peaceful and pure life. They turned away from public affairs and sought refuge in the stern, solitary atmosphere of Stoicism. Yet, Rome, like Greece, left an unparalleled heritage. The stories of Lucretia, Fabius Cunctator, and Brutus taught lessons of devotion and fulfillment of duty that have never been forgotten. Roman fortitude in adversity during the war against Hannibal, Roman uprightness as tragically exemplified by the two Catos, Roman statesmanship as shown by Augustus, and the Roman peace, as it prevailed under a Trajan, Hadrian, or Marcus Aurelius, have remained treasures of Western civilization and symbols of a conquest greater than armies could achieve.

## Selected Readings

Boardman, John, et al., *The Oxford History of the Classical World* (Oxford: Oxford University Press, 1986).

Christ, Karl, *The Romans* (Berkeley: University of California Press, 1984).

Fine, John V. A., *The Ancient Greeks* (Cambridge, Mass.: Harvard University Press, 1983).

Finley, M. I., ed., *The Legacy of Greece* (Oxford: Oxford University Press, 1981).

Ward-Perkins, Bryan, *The Fall of the Rome: and the End of Civilization* (Oxford: Oxford University Press, 2005).

Jenkyns, Richard, ed., *The Legacy of Rome* (Oxford: Oxford University Press, 1992).

Powell, Anton, *Athens and Sparta: Constructing Greek Political and Social History from 478 B.C.* (New York: Routledge, 2001).

McNeill, William H., *The Rise of the West* (Chicago, the University of Chicago Press, 1991).

## Test Yourself

1. The two main historians of ancient Greece were_____.
   A. Homer and Hesiod
   B. Herodotus and Thucydides
   C. Sophocles and Aristotle
   D. Plato and Socrates

2. The basic Greek political unit was _____.
   A. Theocracy
   B. The *polis*
   C. Democracy
   D. Republic

3. The Sophists, the Epicureans, the Stoics, and Cynics are examples of_____.
   A. Greek philosophical schools
   B. Roman political commendatory
   C. Greek forms of architecture
   D. Roman economic policies

4. A major contribution of the Roman Republic to Western Europe was_____.
   A. The idea of government by just laws
   B. Belief in democracy
   C. Rejection of the concept of slavery
   D. Start of the industrial revolution

5. Rome's history is usually divided into the eras of_____.
   A. The Kingdom and the Democracy
   B. The Federation and the Empire
   C. The *polis* and the Republic
   D. The Republic and the Empire

6. Rome's long-term legacy to the development of Western culture included all but_____.
   A. Its law
   B. Its religion
   C. Its language
   D. Its administrative practices

7. One of the most important Roman literary masterpieces is_____.
   A. Homer's *Iliad*
   B. Plato's *Republic*
   C. Virgil's *Aeneid*
   D. Homer's *Odyssey*

8. The Colosseum is an example of _____.
    A. Roman architecture
    B. Greek sports
    C. Mesopotamian market place
    D. Egyptian art

## Answers and Explanations

1. **B.** The two most important Greek historians were Herodotus and Thucydides. Thucydides, for example, was perhaps more conscious of the permanent significance of his work than were the poets (who, while giving expression to lasting thought, addressed themselves to contemporary audiences). As he himself states, he set out to write a history that was to be a treasure for all times.

2. **B.** The basic unit of the Greek society was the city-state, called the *polis*.

3. **A.** The Greeks initiated various philosophical schools, including the Sophists, the Epicureans, the Stoics, and the Cynics. Socrates, Plato, and Aristotle (4th century B.C.E.) created systems of logic and concepts of ethics that have remained as guides ever since their creation. They discovered various ways to direct people in their search for knowledge and drive to action. They recognized that the human mind cannot comprehend everything and that there are limits within which philosophical investigation could move throughout the history of Western civilization.

4. **A.** The idea of government ruled by just laws was the cornerstone of the Roman Republic. Underlying the structure of the mighty empire eventually built by the Romans was a concept of law which, though it had many roots in Greek philosophical thought and derived as well from the many examples provided by the political systems of other Mediterranean nations, was nonetheless unique in the ancient world. The vocabulary of Roman law is still in use, and its procedures serve as models even today. Its stipulations in regard to property, the conduct of business, matters of inheritance, marriage, and divorce, and numerous other fields have influenced codes of justice among all Western nations.

5. **D.** Historians divide Roman history into two major eras: Republic and Empire.

6. **B.** Roman religion left no direct impact on Western civilization. All of the other aspects of Rome's legacy have left enduring impacts on the history of Western civilization. For instance, like the Greek language, Latin made inestimable contributions to the civilization of the modern world. Also, most important among the legacies of Rome are those contributions that have taught the modern world a rational, reasonable approach to political conduct and nation-building. The political genius of Rome, its ability to rule itself and others, to adapt itself to changing conditions, to invent checks and balances in order to avoid excesses, to overcome the threats of social challenges, to regulate "the relationship of man to man," have together constituted an unequaled lesson for future Western civilization.

7. **C.** One of the most important Roman literary masterpieces, Virgil's *Aeneid*, was a work of lasting grandeur which was based on the model of Homer's *Iliad* and *Odyssey*.

8. **A.** The Romans left behind great architectural achievements. They erected triumphal arches, constructed columns celebrating victories, and adorned these structures with inscriptions and representations of Rome's deeds of glory. They built public baths and the Colosseum as well as other large arenas in many Roman cities.

# CHAPTER 2
# The Medieval Heritage

**768-814** Reign of Charlemagne
**825-870** Viking invasion of Europe
**1066** Norman conquest of England
**1054** Schism between Orthodox and Catholic Churches
**1088** Origins of the University of Bologna
**1096-1099** First Crusade
**1147-1149** Second Crusade
**1189-1193** Third Crusade
**1226-1230** The Magna Carta
**1337-1353** Hundred Years War between France and England

*The stories of ancient Greece and Rome are finished. The empires have disappeared; the societies they represented are dead. A cycle was completed. Much of the area where they once flourished passed into the hands of different kinds of people. The story of Western civilization continued, not only in the Mediterranean area, but also in the center of Europe and along Europe's Atlantic borders. Western civilization established new centers in France, Germany, England, Spain, Italy, and other parts of the world. When the ancient world gave way to medieval civilization is a fascinating question: Was it in the 4th or 5th century, or as late as the 7th or 8th century? Our whole attitude toward the problem of survival of civilizations, including our own, may depend on the answer to this question.*

*A new age began somewhere between 475 C.E. to 732 C.E. This new age, the beginning of the "Middle Ages," is not such a closed book as ancient times. The centers of medieval civilization and many institutions of medieval society live on, unlike most of those of the ancient world. No break occurred during the 14th, 15th, and 16th centuries. The Middle Ages evolved almost imperceptibly into modern times. In eastern, western, and northern Europe, new entities were added to old established centers, and in these new areas, the traditions of the old were carried on.*

## ■ MEDIEVAL CONTRIBUTIONS

Four factors mark the fundamental departure of Western medieval civilization from that of ancient times: (1) a geographic shift of the centers of power from the eastern Mediterranean basin northward to Europe; (2) an influx of Germanic ethnic groups into the Roman world and the emergence of new political and social units that carried forward the Germanic heritage in addition to the Roman; (3) an economic transformation following the decline of commercial markets in the Mediterranean Empire and the tran-

*Figure 2-1 Europe during the High Middle Ages, ca. 1400*

sition from a slave-owning, capitalistic society to a society based on a feudal, local economy; and (4) the introduction and impact of Christianity.

## Language

At the beginning of the medieval epoch, not a single modern Western language existed. By its end, almost every one of the Western national languages, all of which would evolve into the languages of today, had emerged. Latin was preserved throughout the Middle Ages as a means of international communication, but by the beginning of modern times, the linguistic tools we use today to form our thoughts had already been shaped. Vocabularies and grammars of present-day languages developed from Latin and Germanic roots and from Slavic sources in the East. Moreover, they had been enriched by numerous new words coined to express new thoughts and designate new instruments or incorporated from other civilizations. By then, the languages spoken by the various peoples or tribes predominated both in daily life and popular literature. The use of these vernacular languages increased among scholars and in religious literature and rites. Thus, modern languages represent one of the chief legacies of the Middle Ages.

## Religion

In addition to the development of modern languages, an outstanding contribution of the Middle Ages was the propagation and preservation of Christianity. The introduction of Christianity to the Western world as the official religion of the Roman Empire coincides with the beginnings of medieval times. By then, the Nicean creed had been formulated, and all major Christian churches have used it ever since. The Bible was translated into Latin, becoming the property of all succeeding generations. Christian ethics were imposed upon pagan views and, even if not entirely triumphant, they have remained ideals toward which the Western world strives. The Church, Catholic or Orthodox, became the dominant social influence upon all the peoples of Europe during the Middle Ages. It permeated every facet of medieval life and thought. With its artistic and educational tenets, its calendar, its law, its ceremonies and its political and economic power, the Church established the pattern for the secular and spiritual conditions that have guided all subsequent ages.

The Church imposed an order and a unity that has never been entirely obliterated, even through later divisions of land areas into nations. The Catholic Church, with its Papacy and organizational hierarchy, created an entity that has survived as a potent factor in modern times. Even the so-called "heresies"—doctrines not approved by the official church—made their contributions. Through the challenges they presented, a constant process of purification was forced upon the Christian church. The Christian faith has continued to be the guiding code in the West for almost 2,000 years and has been enriched by rebellious and defending forces alike.

## Philosophy

Naturally, Christian thought dominated all speculation about transcendental questions. Its influence caused philosophers to engage in a search for ultimate truths, standards of logic, and ethics different from those of the ancient world. Church fathers, such as Augustine, Ambrose, Jerome, John Chrysostom, and others, especially in the 4th century, put medieval philosophy on a new path, but it was only in the 12th and 13th centuries that a complete system of Christian philosophy emerged. Under the guidance of the universities and of those known as "schoolmen," among whom Peter Abelard, Albertus Magnus, and Thomas Aquinas stand out, an attempt was made to preserve or revive the Greek heritage, following the Greeks on the path of logic and rationality, yet not sacrificing any part of the Church's tradition or any of its mysteries and transcendental teachings.

During the 13th century, the scholastic attempt was carried forward by two schools, the "Realists" and the "Nominalists." The former were closer in their thinking to Plato, while the latter relied more on Aristotle. Though neither challenged Christian foundations, the Realists insisted on the primacy of universal ideas and their exclusive "reality," whereas the Nominalists emphasized the role of the "particular" evidences of God's creation in nature and their significance. The Nominalists paved the way for a naturalistic, scientific approach. The long struggle between the two sides forced them to make the greatest of intellectual efforts, which again and again nurtured modern thinking and investigation.

Even apart from scholastic philosophy, the Middle Ages provided a mighty stimulus to modern philosophical pursuits. Scientific speculations about the cosmos and nature by men such as Roger Bacon and, more important for philosophical developments, the mystical views and "experiences" expressed or witnessed by St. Francis and Meister Eckhart have stimulated the speculations of later times. Indeed, the various forces of Scholasticism, of science, of mysticism, and of a revived Classical philosophy constitute lasting contributions of the Middle Ages.

## Learning

Religious thought and philosophical speculation gave direction to all forms of education in medieval times. After several centuries of stagnation in the early Middle Ages, secular knowledge continued on its path toward broader enlightenment. During the Middle Ages, an educational system was gradually created whose aspirations could, at least in part, inspire and form a foundation for developments in the modern world. Primary schooling in medieval times emphasized discipline, which was considered necessary for the formation of character, for the learning of reading and writing, and for Bible studies. This approach was weakened over time, however. The more advanced curriculum of the medieval education system, which provided training in grammar, astronomy, music, and so on, also did not find a permanent home in modern times.

The university, a creation of the 11th century, has been of unique importance. In medieval times, professors and students met, debated, and exchanged ideas in an atmosphere free from outside interference. They devoted themselves to the study of the universe and mankind in their manifold aspects. Their studies embraced the four faculties of theology, law, philosophy, and medicine. Jews and, particularly, Arabs contributed to these studies by their accumulated wisdom in such fields as astronomy, agriculture, classics, science, and medicine. The four faculties of the universities, along with their rites and forms, proved to be of fundamental importance for the progress of Western civilization since their inception. It was largely in the universities that the ever-striving spirit characterizing Western civilization was fostered.

It was also in the universities that training in logical thought was provided. In many instances, this made possible the flowering of all secular activity outside their walls. Thus, receptivity was created for many scientific considerations. Interest grew in the accomplishments of other civilizations, and paper, the compass, and glass were adopted. This heritage, in turn, stimulated original contributions, such as the invention of gunpowder and the printing press that used movable type.

## Art

Medieval art rivals all other medieval accomplishments in its importance for later times. It has exercised an influence at least equal to that of the art created in the ancient world. Just as there is hardly a community in the West in which replication of Greek temples and columns cannot be found, so too there is hardly one in which the round Romanesque arch or, more frequently, the pointed arch of the Gothic cathedral, the stained-glass window, the imagery of Mary and the Christ child, and the paintings of the early Renaissance are not represented, copied, or replicated. The countless wonders of the Gothic style have, indeed, found duplication, often incongruously, in such a variety of modern buildings—churches, universities, private homes, stations, office buildings—that they have become an integral part of our lives.

The more humble artistic achievements of the Middle Ages, those shown by articles made for daily household use, have also left an indelible heritage, and the small arts, the handicrafts in all trades, have excited the imagination of Western cultures.

Mosaics and paintings, created successively in Byzantine, Romanesque, Gothic, and, finally, Renaissance style, are not only on display in museums, where they are the pride of town and nation. They are also to be seen in homes, often transformed in the work of later generations of artists.

Each medieval creation bears witness to the individual genius and detailed, loving care of the individual master. Even if the creations of the early medieval periods with their particular beauty and symbolism are not always meaningful to the uninitiated, those of the Renaissance, of Giotto, Fra Angelico, Botticelli, van Eyck, Memling, and hundreds of others, have become part of the lives of millions who may not be conscious of the names of the paintings or artists.

## Literature

Medieval literature has also made lasting contributions to Western civilization. Twofold were the merits of medieval scholars and writers. They preserved the literary and intellectual accomplishments of ancient Greece and Rome by copying the works with infinite patience and commenting and interpreting them. They then added their own creative work to the ancient heritage. Early in the medieval period, the "minuscule" was developed. This replaced the capital letters used by the Romans with lowercase letters and rendered the labor of writing easier by making it more fluid, which helped to increase the volume of great thought that could be preserved.

Many of the books written or reproduced during this time were prepared with beautiful lettering. Manuscripts with their splendid illuminations are witnesses to the medieval interest in literature, and they are an inspiration to modern endeavors. We possess Church translations and commentaries both in Latin and in later vernacular tongues; mighty hymns, such as *"Ave Maria"* and *"Dies Irae"*; great epics, like *Parzival, Tristan and Iseult,* the *Nibelungenlied,* and *La Chanson de Roland;* histories, chronicles, and scientific treatises; the love songs of troubadours and *minnesangers*; a vast heritage of folk songs; and a not yet sufficiently appreciated body of prose. In the late Middle Ages, individual masterpieces stand out, and towering among them are the works of three Italians: Dante, Petrarch, and Boccaccio.

### Music

Much of the writing and folklore was originally meant to be accompanied by music, but its sound has long since passed, and the voices are dead. We know little about it beyond what parchment or paper can preserve in music notation or what instruments that have survived and been adapted to modern use can tell us. Yet, the oral tradition has not been entirely lost. The sonorous Gregorian chant has come down to us across the centuries, as have thousands of lovely and mysterious folk songs and dances that have been continually repeated, generation after generation. Significantly, in many regions of the West, folklore was not consciously considered a historical heritage until it was 'rediscovered' over the past two centuries.

### Statecraft

During the Middle Ages, most of the great modern European nations emerged as separate entities and within the territorial limits that are approximately the same as those of today. France and Germany became the common heirs of Charlemagne's empire. Britain, conquered and settled by numerous invaders, was fused into the unit it still represents. Russia emerged as a nation with Moscow as its center. By the end of the Middle Ages, the Italians had not yet attained independent statehood, but they possessed a common language and some common national aspirations. Spain had become a united country and Portugal a separate one. The Scandinavian countries were formed. The foundation was laid for Switzerland, Hungary, and other nations. As a whole, medieval times ended the unity that the Western world under Roman rule had once possessed. Notwithstanding the attempts of the Catholic Church to preserve at least a spiritual unity, a multiplicity of states emerged with the separate and identifiable characteristics that are known to us in modern times.

### Law and Legislation

Besides the evolution of nations, the Middle Ages saw other important political changes. While feudal ethics and economics found no acceptance in later times, some aspects of medieval legal developments have been of great significance. The Middle Ages left a threefold legacy to the field of law. The heritage of ancient Rome was preserved, and church canon evolved to remain valid in the Catholic world and extended its influence to other areas. Additionally, the Middle Ages saw the development of what came to be known as "common law."

Originating chiefly from Germanic concepts of justice, which were native to northern and eastern Europe and distinct from those of ancient Rome, common law gradually expanded through the oral tradition and through usage. It came to form an integral part of the mores, ethics, and laws of the modern age. The decisions of courts and judges, as well as the opinions of lawyers and professors of law, established certain principles in conformity with the old spiritual heritage.

Closely linked with the growth of the medieval system of law were a number of political institutions. Most important among them were "diets" and "parliaments," which assumed the right to create public legislation. These institutions left their mark upon all subsequent ages. They were composed of representatives of "estates" or orders. To a large extent, modern social class stratification is partially based on medieval organization. Remnants of the medieval aristocracy and many ruling families have survived into modern times, although their privileged status has been diminished. Titles and privileges can be traced back to medieval patterns, but medieval society also anticipated the broader constitutional rights that were later claimed by the *bourgeoisie*.

## Commerce and Discoveries

The heritage of medieval economic organization has been investigated but, for lack of sources, is not yet sufficiently understood. Yet, both in economic theory and in practical matters of commerce, the Middle Ages passed on a rich legacy. Christian scholars, historians, and chroniclers left treatises that reflect deep insight into the questions of just price, imposing interest fees, monopoly, and profit. Economic theory even forms a part of as fundamental a work as St. Thomas Aquinas's *Summa Theologica.* He and others sought to channel natural human urges like ambition and greed so they would not conflict with the ethical demands of Christianity.

The practical aspects of medieval economic life and economic organization have also been influential. Guilds, developed in the Middle Ages, are still meaningful. Through an awareness of certain moral principles, they sought to limit competition, which was considered a vice. They also promoted high standards and quality of workmanship. The Middle Ages experimented with the organization of communal labor, communal property, and planned production. During medieval times, many of the principles of banking, credit, exchange, and capital formation were either adopted from the East or worked out independently in the West. Numerous achievements in this area influenced later entrepreneurial activity and had an impact on various political experiments, even in the Industrial Age.

One of the major reasons for the continued importance of some elements of the medieval economic system was the vast expansion of European trade that took place during the Middle Ages. Commerce had to adapt to worldwide markets. The enterprises of Italian towns in the Mediterranean area, of the Hanseatic League in the Baltic, the Portuguese ventures to the Far East, and the Spanish explorations into the Atlantic regions were not only precursors, but led to modern business activities. In many respects, these enterprises represented undertakings on the same order as modern entrepreneurship and were subject to very similar conditions. They thus can teach important lessons.

## Cities

Last, the Middle Ages saw the establishment of almost all of the great cities of Europe. By 1500, most of the great commercial centers of Italy, Germany, France, Spain, England, Scandinavia, and Russia, which have played a role in modern times, had been established. The development and rise of towns required methods for organizing them. People had to be attracted, shifting populations had to be managed, special laws and privileges had to be developed, and a division of labor had to be adopted. All of these set the pattern for later times.

## Perspective

*The Middle Ages illuminated the modern world with the faith, scholarship, and beauty they created. The period brought forth ideas, and established ideals that have remained meaningful. The faith and ethics of Christianity, the standards established for learning and philosophy, the works of art and literature, stand as unique examples. They have enriched the modern world to no less a degree than did the highest achievements of ancient Greece and Rome.*

## Selected Readings

Green, V. H. H. *Medieval Civilization in Western Europe* (New York: St. Martin's Press, 1971).
Kitzinger, Ernst. *Early Medieval Art* (1983).
Holmes, George, ed., *The Oxford History of Medieval Europe* (1988).

Littke, Kester K. and Rosenwein, Barbara, eds., *Debating the Middle Ages: Issues and Readings* (Malden, Mass.: Blackwell Publishers, 1998).

Collins, Rogers. *Early Medieval Europe, 300-1000* (New York: St. Martin's Press, 1991).

Peters, Edward. *Europe and the Middle Ages* (Upper Saddle River, N.J.: Prentice-Hall, 1997).

Jordan, William Chester. *Europe and the High Middle Ages* (New York: Penguin Putnam, 2001).

*The New Cambridge Medieval History* (Cambridge, N.Y.: Cambridge University Press, 1995- ).

Hollister, C. Warren. *Medieval Europe* (Boston: McGraw Hill, 1998).

## Test Yourself

1. At the beginning of the Medieval epoch_____.
   A. Not a single modern Western language existed
   B. Spanish and French dominated the family of languages
   C. Spanish and Arabic were the leading languages
   D. None of the above

2. In addition to the development of languages, one of the most outstanding contributions of the Middle Ages was ____.
   A. The preservation and propagation of Christianity
   B. The translation of the Bible into Latin
   C. The development of the Nicean Creed of all major Christian churches
   D. All of the above

3. During the 13th century, the scholastic effort was carried forward by two schools____.
   A. The Realists and the Nominalists
   B. The Realists and the Positivists
   C. The Realists and the Socialists
   D. The Realists and the Gnostics

4. During the Middle Ages, most of the great modern European nations emerged as _____.
   A. Separate entities within territorial limits similar to those of today
   B. France and Germany became the heirs of Charlemagne's empire
   C. Russia became a nation centering around St. Petersburg
   D. A and B

5. Closely connected with the growth of the medieval system of law were a number of political and legal institutions, such as_____.
   A. Diets and parliaments
   B. Congresses and councils
   C. People's assemblies
   D. None of the above

6. One of the most influential medieval economic organizations was____.
   A. The guild
   B. Communal property and labor
   C. Banking, credit and exchange
   D. All of the above

7. Medieval literature was influenced by the earlier intellectual accomplishments of_____.
   A. Egypt and Mesopotamia
   B. Persia
   C. Greece and Rome
   D. The Aztec Empire

8. The medieval university was developed during_____.
    A. The 4th century
    B. The 5th century
    C. The 11th century
    D. The 15th century

## Answers and Explanations

1. **A.** At the beginning of the medieval epoch, not a single modern Western language existed. By its end, almost every one of the Western national languages, all of which would evolve into the languages of today, had emerged. Latin was preserved throughout the Middle Ages as a means of international communication, but by the beginning of modern times, the linguistic tools we use today to form our thoughts had already been shaped.

2. **D.** In addition to the development of modern languages, an outstanding contribution of the Middle Ages was the propagation and preservation of Christianity. The introduction of Christianity to the Western world as the official religion of the Roman Empire coincides with the beginnings of medieval times. By then, the Nicean creed had been formulated, and all major Christian churches have used it ever since. The Bible was translated into Latin, becoming the property of all succeeding generations.

3. **A.** During the 13th century, the scholastic attempt was carried forward by two schools, the "Realists" and the "Nominalists." The former were closer in their thinking to Plato, while the latter relied more on Aristotle. Though neither challenged Christian foundations, the Realists insisted on the primacy of universal ideas and their exclusive "preality," whereas the Nominalists emphasized the role of the "particular" evidences of God's creation in nature and their significance. The Nominalists paved the way for a naturalistic, scientific approach. The long struggle between the two sides forced them to make the greatest of intellectual efforts, which again and again nurtured modern thinking and investigation

4. **D.** During the Middle Ages, most of the great modern European nations emerged as separate entities within territorial limits that approximate those of today. France and Germany were the common heirs of Charlemagne's empire. Britain, conquered and settled by numerous invaders, was fused into the unit it still represents. Russia emerged as a nation with Moscow as its center. As a whole, medieval times put an end to the unity the Western world once possessed under Roman rule. Notwithstanding the attempts of the Catholic Church to preserve at least a spiritual unity, a multiplicity of states emerged with the separate and identifiable characteristics known to us in modern times.

5. **A.** Closely linked with the growth of the medieval system of law were a number of political institutions. Most important among them were "diets" and "parliaments," which assumed the right to make public legislation. These institutions left their mark upon all subsequent ages. They were composed of representatives of "estates" or classes. Remnants of the medieval aristocracy and many ruling families have survived into modern times.

6. **D.** Likewise, practical aspects of medieval economic life and economic organization have been influential. Guilds, developed in the Middle Ages, remain meaningful. Through an awareness of certain moral principles, they sought to limit competition, which was considered a vice. They also promoted high standards and quality of workmanship. The Middle Ages experimented with the organization of communal labor, communal property, and planned production. During medieval times, many of the principles of banking, credit, exchange, and capital formation were adopted from the East or worked out independently in the West. Numerous achievements of this kind guided later entrepreneurial activity and influenced various political experiments, even in the Industrial Age.

7. C. Medieval literature also made lasting contributions to Western civilization. Twofold were the merits of medieval scholars and writers. They preserved the literary and intellectual accomplishments of ancient Greece and Rome, copying their works with infinite patience, adding comments and interpretations. They then added to this ancient heritage their own creativity. Early in the medieval period, the minuscule, lowercase letters that replaced the capital letters used by the Romans, was developed. This made the work of writing easier by making it more fluid, and this helped to preserve the treasure represented by ancient Greek and Roman thought.

8. C. The university was a creation of the 11th century, and it has been of unique importance. Professors and students started meeting in "universities." In an atmosphere free from outside interference, they devoted themselves to the study of the universe and mankind in its manifold aspects. Their studies embraced the four faculties of theology, law, philosophy, and medicine. These four faculties of the universities, as well as their rites and forms, proved to be of fundamental importance for the progress of Western civilization.

# CHAPTER 3
# The Beginning of "The Modern Age" (1492-1517)

**1492** Columbus discovers America
Death of Lorenzo de Medici
End of Muslim Rule in Spain
**1494** France invades Italy
Treaty of Tordesillas
Hanseatic factory in Novgorod closed by Russians
**1495** Leonardo da Vinci, *Last Supper (1503: Mona Lisa)*
**1498** Vasco da Gama reaches India via Cape of Good Hope
Savonarola hanged and burned at stake in Florence
**1503** Death of Pope Alexander V (Borgia)
**1508** Michelangelo, *Ceiling of Sistine Chapel*
**1513** Balboa reaches Pacific shores
Machiavelli, *The Prince*
**1516** Raphael, *Sistine Madonna*
Thomas More, *Utopia*
**1517** Luther, *95 Theses*

*The Modern Age dates from about 1500. This year was not selected arbitrarily. The historical period from 1500 to the present possesses cohesion and a common outlook. Naturalism, individualism, and nationalism give it a special meaning.*

*Moreover, the global expansion of Western civilization constitutes another distinguishing characteristic. While the Classical Period had embraced the evolution of civilizations around the Mediterranean Sea and in the Near East, and while the Medieval Period had enlarged the cultural horizon by including all of Europe as well as most of the Old World, the Modern Age includes the entire globe.*

*The Modern Age had its beginnings in one of the most glorious epochs in Western civilization. As Preserved Smith writes in his* Age of the Reformation *(1920, p. 3): "Though in some sense every age is one of transition and every generation sees the world remodeled, there sometimes comes a change so startling and profound that it seems like the beginning of a new season in the world's great year.... Spring has come."*

*The Modern Age affected most fields of human endeavor and human understanding—exploration and enterprise, science, art, music, literature, religion, and state-building—and some of the most momen-*

*tous works known to history have been created during this time. The first generation of modern times was "great in what it achieved, sublime in what it dreamed; abounding in ripe wisdom and heroic deeds; full of light and of beauty and of life."*

## ■WESTERN SOCIETY AROUND 1500

The society that brought forth such accomplishments was a true reflection of the Renaissance. It was devoted to beauty. It was enterprising and skeptical. It rejected many past religious traditions and authorities and yet was itself religious and reverent. It undertook to penetrate the secrets of nature with unaccustomed curiosity and confidence. Youth played a more important and leading role in society than it does now: Men and sometimes women of 20, 25, 30, even 16 years of age occupied many influential posts and achieved feats of lasting significance. Truly could the young German poet and humanist Ulrich von Hutten sing: "It is a joy to live!"

### Social Aspirations

Unlike the cultural atmosphere of medieval times, when desire for spiritual otherworldliness directed many of the greatest achievements, the spirit of the Renaissance tended toward worldly things—toward the full development of people's natural gifts and a full gratification of the senses through the attractions offered by this world. Among all layers of society we see a thirst to enjoy life and all it could offer in meaningful experience and in transient pleasure. It was a time of great moral, cultural, and spiritual achievement. It was also an age of pleasure seeking, of intemperate eating, drinking, dressing, and lovemaking. Men and women risked life and limb in adventure and enterprise, and behind their lust for life, stood the expectation of pain and early death. Great perils threatened in the form of wars, murders, pestilence, unsanitary surroundings, disasters on the seas, and persecutions by political antagonists or religious fanatics.

### Social Stratification

Changes in the attitudes of people toward their surroundings had a very slow, yet distinct, effect upon societal structure. Orders or "estates" remained essentially as they had been in the past, but an interest in secular matters and, with it, attention to worldly tasks, changed the outlook and occupations of the estates.

### *Clergy*

In the early 16th century, the first estate, the clergy, continued to play the prominent role it had enjoyed throughout the Middle Ages. However, a change in this role was coming. Although there were thousands of higher prelates, humble priests, and monks who devoted themselves with unabated zeal and piety to the service of Christianity, a vast number of them also indulged in worldly occupations. They expanded their economic activities and participated in political struggles as well as secular pleasures and ambitions. Alexander VI, a pope who came from the Borgia family (d. 1503), may be an extreme example of clerical depravity, which is shown by his greed, politics, mistresses, children, and poisons. Many others showed a greater interest in art, devotion to science, ability in languages, perfection in Renaissance manners, and participation in humanistic endeavors than they did in the performance of their religious duties. Soon, low morals, lack of training, and neglect of duty characterized even some reforming groups. Thus, the clergy as a whole lost both respect and its importance.

### *Nobility*

The second estate, the nobility, rivaled the first in its pursuit of worldly interests. The medieval code of honor came to mean little when gunpowder and other inventions undermined the standards formerly

## The Beginning of "The Modern Age" (1492-1517)

Figure 3-1 Voyages of discovery and the claims of Spain and Portugal to overseas empires

set for the conduct of a nobleman, and his military occupations began to play a lesser role. To a large extent, princes had to hire soldiers (mercenaries) to do their fighting for them.

In order to retain their prestige in society, noblemen turned increasingly to the pursuit of industry and trade. Many among the nobles acquired land, using it for the production agricultural crops, exploiting its mineral resources, and participating in business ventures. With the wealth they acquired, they indulged in the entertainments and the advanced secular interests of the age, notably in scholarship, art, literature, and science. A new ideal for the cultured and rich nobles was created. Originating in Italy, the ideal of *virtue,* i.e., of manly activity, intelligence, achievement, and conduct, devoted to all facets of Renaissance life, became the norm.

Significantly, women shared in the interests and activities of the upper classes. Though they were, in some respects and in many instances, still treated with cruelty and abused, some women managed to attain prominent positions. They exercised a greater influence upon political and cultural developments during this period than they had in previous ages. Women ruled as queens, served as regents, diplomats, and administrators of estates, and engaged in professions as doctors, lawyers, and teachers. They excelled as scholars, poets, and arbiters of arts and manners. Chastity was as uncommon among them as among men, and power and luxury were similarly craved.

### The Burgher

In the Age of Discovery, the townspeople, or *burghers*, who formed the "third estate" together with the free peasants, also enjoyed an increase in prestige. Everywhere, merchants and bankers rose to prominence. Owing to the wealth of the burghers, ports such as Cadiz, Lisbon, Antwerp, and London, and trading cities and centers of crafts such as Augsburg and Nuremberg in southern Germany, gained far-reaching influence. The Fugger family of Augsburg, whose interests extended to textile industries, silver and copper mining, wholesale trade, and banking, had a great influence on the emperors and kings of Germany, England, Spain, and Portugal, and was exceptionally powerful. Other businessmen, less wealthy than the Fuggers, could also influence the political fate of great commonwealths. Moreover, artisans gained in influence as a result of the increased demand for new production methods and objects that were useful for the beautification of the surroundings.

Within the burgher class, a differentiation developed between the standards of the wealthy and those of the poor. The rich took the nobility as a model, and they participated in Renaissance pleasures and aspirations. The poor were more limited in their search for pleasure. Among them, emerging new standards of morality emphasized restraint, sobriety, frugality, and duty. This trend was accelerated over the course of the century by the influence of religious reform movements. It was also enhanced by the gradual worsening of economic conditions among the lower classes, which were brought about by unemployment, rising prices, and the beginnings of capitalism. In its early form, capitalism deprived people of security and imposed new economic burdens. Crime increased. Beggars overran the towns, and highwaymen made life unsafe for travelers and merchants.

### The Peasant

Around 1500, the vast majority of the population in Europe was still composed of peasants. This was true even in the Netherlands, a small country that was very active in trade. However, considerable changes also occurred within the peasant class. In the East, especially in Poland and Russia, there was a continued tendency to subject the peasantry to serfdom, while in central and Western Europe, serfdom continued to diminish.

With the growth of towns and trade, there was an increased need for free labor. Simultaneously, changes in agricultural production methods made the institution of serfdom less useful. As a result, many serfs were released from their bondage and left their villages. Those who stayed gained at least partial freedom.

This emancipation movement benefited the peasants to only a limited degree. As the paintings of Pieter Brueghel the Elder, Hieronymus Bosch, and other artists show, many peasants followed the dissipated example of the upper classes and sought particular enjoyment in feasting, which was made possible because the food supply was more ample than ever before. Social evolution imposed new hardships upon the peasants, however. Many who had emigrated to the towns found life there even more difficult than at home. Deprived of security, peasants in many areas revolted, but they could not reverse the trends of the time.

## ■ ECONOMIC CONDITIONS

The most significant factor shaping Western society around 1500 was the expansion of its geographic horizon. New technical means had become available. There were new types of ships, maps, nautical instruments, and superior weapons. Political authority was established to protect them. Scientific experience led to success. A degree of economic organization had been achieved that not only provided financial backing, but also enabled entrepreneurs in various fields to join in common undertakings.

### Geographic Exploration

Men of genius, possessing the material resources and animated by the creative spirit of the age, could transform their long-held dreams into reality. Their incentives were threefold: Gospel, Gold, and Glory—the desire to convert others, to enrich themselves, and to win fame.

Explorers set out in search of new shores. Columbus reached the North American area in 1492. Vasco da Gama sailed to India via the Cape of Good Hope in 1498. Amerigo Vespucci landed on the continent that was named after him, America. Balboa crossed the continent, and in 1513, sighted the Pacific Ocean. The Portuguese explorer, Magellan, with courage and perseverance, performed perhaps the most heroic feat of all. He was the first to attempt the circumnavigation of the globe, and although he himself perished on the trip, one of his five ships actually completed the round trip. John Cabot reached the North American continent near Labrador. In 1521, Hernan Cortes conquered the Aztec Empire in Mexico.

Somewhat later, Pizarro conquered the Inca Empire in Peru for the Spanish. The Portuguese built an empire of their own in the East Indies. Strife over the new possessions was avoided by the Line of Demarcation established by the Pope in 1493. It was altered one year later by the Treaty of Tordesillas, which assigned to Portugal most of the eastern colonies, while Spain retained most of the western colonies.

### *Economic Impact*

The discoveries had a far-reaching influence upon European life. Economically, they provided enormous quantities of coveted gold and silver. The discoveries also secured vast new sources of food, especially fish. Soon, the value of the agricultural resources, game, and fish in many of the colonies overshadowed the resources of mining. Many new products, such as maize and potatoes, were introduced to Europe and changed prevailing food habits.

### *Political Impact*

Politically, the discoveries strengthened the monarchs who enlarged their personal dominions and augmented their wealth. There was a shift of power from old trade centers to new ones in different countries. Eventually, the Atlantic sea routes grew in significance compared with traditional Mediterranean and Baltic trade routes. The redistribution of power resulting from the acquisition of colonies led to new struggles for trade supremacy and to new wars.

## Social Impact

Socially, the discoveries benefited merchants of the burgher class, who gained prestige through the acquisition of new wealth. The discoveries impacted the poorer layers of the population by providing them with food that could be imported, thereby giving them a new means of sustenance. Under these circumstances, populations grew. The newly discovered lands lured the adventurous to emigrate, and as knowledge about the earth increased, old beliefs were given up and thinking habits changed. Last, discoveries led to the transformation not only of the Old World, but also of the new lands, which had to change their own ways of life to be in accordance with European desires and customs.

## Economic Reorganization

Geographical discoveries, combined with the individualistic, enterprising spirit of Renaissance times, fundamentally influenced economic developments.

### Business Organization

The enormous expansion of markets and the development of a money economy, which was strengthened by an ample supply of precious metals flowing from the New World as well as from Europe itself (for example, Hungary), laid the basis for the rise of modem capitalism and private enterprise. The Fugger family of Augsburg represented entrepreneurial activity of a new magnitude and importance. A sharp competitive spirit aiming for personal, monopolistic advantages in production and internal and external trade replaced former social attitudes and economic morals. A greater leniency in the Church toward people who invested capital and received interest, which had formerly been forbidden, aided in a rapid formation of capital in the modern business sense. This, in turn, led to the organization of new business structures.

Best known among these were the so-called "joint-stock companies," which were corporations of merchant adventurers who pooled their resources, at first temporarily for one specific undertaking, but later on a permanent basis for repeated ventures. They chose directors and sea captains to transact the actual business for them, while they restricted their own activities to accumulating gains from their investments. They often secured charters from their governments, which granted them monopolies in certain areas or on certain commodities. The necessary capital was raised for extensive, though often very risky, enterprises.

One of the most famous joint-stock companies was the Muscovy Company in England. Toward the middle of the 16th century, it secured a monopoly over Russian trade. Later, various companies from different countries were founded to carry on trade with the Near East and the East and West Indies. Europe's economic potential was further augmented by provisions for greater credit facilities, such as bills of exchange and paper certificates, new tools applied in the mining and textile industries, and a more rational division of labor through specialization in production methods.

### Expansion of Markets

With the help of the newly created facilities, European producers and traders could reach out for previously untouched markets. They exported horses, cattle, and agricultural products. They established new overseas production centers for Old World products, such as sugar. They introduced such hitherto unknown produce as potatoes, tomatoes, tobacco, maize, and quinine. They also increased the imports of familiar products, such as coffee, rice, silk, and cotton. From Newfoundland, they brought fish; from China, tea. Gold and silver provided not only for monetary funds, but also for a greatly expanded jewelry trade, which made use of Indian pearls and rubies. New "needs" were artificially created. One commodity of special importance contributed to the wealth of the European countries: slaves. Slaves, who were transported from Africa, were used as a labor supply for the New World. Spanish, Portuguese, and, later, English and Dutch traders specialized in slave traffic.

## Philosophy of Mercantilism

Through the new economic practices, conditions evolved to form the underpinnings of the system known to present-day economists as "mercantilism." While some aspects of mercantilism can be traced to ancient and medieval economies, others depended upon conditions evolving in the early modem period. The ideal of the mercantilist philosophers was to strengthen the position of their nations. Believing that the position of a nation depends upon the "bullion" —gold, silver, precious stones—it amassed, these philosophers held that the nation should export more than it imported. This they sought to achieve through increased industrial production, the establishment and exploitation of colonies, monopolization of crucial raw materials, and building up both a merchant marine and a carrying trade that could exclude competitors.

Such measures could, of course, be taken only with the help of a powerful government that backed the commercial enterprises. Mercantilism thus implied a measure of government interference in economic affairs. However, since the bourgeoisie already tended to favor firm, central governmental control, interference by the government was tolerated. Those nations in which centralization under strong rulers advanced became leaders.

## Agricultural Conditions

Inasmuch as mercantilism favored trade and required increased productivity, agriculture also had to adapt to changed conditions. Commercial farming that provided higher yields replaced subsistence farming insofar as tools and organization permitted. Once many peasants began to migrate to the cities, their lands were sold for profit. Large farms were established and worked by an impoverished laboring class. Common lands were taken over by landlords. In Spain and England, many farms were enclosed and used for sheep-grazing and wool production.

# ■THE ARTS AND SCIENCES

Some historians have been inclined to view the economic developments of the Renaissance period as the main reason for the artistic achievement of the early 16th century. According to this view, the wealth and leisure enjoyed by the upper class groups of the population made it possible for great artists to develop their talents and their art to be duly appreciated by a cultivated society. However, such a view cannot be accepted. As always, the primary factor was the genius of individuals. Fortunately, people of outstanding genius lived at the time, and often in the face of grave obstacles, they devoted themselves to achieving what their unique talents inspired and allowed. While others, who were equally prosperous, failed to show similar achievements.

## Painting and Sculpture

Encouraged by popes, princes, and wealthy burghers, Renaissance Italy in particular continued to bring forth an astounding number of the great masters in the fine arts. It suffices to mention painter, architect, and thinker, Leonardo da Vinci *(Mona Lisa, Last Supper);* Raphael *(Sistine Madonna, Madonna of the Chair);* Michelangelo *(Ceiling of the Sistine Chapel, Moses),* equally great as sculptor and painter; Titian *(Charles V);* and the sculptor and goldsmith, Cellini.

No less amazing are the great Germans, including Durer *(Holzschuher; Trent; Knight, Devil, and Death),* Cranach *(Luther),* and Holbein *(Erasmus, Anne of Cleves).* England had little to offer, but in France, there were eminent artists such as Jean Clouet *(Francis 1).* In most countries, many minor painters who, had they lived in different times and been less overshadowed by the greats, would have been considered unique.

What distinguished the paintings of the High Renaissance from those of Byzantine and medieval times were, above, all the natural, realistic forms the great masters gave to the objects and persons in their sculptures and paintings. They paid careful attention to human anatomy. Perspective was introduced, and portrait painting, which had not formerly been practiced, gained in importance. Abandoning the two-dimensional, stylized representations of earlier times and the golden backdrops, artists filled the backgrounds of their paintings with views of beautiful and grand landscapes and castles. Human beings engaged in their daily pursuits appeared more often in paintings. Yet, even when the masters depicted everyday occupations and pleasures, they did not forget the vanity of earthly aspirations. They also produced some of the most beautiful religious paintings and generally set those representing worldly scenes within the framework of the age's spiritual preoccupations.

## Music

The early 16th century, outstanding in art, is also known as a "Golden Age of Song." This century saw the flourishing of the motet and, after 1520, the madrigal. Both were compositions for voices, the former based on sacred text, the latter on secular texts. In many countries, popular song festivals were held, and the art of singing was promoted by guilds (Hans Sachs and the *Meistersinge*). The Catholic Church and religious reformers—especially Luther himself, who composed enduring hymns—competed in beautifying church services with organ music and encouraged singing among the churchgoers. The Dutch composers taught their art and style in many countries. With previously unknown perfection, their instrumentals and works for voice were performed at the courts of princes and nobility as well as in the houses of wealthy burghers.

## Literature

Owing to the mid-15th-century invention of the printing press with movable type, popular education became more widespread. New educational ideals arose. Luther, in particular, favored widespread teaching of the fundamentals of reading and writing. He advocated kindness toward children and encouraged the understanding of pupils in addition to discipline. With the increase in literacy, the demand for books accelerated. The great controversies of the age brought forth a stream of pamphlets, tracts, and brilliant works on classics, history, criticism, education, and politics.

### *Humanism*

The intellectual trend known as *humanism,* with its interest in classical studies and in things human rather than otherworldly, moved from the southern into the northern countries of Europe. One of the greatest humanists of the age was Erasmus of Rotterdam (d. 1536), scholar, promoter of Classical culture and learning, and editor of the Greek text of the Bible. He wrote *In Praise of Folly,* which ridiculed such human weaknesses as avarice, credulity, pedantry, and gluttony. As an advocate of peace and reason, Erasmus opposed the excesses, violence, and coarseness of the age. He admonished princes and churchmen to abandon evil traditions, to reform, be tolerant, and to devote themselves to the true service of Christ. Other leading northern humanists were the statesman Thomas More, the pamphleteer and poet Ulrich von Hutten, and Johann Reuchlin, who compiled a Hebrew grammar for Bible studies and vigorously took part in the controversies of the age.

Numerous French and Scandinavian writers, as well as some Spanish writers, followed the Italian, German, and English example. They combined the pagan and Christian (the Classical and Medieval) heritage and published widely read works of lasting merit. Important histories and biographies of many sorts appeared, including Guicciardini's history of Italy, Gomara's history of America, Vasari's lives of Italian artists, and Benvenuto Cellini's famous autobiography.

### *Luther*

A special place in literary achievement belongs to Luther, whose translation of the Bible into German is a work of beauty and majesty. The dialect that he used prepared the way for the modern High

German tongue as generally spoken today. The English Bible translation by Tyndale was based on Luther's edition.

### *Poetry and Drama*

Compared with the great religious and humanistic literature, however, poetry and drama attained lesser heights. There were few who excelled in literary works of imagination. Perhaps the best known is the Italian, Ariosto (d. 1533). He was widely appreciated and subsequently served as a model for several generations. Popular drama, miracle plays, and poems in the classical style were generally imitative and not inspiring.

### Natural Science

The broadening horizon of Western people, their inquisitiveness and secular interests, directed their attention to closer observation and investigation of natural phenomena. Moreover, the geographical discoveries stirred their minds and enlarged their scientific understanding. Much new knowledge was gained in geography and anthropology. Discoveries brought new inventions and improvements in technique. Additionally, in areas that had no direct connection with geographical discoveries, outstanding advances were also made.

The greatest was perhaps reflected in the work of Copernicus (d. 1543), who showed that the Earth circles the Sun. Rather unwillingly, people came to realize the relative insignificance of their own world within the larger scheme of nature. Of comparable importance was the growing understanding of human physiology. Vesalius (d. 1564) dissected and described the human body. Leonardo da Vinci (d. 1519) examined and charted many of its organs. Servetus (d. 1553) investigated the pulmonary circulation of the blood. Paracelsus (d. 1541) sought new therapeutic methods. Similar interests led Gesner (d. 1565) to compose a history of animals and Agricola (d. 1555) to study mineralogy.

The exact sciences, which were based on rational deduction and observation, still intermingled with pseudo-sciences, which were based on superstition or on the word of accepted authority. Standards were established for scientific work by Leonardo da Vinci, who called for mathematical thinking and experimentation, but these were not generally accepted. Many scientists continued their efforts to solve the mysteries of life and nature with the help of astrology, alchemy, and magic, but since these unscientific methods did not stand the test of time, historians have been inclined to pass them over in their descriptions of what captivated the minds of 16th-century people.

### Political Science

A special place among the endeavors of the age belongs to the numerous political writings. Despite widespread adherence to the theoretical propositions of medieval thinkers, these writings show a clear, realistic approach to political problems. Many works discussed the duties of princes and of upper class ladies. Erasmus wrote such a book. More influential was the internationally consulted *Courtier* by Castiglioni. It was the standard work on courtly manners and Christian behavior in public affairs. The English humanist and statesman Thomas More (d. 1535) wrote *Utopia,* which describes an "ideal commonwealth" based on Christian concepts. Through the nobility of its conception, *Utopia* exercised a strong influence on later political thought.

### *Machiavelli*

However, none of these works compares with the historical influence of Machiavelli (d. 1527), author of *The Prince.* Machiavelli, who as a humanist was well acquainted with classical literature, analyzes with penetrating insight into human psychology the sources of political power and its "demoniac" nature. Drawing upon experience and giving no thought to morality, he counsels princes on how best to gain, maintain, and use power. Self-interest alone, he holds, should dictate their actions. His work has remained unique in the field of rational statecraft.

### Perspective

*Influenced by the great tradition of classical and medieval times, the High Renaissance introduced the Modern Age. The focus of attention was no longer upon sin and salvation, but upon the activities of human beings and the configurations of their natural surroundings. Worldly concerns now occupied the mind. Nobles and burghers engaged in commercial activities and sought wealth, which brought them new power—more than the sword had ever provided. Industries were expanded, which resulted in a greater division of labor, and new class stratifications developed. Wealth allowed princes to participate in new types of warfare. They would hire mercenaries instead of relying on knights bound to them by concepts of honor. It was a time of overwhelming change and upheaval. The great passions evident in all areas of human endeavor led, at times, to cruel behavior in human relationships, but also to astounding cultural achievements. The literature, art, and philosophy of the Renaissance are examples of these achievements.*

### Selected Readings

Burckhardt, Jacob. *The Civilization of the Renaissance in Italy* (London: Phaidon Press, 1960).

Postan, M.M. and Habakku H. J. eds., *Cambridge Economic History of Europe.* 8 vols. (Cambridge: Cambridge University Press, 1966).

Einstein, Alfred. *A Short History of Music* (New York: A. A. Knopf, 1960).

Gardner, Helen. *Art through the Ages* (San Diego: Harcourt Brace Jovanovich, 1986).

Hay, Denys, ed. *The Renaissance Debate* (New York: Holt, Rinehart, and Winston, 1965).

Janson, Horst. *History of Art* (New York: H. N. Abrams, 1986).

Magnus, Laurie. *A Dictionary of European Literature* (London: C. Routledge and Sons, 1926).

McKim, Donald K. The Cambridge Companion to Martin Luther (Cambridge: Cambridge University Press, 2003).

Weber, Max. *Protestant Ethics and the Spirit of Capitalism* (New York: Charles Scribner's Sons, 1958).

## Test Yourself

1. In the early 16th century, the first and the second estates were___.
   A. Clergy and the Nobility
   B. Commoners and Nobility
   C. Bourgeoisie and Commoners
   D. Peasants and Guilds

2. In the Age of Discovery, the townspeople or burghers together with the free peasants formed____.
   A. Guilds
   B. The Third Estate
   C. The Estates General
   D. The Aristocracy

3. Around 1500, the vast majority of the population of Europe was composed of___.
   A. Peasants
   B. Bankers and Lawyers
   C. The Nobility
   D. The Clergy

4. The early conquerors of the Pre-Columbian American societies were motivated by the motto ___.
   A. God, King, and Gold
   B. Gospel, Gold and Glory
   C. Guns, Gold, and Steel
   D. God, Guns, Gold

5. Vasco da Gama sailed to India via the Cape of Good Hope in_____
   A. 1513
   B. 1492
   C. 1498
   D. 1500

6. In 1521, the Aztec Empire in Mexico was conquered by_____
   A. Christopher Columbus
   B. Hernan Cortes
   C. Pedro de Alvarado
   D. Ferdinand Magellan

7. The early 16th century, outstanding in art, is also known in music as_____.
   A. The Golden Age of Song
   B. The Golden Age of Chamber Music
   C. The Silver Age of Chanting
   D. The Golden Age of Opera

8. The author of *The Prince* was _____.
   A. Hernan Cortes
   B. Martin Luther
   C. Niccolo Machiavelli
   D. Boccacio

## Answers and Explanations

1. **A.** In the early 16th century, the first estate, the clergy, continued to play the prominent role it had enjoyed throughout the Middle Ages, and the second estate, the nobility, rivaled the first in the pursuit of worldly interests.

2. **B.** In the Age of Discovery, the townspeople or *burghers*, together with the free peasants, formed the "third estate," which acquired increased prestige.

3. **A.** Around 1500, the vast majority of the population in Europe was still composed of peasants. This was true even in small countries active in trade, such as the Netherlands.

4. **B.** Possessing material resources, men of genius who were animated by the creative spirit of the age could transform their long-held dreams into reality. Their incentives were threefold: Gospel, Gold, and Glory—the desire to convert others, to enrich themselves, and to win fame.

5. **C.** Explorers set out in search of new shores. Vasco da Gama sailed from Portugal to India via the Cape of Good Hope in 1498.

6. **B.** In 1521, Hernan Cortes conquered the Aztec empire in Mexico.

7. **A.** The early 16th century, outstanding in art, is also known for its music. As "The Golden Age of Song," it saw the flourishing of the motet and, after 1520, the madrigal. Both of these are compositions for voices, the former based on sacred text, the latter on secular, texts. In many countries, popular song festivals were held, and the art of singing was promoted by guilds (Hans Sachs and the *Meistersinger*).

8. **C.** None of the 16th century works can compare with the historical influence of Niccolo Machiavelli's *The Prince*. In this book, Machiavelli, a humanist who was well acquainted with classical literature, analyzes with penetrating insight into human psychology the sources of political power and its "demoniac" nature. Drawing upon experience and giving no thought to morality, he counsels princes on how best to gain, maintain, and use power. Self-interest alone, he holds, should dictate their actions. His work remains unique in the field of rational statecraft.

**CHAPTER 4**

# The New Monarchies (1455-1519)

**1455-1483** War of the Roses in England
Birth of Tudor Dynasty
**1461-1483** Reign of Louis XI in France
**1462-1505** Reign of Ivan the Great of Moscovy
**1479** Union of Aragon and Castile under Ferdinand and Isabella
**1492** Columbus discovers America for United Kingdom of Spain
**1517** Charles V becomes King of Spain
**1519** Charles V becomes Holy Roman Emperor

*The atmosphere created by new interests and directions of the active forces in society brought forth a new political organization in Europe. For several centuries, feudal traits had been waning, while tendencies toward greater cohesion within the territories of various national groups appeared. These tendencies were supported by rulers who sought to extend their personal power. They were also advanced due to economic necessities, including increased productivity and the expansion of commerce. These changes necessitated the development of a strong central authority, such as absolutist monarchical forms provided. Thus came into being what were known as the "New Monarchies."*

*In a "New Monarchy," the ruling prince had to overcome the challenge of the feudal nobility. Princes succeeded in concentrating decisive power in their own hands; in reducing the influence of estates, parliaments, and diets; and in controlling the military forces, the jurisdiction, and the finances of their realms. In their endeavors, which put an end to much of the strife of the feudal age, they were usually supported by the burgher class, whose wealth and jealousy of the nobility provided the princes with the means to strengthen their own monarchical rule.*

## ■ WESTERN EUROPE

The development of the "New Monarchies" was much more rapid in Western Europe than in other parts. Owing to the opportunities that the discovery of new lands offered, there was a shift in the center of authority and power away from empire and papacy in Germany and Italy, respectively, to the western monarchies. This shift was paralleled by a corresponding shift in initiative and leadership. The western regions of Europe, which bordered on the Atlantic and profited from the new trade routes to the wealth of Asia and America, adapted their political organization more speedily to the demands of modern times.

## Portugal

A "New Monarchy" developed early in Portugal. It gained strength owing to the acquisition of colonies in the Indies and in Brazil. It benefited from the influx of Oriental products, spices and jewels, income from the slave trade, national strength gained through sea power, and support from merchants and bankers interested in colonial expansion. Lisbon, the capital city of Portugal, soon became more important than the older trading city of Venice, and the Portuguese king assumed a virtual trade monopoly. By concentrating in his hands the lucrative Indian spice trade, he firmly established his power and dominated the nobles and the burghers alike. By allowing foreign participation in Portuguese trade ventures, he also avoided conflict with England.

## Spain

The acquisition of colonies contributed to the greatness of Spain under Ferdinand and Isabella. Gold and silver flowed into the treasury of the rulers, who had held a monopoly on trade with America since 1503. They conferred this monopoly upon a *Casa de Contratacion*. Ships in convoys sailed annually from the ports of Seville and Cadiz to bring colonial products safely home. However, unlike the ruler of Portugal, the Spanish royal house used its position less for the accumulation of bullion than for its own political aggrandizement.

After Isabella's death, Ferdinand secured the domination of southern Italy in addition to the large territories of the New World and controlled trade routes in the western Mediterranean. He built the most powerful and effective army in the world, which was commanded by some of the greatest generals of the time. Piracy and highway robbery were checked, and firm order under strong monarchical supervision was maintained.

King Ferdinand continued the unification of the country, which had started with his marriage. Under central authority, a common and essentially weak parliament *(Cortes),* under royal supervision, was created. Religious dissidents were suppressed. The popes conferred the right to make Church appointments on the Spanish king, and the Inquisition became a tool in his hands. A generally valid code of laws based on Roman law was introduced, and even the nobility had to observe it. Legal studies flourished, and arts were protected. Unfortunately for Spain, commercial interests had generally been the domain of existing brotherhoods of towns *(hermandades),* and the king continued to give these conservative forces his protection. This meant that, with high taxes rigorously levied, a vigorous, enterprising and independent middle class could not develop.

*Figure 4–1 The Union of the Crowns of Castile and Aragon with the Marriage of Queen Isabella and King Ferdinand, 1469*

### France

France, with its seat of government firmly established in Paris, had under King Louis XI made progress on the road toward a "New Monarchy." Under Louis's successors, Charles VIII, Louis XII, and after 1515, Francis I—all of whom belonged to the House of Valois—France continued on the same path. The representative body, the Estates-General, whose functions paralleled those of diets and parliaments elsewhere, was kept in a weakened state, while royal power was augmented in jurisdictional, administrative, financial, and Church matters.

Yet, France's development was slower than that of Spain. It was not successful in securing colonies—despite Cartier's discoveries in the St. Lawrence region—and it did not sufficiently encourage modern economic tendencies. Instead, it pursued wars against the empire in Italy, which Charles VIII, out of expansionist desires, greed, and fear of Hapsburg power, had begun in 1494. Francis I continued the struggle and wasted the resources needed for improving France's internal conditions.

### England

Like other Atlantic seaboard countries, England, with less than a third of the population of France, also entered a stage in which the establishment of a modern nation became possible. Henry VII of the House of Tudor had already reestablished respect for law and order. He favored the merchant class, amassed a large treasury, and secured control of the judiciary. The nobility, decimated in the preceding times of trouble, was deprived of its military power and compelled to obey his wishes. However, the nobility maintained its hold on all important posts. Henry VII's successor, Henry VIII, adhered to the same policy. Parliament continued to function, even though its effectiveness was limited because the political initiative rested with the Crown.

## ■ CENTRAL AND EASTERN EUROPE

In the regions of Europe that did not border on the Atlantic Ocean, the traditions of the past remained strong. Because the politically dominant powers of Central Europe benefited little from the economic shifts occurring in the Age of Discovery, they were forced into a defensive position. This caused them to try to preserve the existing social organization in their countries.

Moreover, their attention was increasingly directed eastward where two new great powers, Turkey and Russia, had emerged. Neither Turkey nor Russia shared in the political evolution of the West, and consequently, neither could set an example of political modernization. Yet, with the vigor of rising nations, both began to make their influence felt on the European political scene, principally on the neighboring German Empire.

### The German Empire

At the beginning of modern times, the empire was still an international organization that extended beyond Germany into areas inhabited by diverse national groups, such as the Dutch, Burgundians, Swiss, Italians, Czechs, and others. The empire was composed of seven electorates, many smaller states, numerous ecclesiastical territories, hundreds of towns, and other areas governed by independent knights. It was held together by imperial authority which, though the office of emperor was elective, remained in the hands of the House of Hapsburg. It had a few federal institutions, such as a diet, which decided questions of finance and common organization that affected all members, and a federal court, but these institutions did not offer an encouraging environment for the evolution of a strong centralized state.

Nevertheless, "new" monarchical trends were not entirely absent. While they did not pervade the empire as a whole, these trends could be found within the larger member states, such as Saxony, Brandenburg, Bavaria, Austria, and others. It would, therefore, be incorrect to speak of the political development of Germany as differing radically from that of the Atlantic nations. It was, however, on a more restricted scale, local rather than national, that the trends toward "New Monarchies" appeared.

Despite its lack of modern political evolution, the German Empire was to achieve early in the 16th century a position of power in the world almost unequaled in any earlier or later period. This was achieved through the shrewd diplomacy of the House of Hapsburg, which concluded numerous advantageous marriage alliances. It was furthered by the enterprising spirit of some individuals, especially the merchants of southern Germany and of the Low Countries. It was also enhanced by the economic opportunities afforded by the proximity of Eastern European production centers and markets with their resources, which included grain in Poland-Lithuania, metals in Tyrol and Hungary, and export markets in Russia and the Balkans. By dominating the central areas that connected the east and west as well as the north and south, the Hapsburgs exploited these advantages.

The Emperor Maximilian I (1489–1519)—an intelligent, chivalrous, well-educated, but weak-spirited man—did not succeed in enforcing his will upon the empire, in improving its cumbersome, outdated judicial and administrative machinery, or in leading the whole country toward unification. He did strengthen its position enormously by securing as dowry the rich Burgundian and Netherlands domains. He then married his son, Philip, to the Spanish princess, Joanna, through whom his grandson, Charles, could claim the entire Spanish Empire. In 1517, upon the death of his grandfather, Ferdinand, this Charles, who was born in Ghent in the Netherlands in 1500, actually became the king of Spain and all its colonies. In 1519, upon the death of his other grandfather, Maximilian, the same Charles was elected German emperor. To win the election, however, it was necessary for him to engage in a bitter contest with Francis I of France. This contest forced him not only to distribute lavish bribes to the electors, but also to make sweeping promises, which went contrary to the trends of the time, to maintain "German liberties." As Charles V, he was to rule for almost 40 years over an empire "on which the sun never set." He was a man of high moral standards, earnestly devoted to his task, slow and wise when making decisions, and shrewd in his judgment of people, but he faced a task that surpassed his strength, even as it would have surpassed that of any other ruler.

## Italy

The only Western country in which the new forms of government made no progress, either on a national or a city-state level, was Italy. No central authority existed there. Individual attempts at making the inhabitants conscious of common links had no practical effect. Emperor, pope, and French and Spanish kings shared with the Medici, Sforza, Este, Gonzaga, and other famous Renaissance princes the rule of the area that, centuries later, was to form the Italian nation. Almost all sectors retained their traditional forms of government.

Moreover, wars fought by the Valois and the Hapsburgs over the disunited country desolated the land. The rivalries of the great powers checked the growth of a modern state system. The commercial importance of the country, which had been based on Italian business connections with the Muslims in the Near East, was diminished by the advance of the Turks and the opening of a direct seaway from Western Europe to India.

## Russia and Turkey

Centralization and absolutism, toward which the European national states developed, had long existed in these two Eastern empires. However, owing to Oriental concepts of despotism and the lack of customary ethical restraints that prevailed in the West, they differed fundamentally from their Western counterparts. The term "New Monarchy" is hardly applicable to the two Eastern empires. Both the Russian *tsar* and the Turkish sultan enjoyed a degree of absolute power unparalleled in the West. Their power extended to politics, law, and economic activity. Despite these differences, both countries began, through war and peace, to move toward closer relations with the West. Diplomatic contacts were established. There was a lively interchange of visitors, travelers, and merchants. Descriptions of Russia and Turkey were broadcast throughout Europe.

## Perspective

*The 16th century saw the rapid development of the nation-state. Spain, France, and England led the way. Each nation developed its own types of institutions, but everywhere a centralized monarchical structure ("New Monarchy") gained ascendancy. The nobility, though retaining many privileges, had to adjust. The three great empires, the German, the Russian, and the Ottoman Turkish, on the other hand, struggled to achieve modern forms of government. Under Emperor Charles V, the German Empire was to reach a pinnacle of prestige and power. However, the kinds of centralized institutions in existence could not prevail over increasingly disruptive forces. Germany did not benefit from the resources of the New World or the Far East, both of which opened great possibilities to the seafaring nations and allowed them to expand their wealth and power.*

## Selected Readings

Guerard, Albert. *France: A Modern History* (Ann Arbor: University of Michigan Press, 1969).

Holborn, Hajo. *A History of Modern Germany* (New York: A. Knopf, 1969).

Roger, P. *A History of Russia* (New York: Palgrave Macmillan, 2005).

Killinger, Charles L. *The History of* Italy (New York: Greenwood Press, 2002).

McNeill, W. H. *The Rise of the West* (Chicago: the University of Chicago Press, 1991).

Payne, Stanly G. *A History of Spain and Portugal* (Madison: University of Wisconsin Press, 1973).

## Test Yourself

1. A "New Monarchy" developed early in Portugal and gained strength owing to the acquisition of ____.
   A. Colonies in the Indies and Brazil
   B. Colonies in North America
   C. Colonies in Asia
   D. None of the above

2. The acquisition of colonies in the early 16$^{th}$ century contributed to the greatness of Spain under the rule of _____.
   A. Henry the Navigator
   B. Ferdinand and Isabella
   C. Elizabeth and Philip
   D. William and Mary

3. By 1500, France had firmly established its seat of government in _____.
   A. Lyon
   B. Versailles
   C. Paris
   D. Madrid

4. Despite its lack of modern political evolution, the German empire was to achieve early in the 16$^{th}$ century _____.
   A. A position of power in the world
   B. Overseas colonies
   C. Economic opportunities in Eastern Europe
   D. None of the above

5. The only western country in which the new forms of government made no progress either on a national or a city-state level was _____.
   A. Germany
   B. Spain
   C. France
   D. Italy

## Answers and Explanations

1. **A.** A "New Monarchy" developed early in Portugal. It gained its strength because of the acquisition of colonies in the Indies and in Brazil. It benefited from the influx of Oriental products, spices and jewels, income from the slave trade, national strength gained through sea power, and support by the merchants and bankers interested in colonial expansion. Lisbon, the capital city of Portugal, soon surpassed the greatest older trading city, Venice, in importance, and the Portuguese king assumed a virtual trade monopoly. By concentrating in his hands the lucrative Indian spice trade, he firmly established his power and dominated the nobility and burghers alike. By allowing foreign participation in Portuguese trade ventures, he also avoided conflict with England.

2. **B.** The acquisition of colonies contributed to the greatness of Spain under Ferdinand and Isabella. Gold and silver flowed into the treasury of the rulers, who had held a monopoly on trade with America since 1503. They conferred this monopoly upon a *Casa de Contratacion*. Ships in convoys sailed annually from the ports of Seville and Cadiz to bring colonial products safely home. However, unlike the ruler of Portugal, the Spanish royal house used its position less for accumulation of bullion than for its own political aggrandizement.

3. **C.** France, with its seat of government firmly established in Paris, had under King Louis XI made progress on the road toward the status of a "New Monarchy." Under Louis's successors, Charles VIII, Louis XII, and, after 1515, Francis I—all of whom belonged to the House of Valois—France continued on the same path.

4. **A.** Despite its lack of modern political evolution, the German Empire was to achieve early in the 16th century a position of power in the world almost unequaled in any earlier or later period. This was achieved through the shrewd diplomacy of the House of Hapsburg, which made numerous, advantageous marriage alliances. It was furthered by the enterprising spirit of some individuals, especially the merchants of southern Germany and of the Low Countries. It was also enhanced by the economic opportunities afforded by its proximity to Eastern European production centers and markets with their resources, including grain in Poland-Lithuania, metals in Tyrol and Hungary, and export markets in Russia and the Balkans. By dominating the central areas that connected the east and west, as well as the north and south, the Hapsburgs exploited these advantages.

5. **D.** The only Western country in which the new forms of government made no progress, either on a national or a city-state level, was Italy. No central authority existed there. Individual attempts at making the inhabitants conscious of common links had no practical effect. Emperor, pope, and French and Spanish kings shared with the Medici, Sforza, Este, Gonzaga, and other famous Renaissance princes the rule of the area that, centuries later, was to form the Italian nation. Almost all sectors retained their traditional forms of government.

# CHAPTER 5
# The Age of the Reformation (1517-1555)

**1518** Zwingli begins work in Zurich
**1519** Charles V becomes German emperor
Cortez begins conquest of Mexico
Magellan begins circumnavigation of the world
**1520** Suleiman the Magnificent becomes sultan of Turkey
**1521** Luther before Diet of Worms
**1523** Sweden leaves Scandinavian Union
Gustavus Vasa becomes king
**1524** Peasants' Revolt in Germany
**1525** Battle of Pavia
Francis I of France made prisoner of Charles V
Death of Jacob Fugger
**1526** Durer, *Four Apostles*
**1527** Rome sacked by troops of Charles V
**1529** Ottoman Turks besiege Vienna
Diet of Speyer ("Protestants")
**1530** Augsburg Confession drawn up
**1532** Pizarro undertakes conquest of Peru
**1533** Reformation begins in England (Henry VIII)
**1534** Rabelais, *Gargantua*
**1536** Erasmus of Rotterdam dies
Calvin, Institutes of the Christian Religion
**1540** Order of Jesuits founded
**1541** Paracelsus dies
**1543** Copernicus, *De Revolutionibus Orbium Coelestium (On the Revolutions of the Heavenly Spheres)*
**1542** Vesalius, *De Humani Corporis Fabrica (The Structure of the Human Body)*
Holbein dies
**1545** Discovery of Potosi silver mines in Bolivia
**1547** Protestants defeated by Charles V at Muhlberg

**1552** Protestants resume war
**1553** Servetus burned at stake in Geneva
**1554** Marriage of Mary Tudor of England and Philip II of Spain
**1555** Religious Peace of Augsburg
  Persecution of Protestants in England
  Muscovy Company founded in England
**1556** Abdication of Charles V

*By far, one the most momentous events of the early modern period was the Reformation. It started as a reform movement within the Catholic Church. Its original objective was no less than a purification of the Christian church and a renewal of Christian morals in European life. Indeed, the leading men of the Reformation were, and remained, theologians. They considered all their reform proposals from a theological point of view, but the effect of their work was soon felt in all areas of European life—in politics, social relationships, the sciences and arts, and in the economic arena as well. For this reason, historians have been tempted to speak of the Reformation as a broad, international revolution—a term that certainly misrepresents the work and aims of the reformers, but that may have a measure of justification because of the movement's wide effects.*

## ■THE REFORMATION

The urgent need of reform in existing religious institutions was generally recognized both outside and inside the Catholic Church. Over the course of the centuries, doctrinal views, which many believed needed revision, had arisen. More important, numerous practical abuses had penetrated all organizational levels of the Catholic Church and threatened the entire institution. Therefore, many of the most devoted Church members, who were concerned primarily with advancing the Christian way of life, joined forces with those who sought reform for selfish economic advantages.

### Church Abuses

The abuses of the Church and the sins of some churchmen were many. Anarchy reigned within the Church. Central authority had been weakened. Kings and nations assumed rights and duties that belonged to the Church. Among popes and bishops, moral corruption existed. Many, greedy and venal, pursued worldly policies and allowed nepotism and simony, the sale of Church offices. Among the clergy, there was a shocking lack of training, and the rank and file found themselves in desperate economic circumstances, while those further up in the hierarchy lived in luxury. Immorality and sexual promiscuity prevailed among many of the churchmen. Church services and the care of Church buildings were neglected by the priests. A large portion of the clergy became more interested in science, art, and economics, than in the salvation of souls.

Adding to the crisis were the constant rivalries and jealousies among members of the hierarchy, among various monastic orders, and between friars and priests. Bishops tried to hold as many lucrative Church offices as possible without fulfilling the corresponding duties. Moreover, errors of faith developed, and these led to errors in conduct. Popes misused indulgences and abused their power to censure and excommunicate. The Church held economic views derived from a period that had an entirely different economic system and needs. The Church insisted on being exempted from taxation and refused to divest itself of "unproductive" lands.

There were many forces at work within the Church attempting to improve external conditions, purify the hearts of its members, and reconcile Christian duties with the humanistic trends of the age, but these forces proved weak. Their effects came too late.

## Early Reform Movements

The greatest figure of the Reformation was Martin Luther. Today, hundreds of years later, the immediate and direct influence of his work is still felt. Many individuals before Luther had urged the Church to reform. Some had attacked the same dogmas that Luther challenged: Ockham, Marsilius, Bradwardine, Wycliffe, Wessel, Huss, and many humanists were among them.

### Savonarola

The last of these was Savonarola, a Florentine who, shocked by the corruption of the Roman Court under the Borgia pope and by the widespread secular interests of the clergy, preached purification and repentance. When he became involved in Florentine political quarrels, his enemies succeeded in having him hanged and burned as a heretic in 1498.

### Luther

Martin Luther was, in a sense, Savonarola's immediate successor. He was born in 1483, the son of a miner. At first, he studied law, then turned to theology and became an Augustine friar. He took his duties most seriously. He prayed, fasted, chastised himself, and made a pilgrimage to Rome. When a new university was founded in Wittenberg, Saxony, his superiors sent him there to teach. Terrified by the corruption he had seen in Rome, doubtful as to many teachings of the Church, and convinced that only faith and the grace of God can lead to salvation, he wrote ninety-five theses in 1517 attacking one of the worst abuses, the sale of indulgences.

Indulgences were designed to bring remittance of the punishment if the sinner showed a contrite heart, confessed, accepted due penalty, and performed good works. However, indulgences were granted and often sold without demanding repentance or good works. The sale of indulgences was a big business, and the profits flowed into the pockets of bankers and bishops. Some of the funds were used for the beautification of Rome.

### Ninety-five Theses (1517)

The publication of theses, statements debating theological questions, was a rather common procedure. Luther's act, however, had extreme repercussions because of the logic and vigor of his statements and his implied challenge to papal authority. Pious Christians everywhere saw in his act the long-desired beginning of reform. Numerous worldly interests saw in it a means to escape some of the judgment and financial demands of the popes. Princes saw in Luther's act a reason to stop the flow of money to Rome, channeling it, instead, into their own pockets. They used the act as an appeal to German national consciousness and sensed in it an opportunity to break entirely with a degraded papacy that was absorbed in politics, whose heirs they themselves wanted to become. Rome reacted vigorously to Luther's action, and a number of disputations and debates were sponsored between Luther and leading Catholic scholars. These debates only served to widen the breach, however.

### Doctrinary Tracts and Luther's Excommunication

In 1520, Luther took a further decisive step by publishing three pamphlets. Again, he described Rome's abuses, demanded reforms in morals and in dogma, and attacked some of the sacraments, including transubstantiation and the worship of saints. He again insisted that the Bible alone, with no additional precepts of the Church, constituted the final authority for a Christian. He emphasized that, on the foundation of God's Word, everyone could be his own priest and master and need be nobody's servant.

The pope threatened Luther with excommunication, but in the presence of applauding Wittenberg students, Luther publicly burned the pope's decree or "bull." He thereby protested in behalf of the individual's inalienable right, as a Christian, to be subject to God alone.

*Figure 5–1 Martin Luther, 1483–1546*

**Diet of Worms (1521) and the Translation of the Bible**

The rebellion against established Church authority started by Luther led to a quick reaction on the part of political authority, as emperors and kings began to fear for their own positions. Charles V, a devout Catholic, invited Luther to attend a diet of the German estates, which was to be held in Worms in 1521. Under safe-conduct, Luther appeared. Before the assembled princes, he courageously restated his position, as "it is neither safe nor right to act against one's conscience."

Charles honored the safe-conduct, but Luther was put under the ban of the German Empire, which deprived him of all legal protection in the empire. His political friends gave him asylum in one of their castles, the Wartburg. There, Luther composed hymns, studied educational methods, and, particularly, worked on his translation of the Bible. Within a year, grave disturbances called him back to Wittenberg.

**Social Consequences**

Luther's attack on authority and tradition had released many revolutionary forces. Numerous preachers and theologians felt that he had not gone far enough. Groups seeking salvation in independent ways, mystics, lay brother-hoods and sisterhoods, and others, had existed before Luther, and now additional ones arose, demanding the abolition of, or substitutions for, all dogmas and sacraments, images, and traditional rites. Often, they also rejected worldly authorities, princely powers, and existing economic and behavior patterns. Some wanted to introduce free love and a completely free, communistic society.

Luther, who himself had rejected celibacy and married in 1525, fought such extreme trends. But the stream of demands could not be stopped. Anabaptists, who were against infant baptism, and other religious radicals caused widespread disturbances. Knights rebelled against their overlords, and eventually—as in Wycliffe's and Huss's times—a great peasant revolt broke out. In "Twelve Articles," the peasants protested against serfdom, illegal and extravagant taxes, restriction of their rights to common lands, and the abolition of customary law in favor of Roman law with its property concepts. They demanded emancipation and the right to worship God in their own chosen ways.

Luther had exhorted the nobles to deal fairly with their peasants and to yield to justified demands. Anticipating John Locke, he advocated the peasants' rights to defend themselves against unjust government, but he was shocked by the violence of the resulting peasant uprising. He gradually became more conservative and turned against the pillaging peasants, using a violence of language not uncommon to his time. This change cost him the support of many. He insisted on the right of God-ordained secular powers to reestablish order and worldly authority by fire and sword. However, the entire social fabric of past ages had been shattered.

## Political Consequences

The political effect of Luther's work was no less significant than the social consequences. In the German Empire, the forces of disintegration became stronger. Many princes, foreseeing an opportunity to confiscate the wealth of the churches and monasteries located in their realms, adhered to the new religion and rebelled against the emperor. In England, on the other hand, the king himself took advantage of religious controversies to improve and enhance his personal rule. In Scandinavia, the conflict caused the Swedes, under the leadership of Gustavus Vasa, to break ties with Denmark and establish an independent kingdom.

In most regions, strife and internecine war resulted. On the international stage, the French used the newly developing dissent for territorial aggrandizement. The papacy was torn between its political ambitions and the desire to see Catholicism restored everywhere.

## Effects on Imperial Politics

Of special consequence was the effect of the reform movement on the position of the German Empire and on the role of empire and papacy in the Western world. Despite numerous struggles, the two powers had always been interdependent, but at this critical moment, when the survival of both was threatened, and unity should have been the first thought, Charles V was deserted by the pope, who feared imperial might more than heresy.

The emperor was forced to meet the problems alone. With fortitude, he sought to stem the tide. He turned, first, against the French, who had once again invaded his possessions in Italy. His Spanish armies decisively defeated them and took their king as a prisoner. Francis was not released until he had promised to keep the peace and to make restitution of conquered lands—a promise which, with the connivance of the pope, he soon broke.

Next, Charles had to use force against the pope himself, the ambitious and luxury-loving Medici, Clement VII. In 1527, Spanish, German, and Swiss mercenaries seized Rome, which they sacked, destroying untold works of art and stripping it of much of its riches. For the time being, papal opposition was eliminated. A measure of cooperation between empire and papacy was established. Then, Charles had to deal with the Ottoman Turks, the arch enemy of Christendom, with whom the king of France had entered into close relations and whom he had enticed to invade the empire. In 1529, the Turks reached the gates of Vienna. They were repulsed, but they did gain dominion over Hungary.

Last, the emperor had to contend with the German princes. Toward them, he tried a policy of moderation. In 1529, a diet was held in Speyer. However, it produced no concession by the Catholic princes, so the Lutherans protested against the decision. The name "Protestants" is derived from this event. In the following year, the Protestants drew up a statement of their faith, the "Augsburg Confession," and reaffirmed their creed, but owing to the mediation of the emperor, a measure of cooperation between Catholics and Protestants was worked out.

## ■THE SPREAD OF THE REFORMATION

Soon, Luther's religious reform movement turned from a principally German development into a European movement. In doing so, it lost some of the parochial character that it had possessed as it comprised a number of specifically German grievances. In spreading news about the work of the reformers, Gutenberg's invention, the printing press with movable type, was a factor of immeasurable importance. An enormous outpouring of books and pamphlets, characteristic for the age, conveyed religious demands and thoughts from all other fields to all parts of Europe, where an increasingly literate public could absorb them.

### Expansion on the Continent

The Reformation reached beyond Germany and spread to the north, particularly Switzerland, the Scandinavian territories, and the British Isles.

### *Switzerland*

In Switzerland, the first country affected by the Reformation in Germany, Luther's initial steps in 1518 had promptly induced a priest, Ulrich Zwingli of Zurich, to advocate similar reforms. Zwingli, like other humanists, was skeptical of traditional, accepted views and demanded that recognition be given

*Figure 5–2 The spread of Lutheranism in Europe.*

only what the original religious sources said should be recognized. He therefore followed Luther in turning to a theological interpretation of the Bible itself rather than to Church traditions.

Zwingli went further in regard to the purification of dogma, however, and did not hesitate to include the sacraments of baptism and communion, whereby he created a breach between his own adherents and those of Luther. Theological disputes between the two men failed to resolve their dogmatic differences. Thus, an early split in the Protestant camp resulted. Zwingli himself was killed in 1531 while accompanying Swiss troops in battle, but his work was carried on by others.

### *Scandinavia*

In Sweden and Denmark, Lutheranism spread early. The Swedes, once they had freed themselves from Denmark and the rule of Christian II, brother-in-law of Charles V, introduced Lutheranism. Shortly thereafter, the Danes themselves revolted against their king because of his economic policies and arbitrary rule. Having driven Christian II out of the country, they, too, accepted the Lutheran faith. They introduced it into Norway as well. The new faith was likewise accepted by large segments of the population, especially townspeople, in Hungary, Lithuania, Livonia, the Netherlands, and even by some converts in France, Spain, and Italy.

### *Expansion in British Isles*

Luther's movement created a special situation in the British Isles. The Reformation was, at first, of little interest to the average British subject. Subsequently, it found adherents both in Scotland and in England. It was not, however, the religious question, but the personal problems of King Henry VIII that caused England's reforms to take on worldwide importance during the 1530s. Henry was a despotic, utterly selfish, though not incompetent, ruler, who achieved little in international relations, but much of importance in internal affairs. He prevented a resurgence of the nobles' power, preserved order, strengthened royal absolutism, and chose to cooperate with Parliament, enlarging its powers rather than to subduing it. He incorporated Wales into England.

Further, he carried out the break with Rome. He had originally attacked Luther, but when the pope refused to give him a dispensation so that he could discard his wife, Catherine of Aragon, a relative of Charles V, and marry his mistress, Anne Boleyn, who he hoped would bear him a son, he decided to make use of the predicament in which the pope found himself in regard to the Protestant movement.

Step by step, with the help of successive advisers, some of whom he executed after they had served his purpose,—Cardinal Wolsey, Sir Thomas More, Thomas Boleyn, John Fisher, Archbishop Cranmer, Thomas Cromwell—Henry separated England from Rome. He had himself recognized as head of the English Church, dissolved the monasteries, confiscated their wealth, and discontinued the payment of taxes to Rome. In 1539, he arranged for Parliament to confirm a statement of faith, the "Six Articles," which, while preserving essential Catholic doctrines, in essence refused to acknowledge papal authority. Thus, a true moral and doctrinal reformation did not occur in Henry VIII's England, but the position of the papacy was undermined. After Henry's death in 1547, the real reform work began.

## ■ OUTBREAK OF RELIGIOUS WARS AND THE RISE OF CALVINISM

The changes under Henry VIII obscured religious issues everywhere in Europe and emphasized the political aspects of the reform movement. In vain did Luther hope for a reestablishment of Christian unity built upon a Church adhering to the doctrine of justification by faith, implying that by faith alone the believer can be saved, and using a simplified service. Until his death in 1546, Luther remained very active, interpreting the Bible, instituting schools and seminaries, installing superintendents, writing numerous works, and giving advice to secular authorities.

The political and economic implications of the reforms and their unavoidable practical effect were enormous. Two distinct leagues, a Catholic and a Protestant one, the latter called the "Schmalkaldic League", had already been formed in Germany. Once Luther died and his authority ended, war broke out between the leagues.

### Schmalkaldic War

This war was the first in a long series of internal struggles between Catholics and Protestants in many countries. It showed that the situation had gone beyond the possibility of compromise. By 1546, this impasse was recognized not only by the Protestants, but also by Charles V. He, too, had worked for a reunion of the faiths and tried to accomplish reunion by convening a general Church Council. The popes, however, opposed a general Council, and even after the death of Clement VII, popes were unwilling to effect moral reform in the Church and consistently withheld their cooperation. In their refusals, they were supported by France, which engaged in one war after another against the Hapsburgs and profited from the split within Germany.

Charles had no alternative but to seek to reestablish unity by force of arms. He declared war on the Protestants, and the first battle, which was fought at Muelberg (1547), brought him startling success. His forces routed the Schmalkaldic League and captured its two chief leaders. The emperor's triumph served only to further frighten the pope and various foreign princes. Although Charles, showing his customary moderation, had imposed only a truce, the so-called "Interim" (1548), and had redoubled his efforts to find a permanent solution through a General Council, no reconciliation was effected. Hence, a few years later, when his chief ally deserted him and his armies were defeated, he finally gave up all hope for the reestablishment of unity.

### Peace of Augsburg (1555)

In 1555, a peace treaty of fundamental importance was signed. It granted each German prince the right to establish, for all his subjects, the religion that he himself professed. Therefore, Lutheran princes, and with them, Lutheran states, gained equal rights and status with Catholic states—even though the peace forbade any future conversion of Catholic bishoprics into secular Protestant states.

### Abdication of Charles V

Charles suffered two other disappointments in addition to his failed unity effort. His troops did not recover territories in Lorraine, which the Catholic French had annexed with the cooperation of Protestant German princes. Also, the marriage of his son, Philip, to the English queen, Mary, daughter of Henry VIII, did not bring the hoped-for union of Spain and England. The marriage did not produce a child who could inherit both thrones.

Exhausted after forty years of trying to guide the fate of the world, Charles finally decided to divest himself of his various crowns. In a series of emotionally charged ceremonies, particularly the one in Brussels in 1556, he installed his son, Philip, as his successor in Spain, Italy, and the Netherlands, and his brother, Ferdinand, in the German Empire and in Hungary. The Hapsburg possessions were thus divided, and he himself retired to a monastery in Spain where he died two years later.

### Rise of Calvinism

By the time the Peace of Augsburg had been concluded, and Charles had abdicated, the split in the Christian Church had, in any case, become irreparable. The Protestant forces had been augmented by another reformatory group, the Calvinists.

John Calvin (1509-1564), a French law student, was influenced early by Luther's thought. He turned to theology and fled France as a result of one of Francis I's sporadic, politically inspired persecutions of heretics. In 1536, he published his fundamental work, the *Institutes of the Christian Religion*. He found asylum in Switzerland, and he eventually established his political and religious leadership in Geneva. Like Luther, Calvin based his teachings on the Bible, rather than Church authority, and like Luther, he preached justification by faith.

He also accepted Zwingli's interpretation of the sacraments, however. He insisted that no man can achieve the Good except by the will of God because God has predestined our actions. Therefore, man should abandon himself entirely to God, who, to a certain extent, reveals his will to man and who allows man to lead a virtuous and possibly prosperous life on earth doing good works.

In the sphere of public affairs, Calvin gave the Church a hierarchical structure and demanded that it be given a leading role in the community. Pastors, teachers, deacons, and elders, constituting a supervisory council, were to direct all action and watch over education, morals, and orthodoxy. Such a Church government was actually established in Geneva. It supervised the abolition of all remnants of Catholic worship, censored books, prohibited all luxuries and most amusements, and emphasized prayer and work. It went so far as to drag the famous scientist Servetus before its tribunal. He had been accused of heresy by the Catholic Church, but he also opposed Calvinist concept of the Trinity. The tribunal in Geneva had Servetus burned at the stake in 1553.

### *Effect of Calvinism*

Calvinism spread even more rapidly than Lutheranism. It was more international in character and was based more on rationalism than on mystical beliefs. It was more in line with the economic trends of the age and more easily reconciled Christian ethics with business points of view. Calvinism described thrift as a virtue and prestige as a sign of moral strength. It also allowed reasonable interest-taking—a fundamental requirement for the development of modern capitalism. It spread rapidly to the Netherlands, France, England, Scotland, and Poland. In many countries, it became a powerful political and economic tool. In Scotland, where the French Catholic influence within the royal family was resented, the fervent preacher John Knox spread the tenets of Calvinism.

## ■ THE COUNTER REFORMATION

Pressed from many sides, the Catholic Church finally initiated reforms, but it was too late to save Western Christian unity. Again and again, the Church had hesitated, deliberately avoiding recourse to the customary means of settling disputes, namely, through the convening of a General Council. The popes feared not only the power of the emperor in a Council, but also a renewal of the struggle between pope and Council for supremacy within the Church. It also feared the opposition of the clergy to the papacy. The popes were wary of the nationalist tendencies all over Europe and anxious to avoid possible losses of authority, funds, and prestige.

### The Beginnings of the Catholic Reformation

Nevertheless, for some time, the reform movement within the Church showed considerable strength. A number of reforming orders, such as the Theatines and Capuchins, were founded, and several reform

**Figure 5–3 John Calvin, 1509–1564**

popes were elected. Most prominent among them was Hadrian VI, teacher and friend of Charles V, a Netherlander, and one of the rare non-Italian popes. His reign was short, however, and he was succeeded by Clement VII, a luxury-loving Medici and typical Renaissance prelate.

Only after Clement's death did the reform movement find new official support. Yet, in 1545 at the insistence of Charles V, a General Council had assembled in Trent; the popes still obstructed its work. Only after Charles V abdicated and Hapsburg power was divided did the moment seem propitious for the popes to support the reform work of the Council.

### The Founding of the Jesuit Order

By the time the Council convened again, the popes were receiving unquestioning obedience and aid from an unexpected source, the newly founded Society of Jesus—the Jesuits. A wounded soldier, the Spaniard Ignatius of Loyola (1491-1556), had turned from his former profession to become a soldier of Christ. He had written a book of *Exercises,* which taught the need for prayer, meditation, self-control, practical moderation, and training of the will to obtain salvation.

He gathered disciples and organized an order, for which he won recognition from the pope and which he placed, like an army, at the pope's absolute disposal. The purposes of the order were to combat heresy, spread Catholic education, and undertake missionary work. For the sake of effective results, the Jesuits underwent rigorous training. Many of them became the most learned members of the Church and of secular society as well. They did not hesitate to ally themselves with the powerful of this earth, to make questionable political compromises, and to employ all practical means—force as well as persuasion, Inquisition as well as prayer—to regain heretical lands. They devoted special attention to the colonies and carried their activities as far as Japan.

### Conclusion of Council of Trent (1563)

Thus strengthened, the popes reconvened the Council, which had held only intermittent sessions, and in 1563, brought it to a conclusion. They achieved what they had set out to do. Since the Protestants did not recognize the authority of the popes or the decisions of any council unless they were based entirely on the Scriptures, a compromise with them was excluded from the outset.

Instead, the Council reasserted the Catholic point of view. It focused its attention on doctrine and ritual. It affirmed that the Scriptures and traditions are equally binding for the faithful and that the supremacy of the pope is incontestable. The Council published an "Index" of books that Catholics were forbidden to read without special dispensation. It refuted heresies and reaffirmed old dogmas. It prescribed measures to improve Church discipline and the morals and training of the clergy. It prohibited malpractice in regard to indulgences and adoration of the saints. It abolished certain administrative abuses and made the Catholic ritual uniform throughout the church, a ritual based on that used in Rome. It was only after the Council of Trent that the term "Roman Catholic" had any meaning.

The Council of Trent thus concluded a reform of the Church from within, and it rejuvenated the Catholic-Christian spirit. Subsequently, in 1582, Pope Gregory XIII even introduced a new calendar, which was named the "Gregorian calendar" after him, to replace the Julian calendar that had been used since the time of Caesar.

### Perspective

*Reformation and Counter Reformation left a deep imprint upon the Western world in the field of religion and beyond. They affected intellectual trends, economics, and national developments. They stimulated education, changed social relationships, and led to new legal concepts and new laws. As two or more different faiths were subsequently to live side by side, a measure of tolerance became necessary, and the possibility emerged that individuals could make a choice in religious matters. Indeed, the cause of*

*Figure 5–4 The Religious Division of Europe, ca. 1560*

*individualism, which the Renaissance, humanism, and capitalistic enterprise had fostered, was also advanced by the Reformation.*

## Selected Readings

Bainton, Roland H. *The Age of the Reformation* (Princeton, N. J. Van Nostrand, 1956).
Cameron, Evan. *The European Reformation* (Oxford: Oxford University Press, 1991).
Collinson, Patrick. *The Reformation* (London: Weidenfeld & Nicolson, 2003).
Cook, Chris. *The Longman Handbook of Early Modern Europe, 1453-1763* (New York: Longmann, 2001).
MacCullock, Diarmaid. *The Reformation* (New York, 2003).
Johnston, Andrew. *The Protestant Reformation in Europe* (London: Longman, 1991).
Mullett, Michael A. *The Catholic Reformation* (New York: Rutledge, 1999).
Reid, W. Stanford, ed. *The Reformation* (1968).
Rice, Eugene F. *The Foundations of Early Modern Europe, 1460-1559* (New York: Norton, 1970).
Spitz, Lewis W. *The Protestant Reformation* (Englewood, N. J. Prentice-Hall, 1966).

## Test Yourself

1. In 1517, Martin Luther published his famous criticisms of the Catholic Church known as_____
   A. The Da Vinci Code
   B. The "Ninety-Five Theses"
   C. The Donation of Constantine
   D. The Diet of Worms

2. In 1527, Spanish, German and Swiss mercenaries under the Holy Roman Emperor seized the city of_____.
   A. Siena
   B. Pisa
   C. Rome
   D. London

3. The first country in Europe affected by the German Reformation was_____.
   A. France
   B. Switzerland
   C. Spain
   D. England

4. Lutheranism was persecuted in Denmark by_____.
   A. Charles V
   B. Constantine
   C. Ferdinand
   D. Christian II

5. Henry VIII brought about a change in religions in the British Isles due to his desire to divorce_____.
   A. Catherine of Aragon
   B. Anne Boleyn
   C. Jane Seymour
   D. Lady Jane Grey

6. This war was the first in a long series of internal struggles between Protestants and Catholics in Europe.
   A. The War of the Roses
   B. The Schmalkaldic War
   C. The Roman War
   D. Habsburg-Valois War

7. In 1555, a peace of fundamental importance was signed and granted each German prince the right to establish the religion for all his subjects_____.

   A. The Peace of Rome

   B. The Peace of Augsburg

   C. The Peace of Wittenburg

   D. The Peace of Paris

8. The Council of Trent in 1563 affirmed that_____.

   A. The Scriptures and traditions are equally binding for the faithful

   B. The supremacy of the pope is uncontestable

   C. The new ideas of Martin Luther were acceptable

   D. A and B

## Answers and Explanations

1. **B.** In 1517, Martin Luther published his "Ninety-Five Theses." The publication of theses, which were statements debating theological questions, was a rather common procedure. Luther's act, however, had extreme repercussions because of the logic and vigor of his statements and his implied challenge to papal authority. Pious Christians everywhere saw his act as the long-desired beginning of reform. Many worldly interests viewed it as a means to escape some of the judgments or financial impositions of the popes. Princes viewed his act as a basis for stopping the flow of money to Rome and channeling it, instead, into their own pockets.

2. **C.** In 1527, Spanish, German, and Swiss mercenaries seized Rome, which they sacked, destroying untold works of art and stripping it of much of its riches. For the time being, papal opposition was eliminated. A measure of cooperation between empire and papacy was established.

3. **B.** Switzerland was the first country affected by the Reformation in Germany. Luther's initial steps in 1518 had promptly induced the priest, Ulrich Zwingli of Zurich, to advocate similar reforms. Zwingli, like other humanists, was skeptical of traditional, accepted views and demanded that only what was said in the original religious sources should be recognized. He, therefore, followed Luther in turning to a theological interpretation of the Bible itself, rather than to Church traditions.

4. **D.** King Christian II was ardently Catholic, and the Danes themselves revolted against their king, mainly because of his economic policies and arbitrary rule. Having driven Christian II out of the country, they, too, accepted the Lutheran faith. They introduced it into Norway as well. The new faith was likewise accepted by large segments of the population, especially townspeople in Hungary, Lithuania, Livonia, the Netherlands, and even by some converts in France, Spain, and Italy.

5. **A.** Further, Henry VIII carried out the break with Rome. He had originally attacked Luther, but when the pope refused to give him a dispensation so that he could discard his wife (Catherine of Aragon, a relative of Charles V) and marry his mistress, Anne Boleyn, who he hoped would bear him a son, he decided to exploit the predicament in which the pope found himself because of the Protestant movement.

6. **B.** This war was the first in a long series of internal struggles between Catholics and Protestants in many countries. It showed that the situation had gone beyond the possibility of compromise. By 1546, this impasse was recognized not only by the Protestants, but also by Charles V. He, too, had worked for a reunion of the faiths—trying to reach it through the convening of a general Church Council. However, the popes opposed a general Council. Even after the death of Clement VII, the popes were unwilling to effect moral reform in the Church and consistently withheld their cooperation. In their refusals, they were supported by France, which engaged in one war after another against the Hapsburgs and profited from the split within Germany.

7. **B.** In 1555, a peace of fundamental importance was signed at the city of Augsburg. It granted each German prince the right to establish for all his subjects the religion that he himself professed. Thereby, Lutheran princes, and with them, Lutheran states, gained equal rights and status with Catholic states—even though the peace forbade any future conversion of Catholic bishoprics into secular Protestant states.

8. D. The Council of Trent in 1563 achieved what it had set out to do. Since the Protestants did not recognize the authority of the popes or the decisions of any council unless they were based entirely on the Scriptures, a compromise with them was excluded from the outset. Instead, the Council reasserted the Catholic point of view. It focused its attention on doctrine and ritual. It affirmed that the Scriptures and traditions are equally binding for the faithful and that the supremacy of the pope is incontestable.

**CHAPTER 6**

# The Aftermath of Renaissance and Reformation (1555-1603)

**1558** England loses Calais, last foothold on Continent
Ivan the Terrible invades Livonia
**1559** Publication of Prayer Book in England (Elizabeth I)
**1562** Beginnings of religious wars in France (Huguenots)
**1563** "Thirty-nine Articles" of the Anglican Church
Council of Trent concluded
**1565** Beginning of risings against Spain in the Netherlands
**1568** Mary, Queen of Scots, flees to England
**1567** Duke of Alba in the Netherlands
**1569** Union of Lublin between Poland and Lithuania
Mercator publishes map of the world
**1571** Battle of Lepanto: Turks defeated
**1572** Beginnings of War of Independence of the Netherlands (William the Silent)
Massacre of the Night of St. Bartholomew in Paris
John Knox, Scottish reformer, dies
**1576** Titian dies
**1580** Montaigne, *Essais*
Russian penetration into Siberia
**1581** Northern Netherlands depose Philip II
**1582** Gregorian calendar introduced
**1584** William of Orange assassinated
**1587** Mary, Queen of Scots, executed
**1588** Spanish Armada destroyed
**1592** Alexander of Parma dies
**1594** Henry IV gains Paris: end of civil wars in France
Palestrina dies
**1595** Dutch colonization of East Indies begins
**1597** Francis Bacon, *Essays*
**1598** Franco-Spanish peace of Vervins: death of Philip II
Edict of Nantes

**1600** Founding of English East India Company
Shakespeare writes *Hamlet*
**1602** Founding of Dutch East India Company
**1603** Death of Elizabeth I of England

*Youthfulness, confidence, enthusiasm, thirst for beauty and manliness (*virtu*), had marked the early 16th century and made possible the achievements of the High Renaissance. These features no longer characterized the second half of the century. In only two parts of Europe, Spain and England (both of which had previously made few contributions to the glory of the age), do we find a sudden flowering of culture. In these countries, the Renaissance took on a more mature, more intellectual, aspect and found its major expression in literature and science. Many of the great Renaissance artists were by then either dead or, like Michelangelo and Titian, in their old age. The great humanists (Erasmus, Reuchlin, More), the religious leaders (Luther, Zwingli, Calvin, Loyola), the mighty Renaissance princes and patrons of culture (the Medici, Sforza, Este, and other families), had passed from the scene, as had Copernicus and Machiavelli. However, on the political stage, in literature and in the natural sciences, the second half of the 16th century brought forth a considerable number of personalities and events inspired by the great age that was coming to a close.*

## ■ THE POLITICAL SCENE

After the abdication of Charles V in 1556, the idea of European Christian unity, as it had been conceived during the Middle Ages since the crowning of Charlemagne in 800 and Otto the Great in 962 was not revived. Spain, France, and Germany made successive attempts to establish some form of unity by imposing their own supremacy and leadership on the rest of the Continent, but in each case, it was national ambition rather than a general European concept that directed their efforts. Indeed, after Charles V's abdication, the history of Western civilization, more than ever before, becomes the story of individual countries.

It is often the character of a ruler that leaves the sharpest imprint upon the civilization of an age. Thus, William the Silent of the Netherlands, Ivan the Terrible of Russia, Philip II of Spain, Elizabeth I of England, and Eric XIV of Sweden lent color and distinction to the second half of the 16th century. Among the dramatic events they witnessed and to which they contributed were the War of Independence of the Netherlands, the struggle over the Baltic question, the Battle of Lepanto, the Night of St. Bartholomew, and the destruction of the Spanish Armada.

### Italy

On the European stage during this period, Italy was a target of action for other nations. The country saw the decline or disappearance of its vigorous city-states and the weakening of the political position in the papal territories. Italy was mostly under Hapsburg domination and served as a bridge between Spain and Germany. The commerce of the Italian cities steadily lost world significance, and the wealth of other countries overshadowed theirs.

### Germany

Despite being located in the heart of Europe, Germany similarly declined in political importance. The Hapsburgs produced no new ruler of the stature of Charles V. Their resources were exhausted by wars to maintain the empire and the Catholic faith. Common institutions like the diets no longer functioned satisfactorily. The independence of the states that comprised the empire grew, and borderlands were lost. Thus, the Netherlands was joined to Spain and, subsequently, its northern regions achieved independence. Livonia fell prey, first, to Russian, then to Swedish and Polish invaders. Western borderlands in Lorraine were annexed by the French, and the bishopric of Basel joined the free Swiss cantons.

The eastern frontiers of the empire were continually exposed to inroads by the Ottoman Turks, who remained in possession of Hungary and its silver mines. Most of the eastern sea-trade routes to the rich grain resources of the Slavic and Baltic countries fell into the hands of enterprising Dutch traders.

However, individual German states (notably Brandenburg, Saxony, Austria, and Bavaria) grew in strength and gained international prestige. Such states increasingly became the centers of German might and German culture, rather than the empire as a whole.

## Spain

The role of leadership in Hapsburg affairs accordingly shifted to the Spanish branch of the house. Philip II (d. 1598) proved to be an outstanding ruler. Philip was a man devoted to the fulfillment of his duties as king. He worked tirelessly and was persistent in all his undertakings. In a sense, he was the first Western ruler to understand, and build, a modern bureaucracy.

### Internal Policies

Under Philip II, Spain's great military tradition was maintained. Arts and literature flourished. Numerous universities were established and attracted Catholic scholars. Geographical studies were advanced. Spanish architecture found its grandest expression in the mighty, somber palace of the Escorial, which was built by Philip. The manners, fashions, and court etiquette and ceremonials developed in Spain served as models for all of Europe.

Yet, the administration of the enormous empire set tasks for which Spain was not equipped. The wealth coming from the colonies, mainly in silver, was largely wasted. It did not stimulate industry, but rather pride, sloth, and luxury. Since the Spanish nobles considered business activities unworthy of their attention, and since the merchant class was small, foreigners were allowed to exploit the country's natural resources. Taxation remained high. Monopolies hindered fruitful economic activities, and currency debasement was unavoidable. The government lost its credit standing through repeated bankruptcies of the treasury.

Simultaneously, agriculture declined, and large estates, which had been given away by the Crown as rewards to nobles, were used mainly for pasture. The population, impoverished, gradually decreased. This process of economic decline was accelerated by the expulsion of the Jews and Moors from the country. These peoples, through their trade and agriculture, had contributed much to the Spain's prosperity.

### Religious Policies

Philip maintained strict absolutism. Though a devout Catholic, he did not permit political influence by the Church. He kept the clergy dependent and used the Jesuits to advance Spanish aims in Europe and America. On one occasion, he even made war on the pope and besieged Rome.

### Colonial Policies

Just as Philip dominated the affairs of the Spanish clergy, so he personally supervised the administration of government in the New World, despite the distance involved. He followed the established policy of appointing viceroys, but, in matters of policy, he kept them subservient to the "Council of the Indies." The *encomienda* system (landholding by the feudal nobility and forced labor by natives) was retained, and large estates were granted to Spanish nobles in the colonies. After Friar Bartolomeo de las Casas intervened with Philip's father, Charles, the Indians were no longer subjected to slavery. Trade with the New World remained a royal monopoly, and large fleets were sent there annually under the protection of convoys that fought off pirates and smugglers.

### Foreign Policies

In foreign policy, Philip pursued the sole aim of defending the Spanish Empire. He was only partially successful. Closely cooperating with the German Hapsburgs, he fought and decisively defeated France. Allied with Venice and the pope, he engaged in war against the Turks. In 1571, he was victorious at Lepanto, one of the greatest naval battles of all times, upsetting Turkish domination in the western Mediterranean. He invaded Portugal in 1580, after the royal family there died out, annexed the country, and thus gained its rich dependencies in Africa and Asia.

Philip sought to retain control of the Spanish and Portuguese links with the colonial empires in vain, however. Throughout his reign, he had to fight the English on the seas. After years of struggle, his ambitious plan to destroy the English navy and end English competition with the help of a great fleet, the "Armada," failed. In 1588, after being defeated by the English, the Armada was destroyed by storms. In all of his costly foreign policies, Philip used and supported Catholicism out of conviction as well as expediency, so it appeared as if the defense of the "old faith" was the main objective of his policies.

## The Netherlands

Despite Philip's great ability and industriousness, his reign was ultimately disastrous for Spain. His failure can be attributed to the crucial mistake he made in the Spanish Netherlands, rather than to the repeated bankruptcies, the loss of the Armada, or the revival of French power.

### Oppression: Duke of Alba

The Netherlands constituted the greatest asset within Philip's realm. He had inherited the region from his father who, being a native, had understood how to retain their loyalty. Philip was dependent upon their wealth, but instead of promoting Dutch and Flemish trade and winning good will, he tried to rectify a catastrophic financial situation in Spain by extending the crippling Spanish sales tax to the Low Countries. He thereby threatened the merchants with ruin. Moreover, through his arbitrary and arrogant nature, he exasperated the Netherlanders, who were accustomed to a large measure of freedom. Finally, using the protection of the Catholic faith, the enforcement of decisions made at the Council of Trent, and the Inquisition, he sharpened the antagonism of the largely Calvinist Dutch toward their Spanish overlords.

When the Netherlanders petitioned for reforms, Philip sent an army under the Duke of Alba. The Duke had shown his genius as a general in campaigns in Africa, Italy, and Miihlberg. Later on, he also showed his skill in the conquest of Portugal. When he sought to enforce Spanish rule and Philip's taxation system, the Netherlands rebelled. Alba crushed the revolt and executed two of the leaders, Egmont and Horn. A third leader, William the Silent of Orange, escaped to become a hero in the great struggle for liberty that ensued.

### War of Independence: William of Orange

The War of Independence of the Low Countries against Spain has remained an inspiration and model throughout the ages. William was a true Machiavellian, and *The Prince* was his constant companion. He was called "the Silent" because he knew how to hide his thoughts behind a flow of diverting conversation. He was successively Catholic, Lutheran, and Calvinist. He married four times—for purposes of expediency. He was French (Orange), German (Nassau), and Dutch.

Under his leadership, the Dutch and the Flemish recovered from their defeats. They equipped a small navy of so-called "Sea Beggars" to harass Spanish shipping. After the recall of the Duke of Alba in 1573, the Dutch and Flemish forced the Spanish army to relinquish most of the country. In 1581, the independence of the Netherlands was declared, but the war was not yet won. When Philip II sent Prince Alessandro Famese of Parma to Flanders, Famese, a man fully the equal of William in political acumen, succeeded in regaining the southern areas of the Low Countries.

In 1584, during the midst of the struggle, William was murdered, but the Netherlanders fought on stubbornly and courageously. They did not succeed in freeing the entire country, however. The country was divided: Its southern portions remained Spanish and Catholic, while the north established itself as an independent republic in which Protestantism was predominant. There, the Orange family provided political leadership. Soon, under merchant, or *bourgeois*, control, the economy again became the most flourishing of Europe.

## France

The internal policy of France centered on the religious problem and the struggle to maintain royal authority. Its foreign policy was guided by opposition to the Hapsburgs and, particularly, to Spain. However, France was in no position to establish good government at home or enforce its will abroad. Not only was it decisively defeated by Spain in 1559, but religious wars ravaged the country and undermined law and order.

### *Rise of the Huguenots*

The dominant issue in France during the second half of the 16th century was the issue of national unity. The Reformation had split the country. Two parties had been formed: the Catholic, directed by the Guise family; and the Protestant, or Huguenot, led by the Calvinist princes of Conde and Navarre and by Admiral Coligny. Periods of persecution of the Huguenots alternated with periods of toleration.

France might have emulated Germany (where, ultimately, both religions were recognized and existed side by side) or Spain (where Catholicism existed exclusively), but it followed neither example. Indeed, the historical importance of the events in France lies in the fact that it was not the religious question, but a political one that became the chief problem. As so often happens, the conflict between the two groups turned into a triangular struggle. A third party, the "*Politiques*," was formed. This party was not greatly concerned about religion, but put nationalistic aims and centralization of government above all other considerations.

Without delay, the queen mother, Catherine de Medici, who had an ambitious and intriguing character, embraced its tenets because they coincided with her own absolutist aims. She played the other two parties against each other. Thus, the country was torn by internal strife. Disorder, unmatched anywhere else, occurred. The climax came when Catherine, faced by the possibility of a Protestant victory, openly turned against the Protestants and instigated the outrage and horror known as the Night of St. Bartholomew in 1572. Under the pretext of reconciliation, she lured the Protestant leaders to Paris, whereupon these men and some 20,000 of their adherents throughout France were massacred.

### *Civil Wars and Religious Settlement*

After the shock of the stunning blow had passed, the events of the Night of St. Bartholomew led to a prolongation of the internal wars. The Politiques now sought to destroy the Catholic party. Politiques, Catholics, and Protestants—each party led by a Henry—continued to fight the other two in ever-shifting alliances (War of the Three Henrys). After utter exhaustion had been reached, the country was impoverished, farms were destroyed, international prestige was lost, and two of the Henrys murdered. The survivor, Henry of Navarre of the House of Bourbon and leader of the Protestants, succeeded in ending the struggle.

Putting the political issue before all others, he made agreements with his opponents. He obtained recognition as king and converted to Catholicism, but he also pleased the Protestants by issuing the Edict of Nantes in 1598. This edict granted the Protestants freedom of conscience (the right to public worship) and the right to hold office. He guaranteed the latter right to the Protestant minority by permitting them to possess and to fortify a number of towns of their own in France as a guarantee of their safety.

## England

The ambitions of individuals, disruption in domestic affairs, and foreign wars brought ruin to France. Meanwhile, a comparatively peaceful era marked by a concentration on its national aims made it possible for England to enjoy a period of prosperity that coincided with the English Renaissance. The term "Renaissance" is possibly somewhat misleading in terms of England, since achievements in such areas as sculpture and painting were scant. Nevertheless, evidence points to typical Renaissance traits in music with the development of the madrigal and in literature with the masterpieces of Tudor poets and dramatists, especially Shakespeare. In the splendor of its court life, the English also began to rival other Renaissance courts.

### *Economic Expansion*

In England during the second half of the 16th century, the enterprising Renaissance spirit asserted itself in commercial affairs and geographical explorations. The shipbuilding industry expanded rapidly. Sea captains and pirates made England the foremost maritime power in the world. Hawkins, Raleigh, and Drake sought trade routes westward. Chancellor established an eastward route to Russia via the northern tip of Europe. Jenkinson initiated English trade with the *tsar* and, indirectly through the *tsar's* realms, with Persia.

Overseas expansion led to industrial expansion and the establishment of joint-stock companies after Italian models. Business enterprises formed by a group of merchants financed these undertakings and charged a captain to carry them out. They were precursors of the modern stock company. To further these enterprises, a regular credit system was created. As in Spain, so, too, in England these activities resulted in a decline in independent farming and the wider introduction of enclosed farms. The shift in land management led to more sheep grazing, which, in turn, stimulated the textile industry. The townspeople and merchants improved their economic position, and the national standard of living reached a higher level.

### *Religious Settlement*

Unlike many of the Continental powers, 16th-century England was spared religious wars. Under Edward VI (d. 1553), who succeeded Henry VIII, the political-religious changes made by Henry were extended into the realm of religious doctrine. Through two successive "Acts of Uniformity," the *Book of Common Prayer* was introduced. Protestant views regarding the authority of the Bible, justification by faith, and the nature of the sacraments were accepted.

Edward's successor, Mary Tudor (d. 1557), favored Catholicism. Her reign brought harsh persecutions of Protestants, hundreds of whom perished. Her own life was tragic, and her rule was short. Married to Philip II of Spain, she embraced not only the Catholic faith, but also the Spanish cause, which was contrary to English commercial interests. Moreover, in 1558 England lost the port of Calais, its last stronghold on the Continent.

In turn, Mary's successor, Elizabeth I (1558-1603), reverting to the policy of Edward VI, reintroduced a Protestant form of worship. Elizabeth accepted the innovations that had been introduced by the Acts of Uniformity, but she modified their anti-Catholic emphasis. The "Thirty-nine Articles" set forth the Anglican confession of faith. A party of so-called "Puritans" desired more far-reaching changes, but, in order to preserve an all-national Church that the ruler could control, they were suppressed. For the same reason, Roman Catholics were now persecuted, perhaps no less than the Protestants had been during Mary's regime.

### *External Affairs*

England's foreign policies under Elizabeth were dominated by rivalry for commercial expansion and by fear of the power of Spain, France, and Scotland. This fact drove the country into sharp conflict with

Catholic nations. It led to a bitter, repressive policy in Ireland, which Spain periodically tried to use as a stepping-stone for an invasion of England. It disturbed relations with Scotland and its Catholic ruling house of Stuart. Indeed, it brought death to Mary Stuart, known as Mary, Queen of Scots. The queen was a fugitive from her own country and a refugee in England. Accused of participating in Jesuit conspiracies against the life of Elizabeth (who was her cousin), Mary was executed in 1587. The religious rivalry led to incessant, though undeclared, war with Spain and constant attacks on Spanish shipping. This situation reached its climax in 1588, when open war broke out, and the Spanish Armada was defeated. On the other hand, opposition to Catholicism—and to Spain—brought cooperation from the rebelling Netherlands. As to France, no consistent policy could be pursued, since English-French relations depended upon the ever-changing French relations with Scotland and Spain.

### Elizabethan Achievements

By the time Elizabeth died, the English treasury was exhausted. Parliament had become restive. Nevertheless, despite the personal shortcomings of the queen, the Elizabethan Age stands out as a glorious era. Through the influence of literature, better education, and science, a gentler spirit had come to pervade England, a country which the Italians and French had long regarded as barbarian. Elizabeth's regime, supported by capable advisers whom the queen chose well, formed the foundation of political power, economic prosperity, and a vigorous, self-reliant body of citizens. Parliament and the bourgeois class, which held the key to the future, emerged strengthened. Additionally the nobility did not shun participation in commercial activities. Coal mining and shipbuilding flourished as did a Church that combined traditionalism with Lutheran and Calvinist reforms and supported national unity under the monarch.

## Scandinavia and Poland

The great issues of the day—the religious struggles, the capitalistic enterprises, and political centralization under a strong ruler—also continued to affect the small nations of northern and eastern Europe. These issues led to a further redistribution of power that affected the entire Baltic area. Yet, for more than a century after the discovery of America, Baltic trade was still more important than the transatlantic traffic.

### Denmark-Norway and Sweden

Denmark-Norway sought to adapt itself to the changed conditions after it lost control over Sweden in 1523. It succeeded in reestablishing order at home and brought religious strife to an end, with consequences favorable to the Lutheran cause. It also built up its economy with the help of the huge income derived from tolls that Denmark levied upon ships passing from the North Sea into the Baltic Sea through the "Sound." This was the only navigable lane available and was a narrow passageway controlled by Denmark. But the kings continued to squander their resources in futile wars against Sweden, however.

The Swedes, on the other hand, made better progress. Having won their independence under the able, cautious, parsimonious Gustavus Vasa, they developed their rich copper and iron mines, increased their production, channeled traffic through their own ports, and built up a large treasury. This policy enabled them (under Gustavus's sons and successors) to survive bitter wars against Denmark, Poland, and Russia. With the conquest of Estonia in 1561, they became the foremost Baltic power. Yet, Sweden, too, lacked the economic resources, the population, and the modern commercial spirit that would have enabled it to compete successfully with the Western trading nations.

### Poland-Lithuania

Like the Swedes, the Poles cherished dreams of a large empire and dominion over the Baltic Sea lanes. In 1525, they had already established their overlordship of Prussia. In 1562, their Lithuanian partners incorporated southern Livonia. Poland compelled Lithuania to accept complete integration in 1569. Poland forced Danzig into submission and, in 1582, after a series of wars against Russia, annexed large Russian territories.

Such diversified holdings demanded an efficient and tolerant central authority. While arts, crafts, and literature flourished, and the upper nobility enjoyed a life of luxury, however, the country as a whole did not develop the necessary progressive spirit and internal cohesion. The generally weak, elective monarchy was motivated after the Council of Trent by the aim of proselytizing in behalf of Catholicism. It failed to control the disruptive nobility which, itself divided, dominated the law-giving institution, the diet or *sejm*. Little was done to promote trade or the development of a merchant class. Nowhere else was the social gulf among classes, nationalities, and religions as great as in Poland. Thus, conquests of territory contributed to the destruction rather than the growth of the commonwealth.

### Russia

In the meantime, Russia was governed by one of its most eminent rulers, Ivan IV (Ivan the Terrible). Ivan IV continued the work of consolidating the Russian realms that had been initiated by his grandfather, Ivan the Great. He succeeded in incorporating the vast territory along the entire course of the Volga River. He attempted to conquer Livonia (Estonia and Latvia) in order to gain ports that would give Russia access to the sea. Failing in this, he established permanent connections with the West by welcoming English merchants who had opened the northern trade route around the North Cape.

Ivan IV brutally suppressed all potential opponents and kept the princes (*boyars*) and the Church under his absolute rule. He personally monopolized many economic activities and surrounded himself with a powerful bureaucracy that was at his complete command. He catered to English and Dutch traders, who increasingly replaced the Hanseatic merchants on the Baltic Sea lanes. He strengthened new links with the West by inviting craftsmen to visit his country, introducing Western techniques, and expanding diplomatic relations.

It was under Ivan the Terrible that Russia started its eastward march across the Urals. A band of intrepid Cossacks, led by Yermak, invaded Siberia in 1581 and began Russia's mighty eastward movement. As a whole, Ivan IV's reign meant rapid progress for Russia, both politically and economically, as well as expansion eastward. It also led to territorial losses in the West, to moral decline, and to the vicious consequences of autocracy, which endangered Russia's internal stability.

## ■THE SOCIAL AND CULTURAL SCENE

With the fading of the great age of the Renaissance in the second half of the 16th century, there began a period that is known as "Mannerism" in art history. This era linked the High Renaissance and the coming Baroque period. Despite the name, this age of transition was not devoid of sincerity and originality. Although works of genius similar to those produced in the two preceding centuries were rare, love for beauty remained, and it resulted in the creation of works of art that fulfilled the Renaissance promise.

### Society

During the course of the Reformation and the consolidation of national states, major changes occurred in society. On one hand, royal courts and their bureaucracies gained additional power. On the other, wealthy burghers and professionals secured an ever-greater influence. As much as 20 percent of the total population in the West now lived in cities—about twice as many than before the Reformation. Those who benefited from the opportunities afforded by towns in regard to commercial and banking activities sought equality in status with the nobility. Skilled craftsmen likewise gained from urbanization, but common laborers sank to even lower levels. The gulf between upper and lower classes deepened.

The peasants also failed to improve their lot. The rebellions to which they often resorted gained them little. New economic conditions brought them somewhat greater freedom, but did not relieve them from their poverty, nor did the peasants benefit from the wealth that poured in from the colonies.

Life expectancy remained low for all classes. Hygienic conditions hardly improved. Medical knowledge and care progressed to some degree, but diseases like syphilis continued to devastate all layers of society. Nature's disasters took their toll everywhere. Ulrich von Hutten had said "it is a joy to live," but a gloomy mood seized the world toward the end of the century.

## The Military

With the age of chivalry disappearing and national armies not yet formed, the military became somewhat of a class unto itself. Mercenaries made up most of the land forces. In the second half of the 16th century, infantry troops comprising mercenaries found employment on the many battlefields from Scotland to Livonia, from the Netherlands to Hungary, from Sweden to Spain and southern Italy. The infantry even fought on the decks of warships after boarding the enemy's vessels. Cavalry was no longer as useful as it had been in earlier times, and knights lost the distinction that the possession of a horse and servants had given them. The mercenaries were fickle. They freely offered their services to those leaders whose victorious records promised rich booty, but they changed sides readily when it was profitable for them. Strategy and tactics were shaped to fit these conditions. Fighters equipped with muskets instead of pikes or swords were needed, and this requirement gave additional power to those who could afford to pay the costs. Artillery became indispensable, especially for attacking fortresses. Scientific work helped to develop weapons, and even great artists like Leonardo da Vinci were commissioned to improve cannons and fortifications. War, as usual, encouraged developments in science and technical occupations. For example, the need for modern weapons required the expansion of mining and industrial production.

## Art

Among the great painters of the age were those of the Venetian school. This school began to flourish later than schools in Florence and Rome, which preserved for the longest duration the traditions of the earlier masters. Elsewhere, craftsmanship marked the work of the leading artists. A younger generation of artists showed their brilliance and mastery. One towering figure is El Greco (d. 1614), a painter who lived in Spain. His works, such as "View of Toledo" and "Great Inquisitor Guevara," show his sense of the tragic, which is expressed in beautiful, somber, and deeply emotional canvases.

## Music

In music, too, a different spirit arose. The fresh and vigorous trends of the early 16th century, which had popular appeal and were enjoyed by a broad audience, gave way to a more delicate style that was in demand in a narrower, refined society that preferred classical features. The Catholic Church was worried because it sensed the worldly, sensual background evident in much of the art during the later stages of the Renaissance. At the Council of Trent, a special session was devoted to music. There, participants warned against the imitation of classical models, condemned the influence of pagan morals, and demanded a purification of music along the lines of Christian tradition, accentuating severity and restraint.

Soon there emerged one of history's outstanding composers, the Italian Palestrina (d. 1594), who had studied under Renaissance masters in the Netherlands. He met the demands of the Council, yet preserved and furthered the stylistic innovations of his predecessors, including their polyphonic style and use of counterpoint. The earnestness, clarity, and tonal purity of his motets and religious Masses were cherished by popes and art patrons alike. Palestrina, his contemporary, Orlando di Lasso, and a school of their followers are regarded as preeminent forces in the development of early modern music.

Simultaneously, secular music was cultivated both in Protestant and Catholic countries. The Netherlands and Germany continued to emphasize harmony and lost the preeminence they had previously. Italy, perfecting instrumental melody, came to the fore and inspired musicians in other countries. Even England, which had excelled in various forms of music, and which, with masters like William Byrd, continued to create independent works of remarkable beauty, fell increasingly under the influence of Italian music.

New and improved instruments, such as the harpsichord and the violin, appeared. Many compositions were written for instruments instead of for voice alone. Furthermore, music was written for theatrical performances. Toward the end of the 16th century, the modern opera was born through a combination of music and drama.

## Literature

Printed books increased in number and influence. Excellent histories were written, such as one centering on Philip II by Cabrera and *Universal History* by De Thou. Other histories—for example, the *Ecclesiastical History of the Magdeburg Centuries* and a history of the times of Charles V by Sleidanus—served propagandistic purposes in favor of religious causes. In Spain, the novel made its appearance. Everywhere, descriptions of travel, such as the accounts collected by the Englishman, Hakluyt, became popular.

With the increase in the availability of books, poetry and drama found an ever-growing audience. Authors such as the Italian Tasso (d. 1595) and the Englishmen, Spenser (d. 1599) and Marlowe (d. 1593), gained fame during their own lifetimes.

France produced two writers of lasting significance. Rabelais (d. 1553), with the aim of entertaining, created in his *Gargantua* a mirror of human weaknesses, full of fantasy and humor. Montaigne (d. 1592), a sensitive, philosophical man of genius, was strongly affected by the skepticism of his age. He expressed doubt that human beings could ever acquire true knowledge, and in a spirit of unaccustomed detachment, wrote the *Essais*, in which he analyzed human nature so well that this work continues to serve as a guide to everyday living.

The two most notable writers of this period were the Spaniard Cervantes (d. 1616), who wrote *Don Quixote*, and the English dramatist and poet, Shakespeare (d. 1616). They probed the depths of human nature and aspirations, with sympathy for human strengths and weaknesses; they portrayed both individual and national character with a mastery that is still unsurpassed.

## Science

In science, the exact and imaginative approach, sober observations, and careful descriptions of nature of the Renaissance masters provided a basis for rapid advancement. No longer were scientists unquestioningly guided by the writings of classical authors who had dominated for so long. When classical views conflicted with observed facts, they were rejected.

In the latter part of the century, the Dane Tycho Brahe (d. 1601) mapped the sky. The fundamental work of Copernicus was furthered by Galileo (d. 1642), who, after perfecting the telescope and making scrupulous observations that led to numerous discoveries, confirmed Copernicus's findings. Galileo realized the importance of insight and imagination, so long as they did not lead to "postulating in advance." He did not hesitate to propose hypotheses, but he based them on mathematical concepts, and then checked the results experimentally. Galileo thus found and described the law of falling bodies and the motion of the pendulum. He enunciated the principle of inertia.

No less stimulating was the work of the English statesman Francis Bacon (d. 1626). Although, in his search for a scientific method, he overemphasized experimentation and observation, and although he lacked necessary mathematical knowledge, he prepared the way for future scientific endeavors by advocating an "inductive method of reasoning." Like Galileo, Bacon insisted on the necessity of doubting traditional concepts and values.

Advances paralleling those in astronomy and physics were made in other subjects. Gilbert of Colchester (d. 1603) made important discoveries in magnetism. In botany and zoology, new and advanced descriptions of plants and animals were published, though much fanciful information still marked such scientific literature. In general, however, belief in pseudo-sciences, magic, alchemy, and astrology continued to dominate in many fields.

## Geography

Progress in geography was particularly aided by the achievements of the preceding half-century. Maps drawn in the second half of the 16th century—for example, those of the German mapmaker Mercator—showed remarkable perfection after more than 1,000 years of comparative stagnation in this craft. Mapmaking profited from the theoretical advances in science that made mathematical projection possible. It also benefited from practical experience gained through explorations and discoveries, which replace the numerous superstitions inherited from ancient and medieval times.

The new maps stimulated further explorations. Although no important new seaways were discovered, distant lands were explored. Large areas in America, Russia, and even Japan were made known to the Western world. Products such as coffee, which Venice began to import on a large scale, and the potato, which was first planted in Europe in 1584, became popular among Europeans.

Much of the work of discovery was undertaken by merchants. Traditionally conservative groups—the Hanseatic and Venetian traders—were pushed more and more into the background by enterprising Portuguese, Dutch, English, and Scotch merchants. The daring undertakings of these newer groups were backed by well-organized, powerful, and rich joint-stock companies. The travelers came home not only with profits, but also with intriguing accounts of the foreign lands they had visited.

## Religion

As people turned their attention increasingly to exploration of the world around them, they lost some of their interest in questions of dogma. No theological works comparable in importance to those of the early 16th century appeared in the second half of the century. Religious passions, however, remained strong, and brought bitter consequences to the nations. The Inquisition's terror lost much of its impact, especially after the outbreak of the War of Independence of the Netherlands, but the number of civil wars increased.

Catholicism recovered and regained strength in many lands. By 1600, the large Protestant minorities had decreased in Poland, Austria, parts of southern and western Germany, the southern Netherlands, and France. In Spain, Portugal, and Italy, Protestant groups had been crushed. Catholicism made inroads in Protestant northern Germany, England, and Scandinavia. Despite political changes in England, Ireland remained faithful to Rome. Moreover, Catholic refugees from England and other Protestant countries founded colleges in other countries to rally compatriots who were persecuted for their religious views. In many respects, the Catholics adjusted more rapidly to the rational trends of the age than the Protestants, who, cherishing a mystical faith, were inclined to adhere to the letter rather than the spirit of the Scriptures.

## Perspective

*In the latter part of the 16th century, differences in the evolution of Western European nations prepared the way for a political redistribution of power. This redistribution was not brought about without terrible convulsions. It was compounded by social and religious conditions. Internal wars shook France for more than 40 years. Warfare ruined the German Empire. Spain lost its predominant place through a drawn-out, vain struggle in the Netherlands and, on the seas, against growing English power. England itself managed to live through a comparatively quiet time—with grave inner turmoil postponed until the next century.*

War raged almost relentlessly in the North between Sweden, Russia, and Poland, centered around the Livonian harbors of Riga, Reval, and Narva, which served as intermediaries for the heavy East-West trade via Baltic sea lanes. When Russia failed to gain access to the Baltic Sea, it turned its attention to the lower Volga region and Siberia, an area in which small bands of adventurers had begun to open to Russian penetration.

Yet, it can be argued that political developments were overshadowed in importance by cultural advances. Science now began to lead the way into a different world.

## Selected Readings

Butterfield, Herbert. *The Origins of Modern Science* (New York: Collier Books, 1962).

Chadwick, H.M. and Chadwick, N. K. *The Growth of Literature* (Cambridge: The University Press, 1969).

Davies, R. T. *The Golden Century of Spain, 1501-1621* (New York: St. Martin's Press, 1954).

Hall, Alfred R. The *Scientific Revolution, 1500-1800* (Longmans, 1966).

Hart-Davis, Duff. *The Armada* (New York: Bantam, 1988).

Pierson, Pieter. *Commander of the Armada* (New Haven: Yale University Press, 1989).

Shapin, Steven. *The Scientific Revolution* (Chicago: The University of Chicago Press), 1996.

Trevor, Aston, ed. *Crisis in Europe, 1560-1660* (New York: Basic Books, 1965).

## Test Yourself

1. Spain's great military tradition was maintained under the reign of_____.
   A. Charles III
   B. Philip II
   C. Henry VIII
   D. Christian II

2. Denmark and Norway lost control over Sweden in_____.
   A. 1521
   B. 1523
   C. 1610
   D. 1527

3. Ivan IV, one of the most powerful Russian rulers during the 16$^{th}$ century, is also known as_____.
   A. Ivan the Great
   B. Ivan the Bald
   C. Ivan the Strong
   D. Ivan the Terrible

4. Among the great painters of the era, the painter of the "View of Toledo" was ____.
   A. Titian
   B. El Greco
   C. Da Vinci
   D. Caravaggio

5. The two most notable writers of the era were_____.
   A. The Italians, Machiavelli and Galileo
   B. The Spaniard Cervantes and the Englishman Shakespeare
   C. The Englishman Francis Bacon and the Frenchman Valois
   D. None of the above

6. The fundamental work of Nicholas Copernicus was carried on by____.
   A. Francis Bacon
   B. Caravaggio
   C. Galileo
   D. Tyco Brahe

7. Gilbert of Colchester made important discoveries in the field of _____.
   A. Electricity
   B. Astronomy
   C. Physics
   D. Magnetism

8. Progress in geography was advanced by maps drawn in the second half of the 16th century, such as those of_____.
   A. The German map maker, Mercator
   B. The Italian mapmaker, Toscanelli
   C. The Tunisian, Ibn Khaldun
   D. The Spaniard, Juan de la Cosa

## Answers and Explanations

1. **B.** The role of leadership in Hapsburg affairs accordingly shifted to the Spanish branch of the house. Philip II (d. 1598) proved to be an outstanding ruler. Philip was a man devoted to the fulfillment of his duties as king. He worked tirelessly and was persistent in all his undertakings. In a sense, he was the first Western ruler to understand, and build, a modern bureaucracy. Under Philip II, Spain's great military tradition was maintained.

2. **B.** Denmark-Norway, having lost control over Sweden in 1523, sought to adapt itself to the changed conditions. It succeeded in reestablishing order at home and brought religious strife to an end with consequences favorable to the Lutheran cause. It also built up its economy with the help of the huge income derived from tolls that Denmark levied upon ships passing from the North Sea into the Baltic Sea through the "Sound." This was the only navigable lane available, a narrow passageway controlled by Denmark. However, the kings continued to squander their resources in futile wars against Sweden.

3. **D.** Russia was governed during the early 16th century by one of its most important rulers, Ivan IV (also known as Ivan the Terrible). Ivan IV continued the work of consolidating the Russian realms, which his grandfather, Ivan the Great, had started. He succeeded in incorporating the vast territory along the entire course of the Volga River. Ivan IV brutally suppressed all potential opponents and kept princes (*boyars*) and the Church under his absolute rule. He personally monopolized many economic activities and surrounded himself with a powerful bureaucracy that was at his complete command. He catered to English and Dutch traders, who increasingly replaced the Hanseatic merchants on the Baltic sea lanes. He strengthened new links with the West by inviting craftsmen to visit his country, by introducing Western techniques, and by expanding diplomatic relations.

4. **B.** Among the great painters, those of the Venetian school, which flourished later than schools in Florence and Rome, preserved for the longest time the tradition of the earlier masters. Elsewhere, craftsmanship marked the work of the leading artists. A younger generation of artists showed their brilliance and mastery. One towering figure was El Greco (1541–1614 C.E.), who lived in Spain. His paintings, such as "View of Toledo" and "Great Inquisitor Guevara" show his sense of the tragic expressed in beautiful, somber, deeply emotional canvases.

5. **B.** The two most notable writers of this period were the Spaniard, Cervantes (d. 1616), who wrote *Don Quixote*, and the English dramatist and poet, Shakespeare (d. 1616). They probed the depths of human nature and aspirations, and with sympathy for human strengths and weaknesses, they portrayed individual and national characters with mastery still unsurpassed.

6. **C.** The fundamental work of Copernicus was carried on by Galileo (d. 1642), who, after perfecting the telescope and making scrupulous observations that led to numerous discoveries, confirmed Copernicus's findings. Galileo realized the importance of insight and imagination, so long as they did not lead to "postulating in advance." He did not hesitate to propose hypotheses, but he based them on mathematical concepts, and then checked the results experimentally. Galileo thus found and described the law of falling bodies and the motion of the pendulum. He enunciated the principle of inertia.

7. **D.** Advances paralleling those in astronomy and physics were made in other subjects. Gilbert of Colchester (d. 1603) made important discoveries in magnetism.

8. A. Progress in geography was aided particularly by the achievements of the preceding half-century. Maps drawn in the second half of the 16th century (for example, those of the German mapmaker Mercator) showed remarkable perfection after more than a thousand years of comparative stagnation in this craft. Mapmaking profited from the theoretical advances in science that made mathematical projection possible. It also profited from the practical experience gained through explorations and discoveries. This replaced the numerous superstitions inherited from ancient and medieval times.

# CHAPTER 7
# The Emergence of the Modern State System (1603-1648)

**1605** Beginning of Times of Trouble in Russia
Cervantes, *Don Quixote*
**1607** Jamestown settlement in Virginia founded
**1609** Galileo: Law of Falling Bodies
Kepler publishes his first two laws of planetary motion
**1610** Henry IV of France assassinated
**1614** Invention of logarithms
**1616** Richelieu becomes minister in France
**1618** Beginning of Thirty Years' War
**1619** Kepler published his third law of planetary motion
**1620** Settlement in New Plymouth founded *(Mayflower)*
Francis Bacon, *Novum Organum*
**1624** English settlements in East India
Dutch settlements in Indonesia
Decline of Portugal
**1625** Grotius, *De Jure Belli et Pacis (Law of War and Peace)*
**1626** Dutch settlement on Hudson
**1628** Petition of Rights submitted to Charles I of England
Surrender of Huguenot-held La Rochelle to Richelieu
Harvey's treatise on circulation of blood published
**1629** Edict of Restitution
**1630** Theory of mercantilism (Thomas Mun's treatises published in 1664)
Swedish intervention in Thirty Years' War (Gustavus Adolphus)
**1632** Battle of Lutzen
Rembrandt, Anatomy
**1634** Assassination of Wallenstein
**1636** Corneille, *Le Cid (The Cid)*
Harvard College established
**1637** Descartes, *Discours de la Methode (Discourse on Method)*

**1642** Civil War breaks out in England
Death of Richelieu
**1648** Peace of Westphalia

*The 17th century saw the development of trends that were to culminate during the 18th century in the so-called "Age of Reason." The passions and religious fervor of the preceding century were overshadowed by increasingly rational attitudes toward life. Even the 17th-century "preligious" wars, which witnessed strange alliances between opposing creeds, reflect new political concepts rather than a concern about dogma and faith. New power relationships emerged. New aims, differing from those of the Renaissance and bearing witness to heightened national feelings, were pursued. A new type of diplomacy developed, one that was to endure until the 20th century.*

## ■THE INTERNATIONAL SCENE

Two factors stand out in the political history of the 17th century: the rise of France in Europe, and the rise of England in overseas territories. The chief loser was the House of Hapsburg, both in Spain and in the empire. The position of superior power that Spain had held in the period following the discovery of America had actually rested on shaky foundations; the maintenance of that position had overtaxed the material and spiritual resources of the country. Similarly in the empire, the Hapsburgs lacked both the military and the economic bases for the preservation of imperial authority and the bureaucracy needed for serving the central government. Meanwhile, France and England could build on structures adapted to the modern world that was emerging from the Renaissance. Furthermore, there was a third area of wide political importance—its role indistinct during the 17th century, but already marked by signs of future greatness. This area comprised the colonial territories in America, to which European civilization was transplanted.

### Expansion of Europe

The drive of the Modern Age of Western Civilization, expressed in Europe's worldwide undertakings, is without parallel. The process of "Europeanization" of the world represents one of the most significant phenomena in modern times. The principal elements of European culture (religions, law concepts, political thought, languages, industrial techniques, customs and manners—the entire classical and medieval heritage) gradually spread everywhere. While the colonies and Eastern civilizations also made substantial contributions to life in Europe, the contributions Europe made to them were more significant.

### Settlement of America

Settlement of the American continent was the most important phase of European expansion. The settlers came principally from four centers: Spain, Portugal, France, and England. During the 17th century, Spain tried both to consolidate and to extend its holdings, while France and England, joined by Holland, Sweden, and Denmark, not only established themselves in the northern parts of the continent, but also began to seize some of the Spanish possessions.

### Spanish America

Under Charles and Philip II, Spain developed an administrative system for its colonies; later rulers did little to change it. The policy was conservative. Government in America remained in the hands of viceroys, who were responsible to the home government. The *encomienda* system was also preserved.

With the gradual exhaustion of the easily accessible mining resources, more attention was paid to the agricultural wealth and opportunities of the New World.

Spanish colonization was greatly aided by the Catholic Church, which enlarged its missionary activities and helped to expand Spanish rule to American lands. In Mexico, Peru, the La Plata region, Portuguese Brazil, Colombia, and Paraguay, the Dominicans, Franciscans, and, especially, the Jesuits dominated in cultural and, sometimes, in political affairs. They adapted themselves to new surroundings and allied themselves with native ruling groups. They undertook programs of education, which gave them influence over the children and thereby opened the gates for an influx of European institutions and customs.

The missionaries were also interested in the economic welfare of the natives, and they tried to protect the weak against exploitation. In Paraguay, they went so far as to encourage communistic institutions. Of course, the civilization they introduced indirectly benefited the home countries, which gained a large labor force and could use it to exploit the natural resources of the colonies.

### *French America*

In American territory claimed by France, European culture was less pervasive than it was in the Spanish areas. French colonization focused on Canada, beginning around 1603 when De Champlain was made the first governor of Canada. This was followed by the founding of Quebec in 1608. Canada was a sparsely populated region and lacked readily available natural resources, except for furs and timber. Consequently, compared with Spain, France showed much less interest in America. Emigration from France to the New World was negligible. Further, the French did not organize any nationally important trading companies for their colonies.

As a result, political and social conditions developed that were markedly different from those in Spanish America. The home government did not set up any elaborate administration, nor did it maintain close relations with the colonists and natives. Both groups were equally subject to the laws. In Canada, the precepts and influences of Catholic Orders were dominant.

### *English America*

England proved to be more active than either Spain or France. Its colonies in North America, which for a time had to compete with Swedish and Dutch settlements, were largely occupied by Protestants. At an early date, the English colonies set a pattern that differed sharply from those set by the French and the Spanish.

The English settled in Virginia, beginning with the Jamestown colony in 1607. Eventually, despite severe hardships and early political difficulties, they succeeded in establishing prosperous agricultural enterprises. Virginian wealth was based largely upon the production of tobacco, for which the English, following the Spanish example, found it advantageous to make use of black slaves. A trading company in England, the Virginia Company, was granted proprietary rights, but the actual administration of affairs was quickly taken over by a local representative assembly of settlers.

In 1620, another colony, even more independent of the home country as a result of its dissenting religious beliefs, was founded in Massachusetts by Puritan emigres. In accordance with the Mayflower Compact, an agreement entered into by passengers on the ship *Mayflower* during the journey to America, a representative assembly of all free men held the reins of government. In New England, during the early period of settlement, the problem of survival was even more difficult than it had been in Virginia. The settlers faced similar disadvantages of climate and soil and, in addition, continuous internal dissension and the hostility of the Native Americans. The success of the colonists can be attributed to their habit of hard work, their united but often brutal defense against the natives, and their conviction as to the righteousness and eventual victory of their cause. During the 1630s, immigration to the New England colonies assumed substantial dimensions, and, in 1634, an English colony was founded in Maryland.

### Expansion into Asia

The 17th-century establishment of European dominance in America was not matched by comparable expansion into Asia. The Europeans established themselves in numerous ports and some inland trading places, and they entered into lucrative commercial relations, but no territories could be occupied as in America. No populations could be subjugated nor could their resources be exploited.

The Europeans were unable to permanently introduce Western religious beliefs and social patterns. In the 16th century, Loyola's Jesuit colleague, Francis Xavier, had spread the Catholic faith into Southeast Asia. Early in the 17th century, Catholics in Japan may have numbered half a million, and even in China, converts had been made. However, owing to the vigor of the old, indigenous civilizations in the East and to the strength of their economic, social, and religious institutions, the process of Europeanization, which was already rendered difficult by strife among the Europeans themselves, was held back. The contributions of missionaries, traders, and soldiers had little effect. Even this limited influence was restricted chiefly to southern Asia and failed to leave significant traces in China and Japan.

## ■ EUROPE'S POLITICAL SCENE

It was during the 17th century that European expansion, especially in lands across the Atlantic, produced the changes in Europe's political power that had been foreshadowed in the Age of Discovery. Spain and Portugal, which had been the first to explore and settle the New World, however, did not benefit permanently from their achievements. Whether for reasons of geographical location and climate or for reasons of individual ability and spirit of enterprise, it was not the Latin countries in the south of Europe that reaped the fruits of colonization, but the seafaring nations in the north. Germany itself did not share in this development, nor did the Slavic parts of Europe which, far removed from the Atlantic sea lanes, continued along their own independent cultural paths.

### Decline of Spain and Portugal

The death of Philip II in 1598 marked a decisive turn in Spain's role. Literature, music, and the arts continued to flourish, and the country entered what has come to be known as its "Golden Age." However, economic conditions deteriorated. Despite the work of the capable minister Olivares, the nobility, profiting from the weakness of Philip II's successors, regained their former influence.

The administration of the colonies became increasingly costly, while the wealth of the colonies was squandered for luxuries, prestige, and war. Increasingly desperate efforts were required to keep the sea lanes open, especially in the struggle with England. Prices continued to rise. Initiative was lacking. Emigration and wars checked population growth. The remnants of the Moorish and Jewish populations were eliminated in fearful persecutions. The army decayed and, under incompetent kings, the bureaucracy failed to function satisfactorily. In 1639, the French took advantage of an uprising in Catalonia and invaded the country, further weakening Spain.

By then, Portugal, too, was engulfed in the general economic and political decline. By the middle of the century, when income from the East and the New World began to dwindle—partly because of the exhaustion of the great silver mines worked since 1545—power shifted from the Iberian domains of the Hapsburgs to the lands of rival dynasties in the north.

### The German Empire

The possessions of the Austrian Hapsburgs, and with them the whole German Empire, underwent a similar decline, but for different reasons. Germany suffered from political fragmentation and lack of central authority. Trade decreased in the Mediterranean area, as did the commerce across the Alps, which fed the great southern German centers. Germany lacked the harbors necessary to develop transatlantic trade.

It was also damaged by the conservatism of both the southern German bankers and the northern German merchants of the once-powerful Hanse.

Leaders of genius became a rarity in the intellectual, political, religious, and business spheres. Moreover, the Peace of Augsburg was often violated. The balance of power continued its shift due to the growth of Lutheranism in some regions and the strength of the Counter Reformation in others. Foreign powers—England, Spain, and France—saw opportunities to further their political objectives by interfering in German affairs and by helping one side and then its opponents.

### Thirty Years' War (1618-1648)

As a result, a terrible civil war broke out in 1618. It began as a religious war between Catholics and Protestants when, during negotiations, Emperor Ferdinand II's ambassadors to Bohemia were hurled out of a window in Prague ("defenestration"). This war quickly involved foreign nations because the Bohemians promptly deposed Ferdinand, who wanted to reintroduce Catholicism. They replaced him with a Protestant, the Elector Frederick of the Palatinate, who was a relative of the English king. Frederick suffered a major military defeat in 1620.

Shortly thereafter, Protestant Denmark came to Frederick's aid, but the imperial and Catholic forces again proved their superiority. Under the leadership of two great generals, Wallenstein and Tilly, the imperial armies forced the Danes and their Protestant allies to retreat. In 1629, the first two phases (Bohemian and Danish) of the war ended. Ferdinand regained the crown of Bohemia, and in the same year, promulgated an Edict of Restitution, which cost the Protestants all the Church lands they had secularized and taken over since 1555.

In fact, it appeared that the war would end with the triumph of the Catholics. However, fearful of this eventuality, the foes of the Hapsburgs combined their efforts. They found a capable standard bearer in Gustavus Adolphus, king of Sweden, devout Protestant, wise and generous statesman, and a leader who was shrewdly aware of Sweden's interests. Soon after his accession to the throne, he entered the long struggle for Baltic hegemony and proved his generalship by conquering the Polish possessions in Livonia. He then saw a chance to help his Lutheran brethren while simultaneously completing his domination of Baltic shipping by conquering Germany's Baltic coast.

As these aims implied war on the Hapsburgs, he obtained subsidies from Catholic France, whereupon a third phase (Swedish) of the war began. At the head of a splendid army, well equipped with artillery, he pushed deep into the heart of the empire. In his plight, the emperor had to recall Wallenstein, whom he had ungratefully dismissed. Wallenstein had enormous wealth and was in control of an army he recruited and, therefore, he was indispensable to the Catholic side.

In 1632, a decisive battle was fought at Liitzen in Saxony. Wallenstein was defeated, and Protestantism was saved, but Gustavus Adolphus was killed. Without him, the Swedes were reluctant to continue the war. Wallenstein's star commenced to rise again. When he began secret preparations for making himself ruler of a centralized German national state, however, he was murdered (in 1634), a turn of events that the emperor did not regret.

In 1635, Ferdinand consented to a compromise peace, which was concluded in Prague. He revoked the Edict of Restitution, the main object of contention. Since Hapsburg power was not yet finished, the French stirred up the Swedes anew. Moreover, they persuaded the Dutch to attack the Spanish Netherlands, induced the state of Savoy to seize the Hapsburg possessions in Italy, and put troops of their own into the field. Thus, the devastating war continued during a fourth period, which lasted another thirteen years.

### Peace of Westphalia (1648)

Peace was concluded in 1648 at Munster and Osnabruck, two towns in Westphalia. The empire survived, and the Hapsburg influence remained an important factor in European affairs, although its impe-

*Figure 7–1 The 1648 Peace of Westphalia, recognizing the new boundaries of European States.*

rial authority was greatly reduced. The central administration of the German Empire was further weakened, and its more than 300 component states were accorded almost total independence.

Some of the individual states, such as Brandenburg and Saxony, gained territory and achieved status as European powers. The independence of Switzerland and Holland was recognized. Calvinists gained equal rights with Catholics and Lutherans. The claim of France to the western territories of the empire in Lorraine, which it had annexed, was confirmed. So, too, was the claim of Sweden to the Northern provinces along the Baltic Sea and the mouths of Germany's rivers.

The real winners of the war were France, which reached the peak of its power in Europe, and Sweden. Germany was devastated; in some regions, the population had declined by a third or more. Towns and villages had to be rebuilt, agriculture had to be reestablished, and the intellectual centers had to be revived.

The Peace of Westphalia was supplemented by two additional treaties: one between France and Spain (the Peace of the Pyrenees, 1659), and another among Sweden, Poland, and Brandenburg (the Peace of Oliva, 1660).

With its long negotiations and numerous provisions, the Peace of Westphalia marks one of the most significant moments in the history of Western civilization because it confirmed, and in a sense codified, the changes that had taken place in the political system of Europe. The aspirations for an international organization represented by the "Holy Roman Empire" were not revived. The "national state," exemplified by France, triumphed. Future interrelationships in Europe had to be based on the fact that, in the diplomacy of the several countries, religious considerations would be subordinated to those of national self-interest. Loyalty to the state replaced loyalty to religious institutions. During the Westphalian peace negotiations, new procedures and methods of diplomacy were devised that were to persist for almost two centuries.

## Russia

While Hapsburg power and the role of central Europe were on the decline, the countries on the flanks of the Continent were gaining strength and prestige. Russia emerged from a struggle with Poland to become the leading power in the East. Toward the turn of the century, Russia's ruling dynasty became extinct. Boris Godunov, the last tsar's chief adviser, had himself elected as successor. He proved to be a capable, far-sighted ruler who was oriented toward the west, but as a "usurper," accused of having eliminated the rightful heir to the throne, he never gained the allegiance of the nobility or the trust of the people. A terrible drought in 1603-1604 added to his difficulties.

After Godunov's death in 1605, Russia went through a disastrous period of social revolution, political disintegration, dynastic rivalry, invasion by the Poles, who wanted to put a Pole on Russia's throne, and external war (the "Times of Trouble," 1605–1613). Out of this upheaval emerged a new autocratic regime and a new dynasty, the Romanovs. Only with their election in 1613 was internal peace restored.

The Romanovs ruled with the help of a new "service nobility." Through their holdings of land and serfs, the new nobility controlled the wealth of the country; simultaneously, it formed the backbone of the administration. The reorganization was achieved at the expense of the old, independent nobility, which was rendered powerless; of the peasantry, which was reduced to complete serfdom; and, eventually, of the Church, which was brought under tsarist control. A new legal code was published in 1649. Of great importance was the fact that the Ukraine, largely inhabited by Cossacks, was conquered.

Thus, Russia expanded westward. Closer contacts with Western nations were established. The balance of power between Russia and Poland was permanently changed in favor of Russia. Immigration, especially that of the Germans, English, and Dutch, was encouraged. European techniques, knowledge, artisanship, and luxury goods increasingly infiltrated the country.

## The Netherlands

The increased power of the large nation on the eastern flank of Europe was matched by the corresponding, if not greater, rise of Western Europe. In the West, economic rather than military power formed the basis for growth and preeminence. Hence, a small country, such as Holland, was able to become a great power. While Antwerp had been ruined during the wars for independence, Amsterdam had become the financial center of the West.

The advantages gained by the Dutch as a result of this shift were augmented by a policy of tolerance. Refugees from various lands—including Jews and especially those expelled from Spanish dominions—were readily accepted. They helped to establish wide-ranging trade connections. Owing to their industry and skills, the immigrants contributed to Holland's economic prosperity. The government was run by the wealthy burghers, who kept taxation low. Agriculture, fishing, the textile industries, shipbuilding, and transportation flourished. There was less class distinction than elsewhere, and the level of cultural activity was high. Holland became a center of the expanding book trade. New universities were founded. Scholars and artists could do their work in an atmosphere of comparative freedom and tolerance.

## England

In the Netherlands, the assumption of political power by the wealthy bourgeoisie and the subordination of military goals to economic objectives took place without grave internal crises, despite continued opposition of various groups to the landholding nobility. The necessary adjustments in the other great maritime nation of the north, England, encountered much greater difficulties.

## The Stuarts

After the loss of its Continental possessions, England became an insular power, restricted to its island. This brought unexpected security. Dynastic expansion was no longer directed toward European lands, but toward overseas colonies. However, internal tensions developed. Elizabeth, who had refused to marry, was succeeded in 1603 by James I of the House of Stuart. Under his rule and that of his successor, Charles I, the controversial issues concerning the condition and control of the Church and the immunities and rights of Parliament, all of which had been deferred during the reign of Elizabeth, were reopened. These issues were complicated by various factors, including inflation, the growing costs of government, the heavy expenditures incurred by English diplomacy as carried on since the time of Elizabeth, and the wasteful, factional strife at the Stuart court.

To meet this emergency, the king was compelled to increase taxes and customs duties and to sell administrative offices. In view of the accumulated debt, he had to pursue financial policies repugnant to a Parliament that desired, above all else, to maintain economic stability and prosperity. As parliamentary opposition grew, the king became more and more arbitrary, further increasing the general feeling of dissatisfaction.

Soon, every powerful group in the country was antagonized. Even a large part of the landholding nobility resented the king's rule, in spite of the fact that the Stuarts seemed to have special sympathy for them. They also held all major administrative offices and dominated in Parliament. Eventually, the opposition, though divided as to its ultimate aims, was united by a desire to limit the power of the Crown and to participate in policymaking. The ensuing deadlock was reinforced by the friendly attitude of the Stuarts toward Catholicism and their pro-Spanish point of view, which impeded the realization of English nationalistic and mercantile aims.

## Revolution

The widespread discontent was intensified by the unpopularity of the advisers appointed by Charles I and by his failure in foreign affairs. Finally, Parliament was induced to draw up a "Petition of Right" in 1628. This petition demanded an end to taxation without act of Parliament. It also opposed arbitrary imprisonment, billeting of soldiers in private houses, and martial law in time of peace. The king, though he insisted upon his "divine right," signed the petition. In the following year, however, he dissolved Parliament and ruled without it for eleven years, during which time the country prospered.

Opposition to royal absolutism again developed when the king, who was in dire need of new funds to combat piracy in the English Channel, tried to levy additional taxes. His right to do so was challenged by a burgher, John Hampden, but it was sustained by subservient judges. Popular passions were further aroused by the king's conciliatory policies toward Catholics and by the harsh treatment which he and his archbishop, Laud, directed against nonconformist Puritans. This religious issue, plus the numerous other grievances, brought matters to a head. When Charles insisted on forcing the sects to accept the Anglican service, they took up arms in rebellion.

The king had to summon Parliament (in 1640) in order to recruit troops. Once reassembled, this "Long Parliament," which lasted until 1653, presented demands; namely, that the king must not be allowed to dissolve the assembly at will, that meetings must be held regularly, and that all special jurisdiction claimed by the kings since Tudor times must be relinquished. Parliament insisted that it must control all income. Eventually, it ordered the arrest and execution of some of the king's closest advisers, including Archbishop Laud.

## Civil War

These demands and actions failed to solve the problem, for Parliament itself was divided. One party was sympathetic to royal absolutism; another favored the interests of the rich entrepreneurs; and still another supported the cause of the poorer parts of the population. There were still other groups, including the so-called "Levelers," who espoused communistic principles. In addition, Parliament was split by the religious issue. Anglicans, Calvinists, and Catholics disagreed about religious tolerance and state control over the Church.

The various economic and religious groups kept shifting their positions and loyalties in accordance with swiftly changing political circumstances. Thus, no clear alignment of sides had been established when, in 1641, a revolution broke out in Ireland over the question of settling Protestants in Northern Ireland (Ulster). In 1642, the king himself, believing that the time to reestablish his own authority had arrived, took up arms against Parliament. Civil war began.

Twice beaten in battle, Charles I fled to Scotland, but was extradited and handed over to Parliament. Even at this point, he took advantage of the divisions within Parliament and was able to defy the opposition until a determined Puritan minority under Oliver Cromwell organized a staunch and fanatical army that defeated the royal forces. The Puritans then reassembled the legislature as a "Rump" Parliament (purged of all members unsympathetic to their cause), which brought the king to trial. In 1649, having been adjudged guilty of treason, Charles was executed. Under Oliver Cromwell's leadership, the Rump Parliament set up a new government.

## France

While civil war prevented the establishment of royal absolutism in England, absolutism in France reached its peak of development. Intelligent rulers, such as Henry IV (assassinated in 1610), and a long succession of unusually able ministers who supported royal power, contributed to its success.

### Sully

The first of the great ministers was Sully, an intelligent, honest, and efficient Calvinist in the service of Henry IV. Under his guidance, a great deal was done to repair the damage sustained from a half-century of civil war. Brigandage and highway robbery were suppressed, and most of the dissolute army units were disbanded. Peace was maintained both within the country and in foreign affairs. The privileges of the nobility were severely restricted, and more officials were appointed from among the bourgeoisie.

The treasury was restored to a healthy condition by measures such as the farming out of tax collections, which meant that the right to collect certain taxes was sold to the highest bidder. This bidder then paid an agreed sum into the treasury and kept for himself what he was able to collect in taxes. The new system of tax collection provided the treasury with a small but certain income and was used mainly to collect the *taille,* a property tax levied upon all landowners outside the ranks of the nobility. Sully put a stop to tax abuses, especially the imposition of illegal taxes, and he made certain that the royal domain was managed on a profitable basis.

### Absolutism and Mercantilism

As there was widespread satisfaction with a system that had reestablished security and order, there was no need for action by the Estates-General, which represented the people. The king and his first minister made all decisions. In economic affairs, they adopted mercantilist policies with the principal aim of increasing production and accumulating bullion, i.e., precious metals, and strengthening exports. They facilitated trade by building roads, canals, and bridges, clearing land, and draining marshes. By means of subsidies and granting of monopolies, they aided long-established industries (e.g., paper and textiles) as well as new industries (e.g., silk manufacturing). By selling offices, they secured a large income for the Crown. They sent explorers out to lay claim to new colonies, especially in Canada. They also enacted new navigation laws to prevent ships owned by foreigners from transporting goods to French possessions. In foreign affairs, they adhered to a traditional anti-Hapsburg policy, but avoided war.

### *Richelieu*

The same policies which had been formulated by the stern and austere Calvinist, Sully, were pursued by the luxury-loving Catholic, Cardinal Richelieu, who became chief minister under Louis XIII, the son of Henry IV, in 1624. Richelieu was a learned man with broad cultural interests. He possessed an iron will, vast ambition, and a realistic understanding of politics. He put an end to the political irresponsibility and wasteful practices that had marked the period following the death of Henry IV and sought to strengthen the rights of the Crown.

Richelieu refused to convene the Estates-General, which had feebly attempted to regain its authority; it did not convene again for 150 years. He deprived the nobility of most of its remaining powers and ordered the royal forces to both seize its strongholds and execute some of its leaders. By means of hard-fought military campaigns, he forced the Huguenots to surrender their fortified towns, even though this had been stipulated as inviolable by the Edict of Nantes.

The Cardinal did not, however, destroy the Huguenots' religious freedom, for he was mainly interested in political matters. In fact, Protestant forces were Richelieu's chief allies against the Hapsburgs during the Thirty Years' War. Reforms were introduced in the army and the navy, enabling them to provide adequate protection for the colonies.

As in Sully's time, most of the government's officials were recruited from the middle class. Provincial administrators *(intendants),* judges, and other high officials constituted a new social group, which consisted largely of commoners who derived their new status from office rather than from birth. It was called the *noblesse de la robe.* This bureaucracy remained the most politically influential segment of the population until the Revolution of 1789.

Most of Richelieu's measures were designed to maintain French prestige abroad and Bourbon absolutism at home. When Richelieu died in 1642, France was, indeed, on the road to supreme power in Europe. His very able successor, Cardinal Mazarin (d. 1661), who resembled Richelieu in his vanity, greed, ambition, and shrewdness, was just the man to preserve what Richelieu had built and to augment it. Mazarin's career ushered in the "Age of Louis XIV."

## ■ PHILOSOPHY AND ARTS

The Peace of Westphalia, which ended the intense religious and political conflicts engendered by the Reformation, laid the legal basis for the modern European state system. At about the same time, the works of the great thinkers on the Continent determined the future direction of Western intellectual endeavors. More and more, Europeans devoted themselves to scientific investigations of nature, and this had a profound impact on their philosophy. Thus, both in the political and in the intellectual spheres, the mid-17th century is correctly regarded as the dividing line between two major periods in the history of Western civilization.

### Science and Philosophy

Among the scientists and philosophers representing the new spirit of inquiry that was to modify Western culture for centuries, three men stand out: Kepler, Galileo, and Descartes. Kepler (d. 1630) devoted much attention to problems of medieval scholarship and to astrology and other pseudo-sciences. However, he made one of the greatest contributions to the understanding of nature in formulating his famous three laws ("Kepler's laws"), which accurately described the motion of the planets. Galileo (d. 1642), notwithstanding persecution and house arrest by the Catholic Church, continued the work in physics and astronomy that he had started in the previous century. Descartes (d. 1650) was a mathematician and philosopher who spent most of his mature life in Holland and became the foremost precursor of the "Age of Reason." He occupied himself with an investigation of our ability to "know" and the limits of knowledge. He postulated the "self-evident" fact, *Cogito, ergo sum* (I think, therefore I am). From this fact, he proceeded rationally and logically to draw conclusions. He occupied himself with "truth" and ethics. To him, a steadfast son of the Catholic Church, God appeared as the "First Cause," but mechanistic laws ruled in nature. Cause-and-effect determined everything that occurred in the universe, and a dualistic reality existed—a dualism of mind and matter. It is noteworthy that Descartes also developed the principles of analytic geometry and contributed to other sciences, such as optics.

### *Other Contributions*

The work of 17th-century cosmologists and philosophers was greatly aided by new developments in mathematics, anatomy, and physiology, and social sciences such as law. Contributions to mathematics included the invention of logarithms by the Scotsman John Napier in 1614. In anatomy, a notable contributor was the Englishman William Harvey (d. 1657), who correctly described the system of blood circulation and thus paved the way for the development of modern physiology. In law, the scientific trend inspired the Dutchman Hugo Grotius (d. 1645) to formulate proposals for a body of international law relating particularly to war and peace.

## Education

Progress in science was closely connected with improved standards in education. New universities were founded in both Catholic and Protestant strongholds—e.g., in Catholic South America and in the Protestant Netherlands. The first college (Harvard, 1636) was established in North America. Among the leaders in the advancement of education during the 16th and 17th centuries were the Jesuit colleges. They had originally been designed to expound the decisions of the Council of Trent, to further the Counter Reformation, and to purge the schools of secular Renaissance influences and immoral authors.

The influence of the Jesuit colleges spread widely. They helped to improve the training of the clergy so that the priests would not only deliver better sermons, but would also more conscientiously fulfill other religious tasks. They promoted humanitarian activities within their own institutions and throughout the community. Francis de Sales and, especially, Vincent de Paul were among those who, influenced by their aims, earned lasting fame by caring for the sick and the aged and building charitable institutions. The Jesuit colleges became important centers of all types of learning, successfully applying new pedagogical principles and encouraging the accumulation of facts in many fields of knowledge.

## Literature

In literature, the towering figure of Shakespeare still dominated in the first decade of the 17th century. He was followed by important, though less universally influential, poets such as John Donne (d. 1631) and Ben Jonson (d. 1637). Donne's lyrics show great originality and warmth of feeling. Jonson's comedies are less illustrative of the passions that marked the age of the High Renaissance. Instead, they display the more moderate, rational, and reflective style of the Baroque period. The latter is also true about the works of the famous writers in Spain's "Golden Age"—the dramatists Lope de Vega (d. 1635) and Calderon (d. 1681). While their works reflect the spiritual fervor the preceding century had shown, they, too, show rational tendencies, stylistic restraint, and a strong emphasis on form.

## Art

In painting, sculpture, and architecture, the first half of the 17th century saw the Baroque style come into full bloom. It flourished in all countries, especially in the Catholic regions. As in the case of other major movements in art history, the Baroque style (1600–1750) went through several stages of development. Many of the qualities associated with the term "baroque"— theatricality, excessive ornamentation, sentimentality, and bombast are derived from its later evolution. These characteristics, with their appeal to the senses, do not constitute the only, or even the most important, element of the Baroque style. Like all art of the 17th century, the Baroque was marked by dynamism, orderliness in spite of its exuberance, an assertion of life and faith, and a mastery of form that has given it permanent value. A certain balance and harmony remained which, while reacting to the individualism of the High Renaissance, emphasized intellectual strength and linked the art of the 17th century with the rational tendencies of the age.

Spain produced perhaps the greatest master of the Baroque, the painter Velasquez (d. 1660). The Baroque style was introduced in the north by the Flemish painter Rubens (d. 1640) and his school, which, even though it adhered to some traditional attitudes, opposed the Puritan trends of Calvinism and post-Trent Catholicism. Rubens was followed by a new, more serene school of painting, which included his pupil, the famous portrait painter, Van Dyke (d. 1641).

In sculpture and architecture, Giovanni Bernini (d. 1680) stood out as the foremost representative of the Baroque style. He designed the colonnades for the church of St. Peter in Rome.

## Music

The Baroque style in the visual arts was also evident in the music of the 17th century. To some extent, the free inventiveness of the preceding period made room for compositions where inventiveness, no matter how intense the feelings, had to be reconciled with demands for a strictly formal frame. The structure of music had to correspond to an elaborate system and to possess a balance such as the taste the period demanded. Even ornamentation became stylized. The polyphonic style was supplemented in what was termed "The New Music" (after an Italian composition published in 1602) by "monody"—compositions where only one voice carries the melody. Instrumental music, owing much of its inspiration to the songs of the 16th century, became popular, and different types of string instruments came into use. The sonata form was created.

Italian opera made further progress and spread to the northern countries of Europe. In Germany, Protestant religious music flourished. It offered beautiful choral preludes and other compositions, especially written for the organ. The three outstanding masters of the period were Claudio Monteverdi (d. 1643) and Alessandro Scarlatti (d. 1725) in Italy, and Heinrich Schutz (d. 1672) in Germany. Thus, the period which saw the terrors of the Thirty Years' War and of the civil war in England, the Times of Trouble in Russia, and mass expulsions in Spain was by no means devoid of beautiful and inspiring achievements.

## Perspective

*The first part of the 17th century presents as dismal a scene in the political arena as did the last part of the 16th. The climax came with the Thirty Years' War, which began with religious strife and brought death to millions, destruction of towns, and widespread misery in its wake. Soon, the religious issues faded and, ultimately, neither ideological nor major national aims were involved, only dynastic interests unrelated to the needs of the people. Ambitious "absolute" rulers were the ones who benefited.*

*On the other hand, the basis for a new direction in Western civilization's cultural evolution was laid in the preceding century. Philosophy and science, regardless of what happened politically, became the focus of a world that searched for truth on the basis of observation and knowledge based on logic. Questions of ethics and of metaphysics were by no means neglected, but doubt led to the application of reason and enhanced the need for experimentation. Great strides were made in mathematics, physics, cosmology, and biology.*

## Selected Readings

Nordstrom, Byron. *The History of Sweden* (Westport, Conn.: Greenwood Press, 2002).

Goodman, Paul. *The Americans: Colonial Experience* (New York: Holt, Rinehart and Winston, 1958).

Friedrich, Carl J. *The Age of the Baroque* (New York: Harper, 1952).

Kamen, Henry. *The Iron Century: Social Change in Europe, 1550–1660.* (New York, Praeger, 1972)

Barton, Simon. *A History of Spain* (New York: Palgrave Macmillan, 2004).

Lossky, Andrew. *Louis XIV and the French Revolution* (New Brunswick, N.J.: Rutgers University Press, 1994).

Marsak, Leonard M., ed., *The Enlightenment* (New York, Wiley, 1970).

Bunch, Bryan. *The History of Science and Technology* (Boston: Houghton Mifflin, 2004).

Rabb, Theodore. *Struggle for Stability in Early Modern Europe* (New York: Oxford University Press, 1975).

Wedgwood, Cicely W. *The Thirty Years' War* (New York: Doubleday, 1961).

## Test Yourself

1. Spanish colonization in the Americas was greatly aided by ____.
   A. France and England
   B. The Catholic Church
   C. Islamic science
   D. All of the above

2. The first English settlement in the Virginia colony was at Jamestown in____.
   A. 1600
   B. 1575
   C. 1610
   D. 1607

3. The Thirty-Years' War ended by a treaty in 1648 known as____.
   A. The Peace of Augsburg
   B. The Peace of Paris
   C. The Peace of Westphalia
   D. The Peace of Wurzburg

4. The English "Petition of Right" in 1628 demanded____.
   A. An end to taxation without act of parliament
   B. An end to arbitrary imprisonment
   C. Martial law in times of peace
   D. All of the above

5. In 1649, having been adjudged guilty of treason,____.
   A. Charles I was executed
   B. Oliver Cromwell was executed
   C. Mary Queen of Scots was imprisoned
   D. Henry IV was assassinated

6. The *taille* is the equivalent of____.
   A. A poll tax
   B. A church tax
   C. A property tax
   D. An income tax

7. Spain produced perhaps the greatest master of the Baroque style (1600-1750), the painter_____.
   A. Titian
   B. Caravaggio
   C. Van Dyke
   D. Velazquez

8. The colonnades of the Church of St. Peter in Rome were designed by _____.
   A. Caravaggio
   B. Giovanni Bernini
   C. Michelangelo
   D. Peter Paul Rubens

## Answers and Explanations

1. **B.** Spanish colonization was greatly aided by the Catholic Church, which enlarged its missionary activities and helped to expand Spanish rule to American lands. In Mexico, Peru, the La Plata region, Portuguese Brazil, Colombia, and Paraguay, the Dominicans, Franciscans, and, Jesuits dominated in cultural and, sometimes, in political affairs. They adapted themselves to new surroundings, allied themselves with native ruling groups, and undertook programs of education, which gave them influence over the children. They thereby opened the gates for the influx of European institutions and customs.

2. **D.** The first English settlement in Virginia was the Jamestown colony in 1607. Eventually, despite severe hardships and early political difficulties, they succeeded in establishing prosperous agricultural enterprises. Virginian wealth was based largely upon the production of tobacco, for which the English, following the Spanish example, found it advantageous to make use of black slaves. A trading company in England, the Virginia Company, was granted proprietary rights, but the actual administration of affairs was quickly taken over by a local representative assembly of the settlers.

3. **C.** Peace was concluded in 1648 at Munster and Osnabruck, two towns in Westphalia, in what has come to be known as the Peace of Westphalia. The empire survived, and Hapsburg influence remained an important factor in European affairs; but imperial authority was greatly reduced. The central administration of the German Empire was further weakened, and its more than 300 component states were accorded almost complete independence. Some of the individual states, such as Brandenburg and Saxony, gained territory and achieved status as European powers. The independence of Switzerland and of Holland was recognized. Calvinists gained equal rights with Catholics and Lutherans. The claim of France to the western territories of the empire in Lorraine, which it had annexed, was confirmed. So, too, was the claim of Sweden to the Northern provinces along the Baltic Sea and the mouths of Germany's rivers.

4. **D.** The widespread discontent was intensified by the unpopularity of the advisers appointed by Charles I and by his failure in foreign affairs. Finally, Parliament was induced to draw up a "Petition of Right" in 1628. This petition demanded an end to taxation without an act of Parliament. It also opposed arbitrary imprisonment, billeting of soldiers in private houses, and martial law in time of peace. The king, though he insisted upon his "divine right," signed the petition. In the following year, he dissolved Parliament and ruled without it for eleven years, during which time the country prospered.

5. **A.** Twice beaten in battle, Charles I fled to Scotland, but was extradited and handed over to Parliament. Even at this point, by taking advantage of the divisions within Parliament, he was able to defy the opposition until a determined Puritan minority under Oliver Cromwell organized a staunch and fanatical army that defeated the royal forces. The Puritans then reassembled the legislature as a "Rump" Parliament (purged of all members unsympathetic to their cause), which brought the king to trial. In 1649, having been adjudged guilty of treason, Charles was executed. Under Oliver Cromwell's leadership, the Rump Parliament set up a new government.

6. **C.** The new system of tax collection, providing the treasury with a small but certain income, was used mainly to collect the *taille,* a property tax levied upon all landowners outside the ranks of the nobility. Sully put a stop to tax abuses, especially the imposition of illegal taxes. He made certain that the royal domain was managed on a profitable basis.

7. D. As in the case of other major movements in art history, the Baroque style (1600–1750) went through several stages of development. Many of the qualities associated with the term "baroque"— in particular, those of theatricality, excessive ornamentation, sentimentality, and bombast are derived from its later evolution. These characteristics, with their appeal to the senses, do not constitute the only, or even the most important, elements of the Baroque style. Like all art of the 17th century, the Baroque was marked by dynamism, orderliness despite exuberance, an assertion of life and faith, and a mastery of form that has given it permanent value. Spain produced perhaps the greatest master of the Baroque, the painter Velasquez (d. 1660).

8. B. In sculpture and architecture, Giovanni Bernini (d. 1680) stood out as the foremost representative of the baroque style. He designed the colonnades for the church of St. Peter in Rome.

# CHAPTER 8
# The Age of Louis XIV (1643-1715)

**1649** English King Charles I executed
**1651** First English Navigation Act
Hobbes, *Leviathan*
**1653** End of Fronde
Cromwell becomes Lord Protector
**1656** Russia incorporates Ukraine
**1658** Death of Cromwell
**1659** Peace of the Pyrenees
**1660** Restoration of Charles II in England
Peace of Oliva
Death of Velasquez
**1661** Death of Mazarin: Colbert named controller-general
**1665** Plague and Great Fire in London
**1666** Death of Frans Hals
**1667** Milton, *Paradise Lost*
Beginning of War of Devolution
**1669** Death of Rembrandt
**1670** Pascal, *Pensees*
**1672** Jean de Witt assassinated
**1673** Test Act in England
**1675** Spinoza, *Ethics*
Leibnitz publishes method of differential calculus
**1678** Peace of Nijmwegen
Bunyan, *Pilgrim's Progress*
**1681** Strasbourg annexed by France
**1682** La Salle in Mississippi Valley
**1683** Ottoman Turks besiege Vienna
William Penn in Pennsylvania (Philadelphia)
Death of Colbert
Newton formulates the law of gravitation
**1685** Revocation of Edict of Nantes
**1687** Newton, *Philosophiae Naturalis Principia Mathematica*

**1688** English Glorious Revolution
Death of Frederick William, "Great Elector" of Brandenburg
**1689** Act of Toleration
Bill of Rights
**1690** Huyghens promulgates theory of light
Locke, *Essay concerning Human Understanding*
**1697** Peace of Ryswick
**1699** Peace of Karlowitz
**1700** Charles XII of Sweden defeats Russians at Narva
**1701** Beginning of War of Spanish Succession
**1703** St. Petersburg founded
**1704** Newton, *Optics*
Newcomen builds steam engine
**1707** Union of England and Scotland established
**1709** Peter the Great defeats Swedes at Poltava
**1713** Peace of Utrecht
England gains *asiento*
**1714** Peace of Rastatt and Baden Leibnitz, *Monadology*
**1715** Death of Louis XIV: regency of Duke d'Orleans

*The second half of the 17th century was not so much a period of new dynamic events as one of consolidation and gradual evolution. In political affairs, it witnessed the continuation of absolutism in France and an opposite trend toward a parliamentary regime in England. It brought the rise of Brandenburg and continued progress in the Westernization of Russia. It also witnessed the growth of European civilization in the centers established earlier on other continents—especially North America.*

*Its truly great and lasting contributions were made in philosophy, science, and art. The age named for Louis XIV is not renowned because of the king's political exploits or for the economic developments of his time. It is famous for the achievements of great philosophers, writers, and scientists. Their rational approach to life and nature brought to maturity the ideological trends that had been growing in Europe since the views of the Nominalists prevailed over those of the Realists during the late Middle Ages. The characteristics of the Baroque, particularly its intellectuality and harmony, pervaded the cultural sphere. Since these characteristics developed most fully in France and were spread by the example set by France, they provided the justification for naming the period the "Age of Louis XIV."*

## ■ THE POLITICAL SCENE

The Peace of Westphalia (1648) had signified an open acknowledgment by the European powers of what had long been a fact; namely, that the supreme position of emperor of the "Holy Roman Empire of the German Nation" no longer commanded wide respect. It had become essentially a shadowy honor, devoid of practical significance. Even the etiquette of diplomacy was revised in accordance with the actual distribution of power. Special consideration was accorded not only to France, but also to newly emergent nations, such as Sweden and England.

### France

When he came to the throne one year after Richelieu's death, Louis XIV was only five years old. He was ten at the conclusion of the Peace of Westphalia, 23 when he took the reins of government into his own hands, and almost 77 when he died. Even if he had not had such a strong personality, this long term as a ruler—the longest of any monarch in European history—could not have failed to leave a deep imprint, especially since he ruled during an age of "absolutism."

*Figure 8–1 France under the Reign of Louis XIV*

## Mazarin

During the first 18 years of Louis XIV's reign, the direction of French affairs was entrusted to Cardinal Mazarin. It was Mazarin, a shrewd diplomat, who concluded the Peace of Westphalia, whereby France took the preeminent position among European countries. It was also Mazarin who sealed the fate of the French nobility. Seeking to profit from the financial straits in which the young king found himself in 1648, the nobility staged a rebellion, the so-called "Fronde." The rebellion sought to reduce the powers of the bureaucrats appointed by the king. It was abetted by the highest court of law, the Parliament of Paris, which was subservient to the nobility's interests. The Parliament demanded for itself the right to control taxation, appoint *intendants* (provincial governors), and supervise legislation. This last right could be exercised by refusing to "register" any laws Parliament deemed to be contrary to custom or that infringed upon existing privileges. Had it succeeded, development toward a parliamentary government would have been unavoidable, although, owing to the composition and the policies of the Parliament, the traditional privileged classes would have gained more than the commercial interests.

However, Mazarin energetically opposed the Parliament. He brutally suppressed the Fronde along with peasant uprisings. At the same time, he lent his hand, for the sake of unity, to the suppression of a puritanical movement within the Catholic Church known as "Jansenism." This movement had had considerable influence on education. Though Catholic, it tended in the direction of Calvinism and was bitterly opposed by the Jesuits. When Mazarin died in 1661, Louis XIV took personal control, and the concentration of power in the hands of the king was such that it could not be challenged.

## Louis XIV

Louis was a man of contradictions: conceited and selfish, but industrious, persistent, noble in bearing, and inspiring. He never called a meeting of the Estates-General, nor did he permit the Estates to obstruct his legislation. Whatever decision he personally made was final. He took counsel only with advisers of his own choice and continued to rely on the *noblesse de la robe* in his administration and his law courts. Justice became somewhat more equable than under his predecessors, but corruption persisted.

*Figure 8–2  Louis XIV, 1638–1715*

Louis was a liberal and understanding patron of the arts and sciences, as long as they glorified him. Architectural projects, in particular, were enthusiastically supported, although at an excessive cost to the country. One example is the enormous castle of Versailles with its famous gardens. French court life established a model for all Europe, and French etiquette supplanted the Spanish court fashions. French elegance was imitated everywhere as were French manners. Yet court morality, which accepted mistresses and bastard children, was already out of tune with the standards the puritanical Calvinistic and Counter-Reformatory trends propagated by the middle class.

## Colbert

Inasmuch as Louis XIV's glory was the chief political objective, all policies were keyed to its promotion. In the early part of his reign, Louis had the good fortune to find an unusually capable minister in Colbert (d. 1683). Colbert was a mercantilist who promoted industry through loans, bounties, tax exemptions, and scientific research. He sponsored the building of canals, ports, and ships, and he simplified the customs system. In order to provide an ample labor force, he offered subsidies to encourage the French people to have large families.

Colbert opposed idleness in the Church and in the lay populations. He abolished internal tolls. Through his support of commercial enterprises, such as the silk industry, and through his honest handling of funds, he greatly increased tax receipts. He accomplished this in spite of the continuation of the inefficient "farming-out" system and despite the shortcomings of an economy that imposed its main burdens upon the commercial and laboring classes, while exempting the rich nobility and the Church. Colbert also promoted colonizing activities. In his time, Marquette, Joliet, and La Salle explored the Mississippi region, which resulted in the development of a substantial fur trade. In India, the French colony of Pondichery was founded.

After Colbert's death, Louis XIV erased many of Colbert's achievements through wars, wasteful financing, and unproductive construction. Taxes stifled industry, and excessive government controls discouraged merchants and industrialists. Schools had to be closed. The population began to decline, and a terrible famine in 1709 added to the woes of the population. Worst of all, Louis XIV, motivated by religious bigotry and his desire to eliminate any dissenting and possibly rebellious groups in order to guarantee stability and unity, revoked the Edict of Nantes in 1685. Attempts at converting the Huguenots to the religion followed by the king and most of the population met with limited success, and a policy of persecution was implemented. Hundreds of thousands of Huguenots were forced to emigrate, which represented a loss to France, but a benefit to the German states, Holland, England, and the other countries that welcomed them.

## French External Policies

Equally ruinous were Louis's foreign policies. Numerous wars were provoked merely for his personal "glory." The economic interests of the country were important factors only in the first war, the purpose of which was to further the mercantilist policies of Colbert, and in the last war, which was fought to establish hegemony overseas. All the other wars went against the economic interests of France.

Enormous sums were expended to build an army superior to that of Spain, an undertaking that was achieved thanks to the ability of men such as Louvois, Vauban, and Turenne. More money went into subsidizing allies, who were lured with promises of territory that would be seized from the Hapsburgs. The idea that the natural borders of France were the Rhine River, the Alps, and the Pyrenees served as an excuse for a policy of ruthless French expansion into Holland, Germany, Italy, and Spain. Ultimately, these wars of expansion proved exceedingly costly.

The first, the "War of Devolution," was fought against a Triple Alliance of Holland, England, and Sweden for the possession of the Netherlands. When peace was made at Aix-la-Chapelle (1668), France's frontiers were extended northward. A second war, undertaken against the Dutch, failed to bring any gains in territory. Initial victories were followed by defeats, and the Peace of Nijmwegen (1678) constituted a draw. In the following years, subsequent to certain sham legal procedures by so-called "Chambres de Reunion," the German territory and city of Strassburg and several Italian towns were annexed.

These annexations provided long-term gains, but, at the time, they merely served to arouse so much apprehension that in 1686 another defensive coalition, which included nearly all the European powers, was formed against France. A third war, the highly destructive "War of the League of Augsburg," lasted until 1697. Then, in the Peace of Ryswick, Louis was forced to surrender some of his earlier conquests and to grant commercial advantages to the maritime nations.

Shortly thereafter, the Spanish line of the Hapsburgs died out. In an effort to prevent any further Austrian-Spanish family links or cooperation, Louis put forward the candidacy of his grandson for the throne. As a result, in a fourth war, that of the Spanish Succession broke out 1701. Again a "Grand Alliance" of most of the European powers was formed. Able generals, such as the Austrian Prince Eugene of Savoy and Marlborough of England, defeated the French armies. Louis was saved from utter ruin by the death of the allied Hapsburg candidate for the Spanish throne and the French diplomatic victories that occurred at the very end of the war.

### Peace of Utrecht (1713)

Finally, in the years 1713 to 1715, peace treaties were concluded at Utrecht, Rastatt, and Baden. Austria thereby gained territories in the southern Netherlands and Italy. England secured vast colonial and commercial advantages, including the rights to the lucrative slave trade (the *asiento*) in the Spanish colonies. Prussia increased its domain. The Dutch obtained land, fortified positions, and commercial rights in areas along their southern frontier.

France maintained its role as a great power. A French prince was allowed to keep the Spanish throne, although subject to restrictions. Thus, when Louis XIV died, cursed by the population, in 1715, the glory of France, even in the political arena, was not seriously impaired. Yet, Louis XIV's love of war, his extravagances in construction, the style of life at his court, and his exploitation of the population boded ill for the future of France.

## England

French policies in the second half of the 17th century added to the nation's prestige and left a lasting impression everywhere on the Continent. On the other hand, England's attention focused on its own insular affairs. By concentrating on immediate practical tasks, the English succeeded not only in overcoming the dangers of revolution and civil war, but also in laying a firm foundation for their future as a world power.

### Cromwell

Four years after the execution of Charles I, Oliver Cromwell made himself "Lord Protector." During his administration, considerable political and economic progress was made, despite the fact that Parliament had played a role subordinate to Cromwell and the army since 1648. New elections were not held because Cromwell, whose backers were in the minority, could not risk them. Revolts were organized by royalists who were eager to put the son of the decapitated king on the throne. Other rebellions were instigated by the Scots, whom Cromwell sought to reconcile, and still others were organized by the Irish, who were brutally oppressed. No basis for a new, legal form of authority was developed.

Yet, Cromwell proved to be a capable ruler. Merchants benefited from the enforcement of navigation acts designed to exclude foreign ships from English ports. They profited from the fight against Dutch competitors and from the stimulation of British shipping. Prosperous trade, in turn, encouraged growth in industry, especially in coal mining and shipbuilding. Cromwell successfully defended the colonial

*Figure 8–2  Oliver Cromwell, 1599–1658*

possessions, organized new colonies, and defeated Holland and Spain—all of which helped to expand British trade. In the religious sphere, the Lord Protector, despite his strict Calvinist leanings, tried to avoid trouble by means of a moderately tolerant policy.

### *Restoration*

Notwithstanding its many successes, the government of Cromwell inspired hatred from the people because of its revolutionary origins, its absolutist trends, its Calvinistic morality, and its program of heavy taxes, which favored the military caste and the overseas merchants. Powerful conservative forces were especially resentful. Consequently, within two years of Cromwell's death in 1658, the Stuart royal line was reestablished.

Charles II was recalled from exile, but before his "restoration," he had to agree to Parliamentary elections. The new Parliament restored the dominant position of the Anglican Church, proclaimed amnesty for political opponents, and assumed supervision of the king's activities, including his foreign policy, choice of advisers, expenditures, and military forces.

### *Charles II*

The reign of Charles II was colorful. Despite disasters, such as the plague and a terrible fire that consumed large areas of London, it was marked by gaiety and artistic and literary achievements. It was an age of extravagance and immorality in which the king and court, imitating France, set an example. During this regime, wealthy individuals gained more national influence, and some of the long-established feudal rights were abolished.

Political parties began to form, including the Whig party, which favored representative government and middle-class commercial interests, and the Tory party, which supported royal rights, the Anglican Church, and the interests of the landed aristocracy. Yet, both parties, despite dissent and corruption, followed policies designed to strengthen the country as a whole. Living conditions gradually improved.

### *The Glorious Revolution (1688)*

The formation of political parties gave the king an opportunity during his last years to increase his influence on the government and to secure the succession of his brother, James II. James, who was a

Catholic, showed more tolerance to Catholics, who had been barred from public office by the Test Act of 1673, and intolerance of Catholics continued undiminished in Parliament and in the community at large. James encouraged the return of absolutist trends. He also entered into close, economically undesirable political alliances with Spain, France, and other Catholic nations.

The English consoled themselves with the hope that, since the old king had no sons, these trends would constitute no more than a brief setback. However, the king ultimately did beget a son, and this gave rise to new fears about Catholic influence. In 1688, a revolt known as the "Glorious Revolution" began. James fled before blood was shed, however.

Mary, his Protestant daughter, and her husband, William of Orange, governor of the Netherlands, were invited by Parliament to take over the reins of government. Parliament reasoned that the Protestant cause and English international interests would be served by their rule. Holland would be brought into a firm alliance and could provide a bulwark against France. Yet, Parliament was careful to impose certain conditions to which the new rulers and their successors would have to submit. These were specified in the "Bill of Rights." Under these conditions, Parliament would decide all matters of taxation, control the army, and supervise legislation. Free elections were to be held regularly. A right of petition was to be guaranteed to all subjects. No excessive bail or excessive fines were to be imposed. No Catholic was to be ruler of England. By an Act of Toleration passed in 1689, Protestant dissenters gained the right to freely exercise their religion, although, like Catholics, they were still deprived of political rights and excluded from public service.

### Results of the Revolution

Absolutism was thus defeated in England, and Parliament emerged supreme. Parliament was not a democracy, however. Parliament suffered from traditional weaknesses, untrained representatives, and perpetual corruption. Furthermore, only men of wealth were eligible for membership, and the government continued to be controlled by the landholding aristocracy. These men were wise enough to consider the interests of the commercial classes so that business enterprises prospered.

Neither William (d. 1702) and Mary (d. 1694), nor their successor, Queen Anne (d. 1714), attempted to interfere with the functions of Parliament as set forth in the Bill of Rights. A union with Scotland, long desired by the English, was consummated in 1707. From then on, Scottish representatives sat in the same Parliament with Englishmen.

### English Foreign Policy

The direction of England's external affairs during the entire period from Cromwell through Queen Anne's reign depended upon the maneuvers of Louis XIV. Accordingly, England was forced alternately into alliances with Holland, France, and Spain. The constant instability in foreign policy was intensified by divergent interests within England. On one occasion, Charles II (d. 1685) himself accepted bribes from Louis XIV.

But underlying all the shifts of policy were three steadfast aims: eliminating competition in colonization; opposing Catholicism, and supporting the weaker powers on the Continent in order to counterbalance the stronger powers. These aims were largely achieved. With the help of a navy, which was greatly strengthened during Cromwell's time, the English eliminated the Dutch as serious colonial rivals and annexed their American colonies. England replaced Spain as the premier maritime power and seized Spain's territories abroad.

England encouraged opposition to any Catholic rulers who tried to spread their religion beyond their borders and welcomed refugees from Catholic countries. Alliances with small nations made it possible for the English to join in resisting Louis XIV until France was defeated and its bid for European hegemony was thwarted.

## Holland and Spain

The rise of England paralleled the decline of the two other great maritime powers: Holland and Spain. After fighting the English in three wars between 1652 and 1674, the Dutch lost their leading position in world affairs. Their merchant marine, which had been many times larger than England's, was severely compromised. The three factors that contributed most significantly to this decline were the continuous wars, the conservatism of Holland's wealthy ruling merchants, and the weakness of the central government, which resulted from political strife.

In opposition to the House of Orange, which favored a unified and centralized country, there was another party led by men like De Witt, which favored provincial independence. Holland remained among the leaders in finance, transportation, fishing, and agriculture—especially vegetable gardening and floriculture. It also maintained its prestige in scholarship, science, and the arts.

Spain, too, still excelled in literature and art, but its political and economic decline was very rapid. Poverty was widespread. The population of the third estate increased very slowly. The masses had no influence on the royal, absolutist regime, which was backed by a wasteful, ambitious, landed aristocracy. Wars, both in the colonial areas and on the Continent, continued to drain the treasury and resulted only in loss of territory in the New World, especially in the Caribbean, and in Europe along the Pyrenees.

## Austria

The other Hapsburg power, Austria, understood better than Spain how to adjust to changing conditions. In fact, the Austrian Hapsburgs recovered rather quickly from the consequences of the Thirty Years' War. What they lost through the lack of German unity they made up by increasing their personal holdings, their *Hausmacht*. Despite the westward shift of economic and commercial centers, Austria recovered a key position in European international affairs. It resumed expansionist policies.

In 1683, Austria's most dangerous enemy, the Ottoman Turks, regained their strength under the able leadership of the vizier Ahmed Kuprili, and once again reached the gates of Vienna. The Austrians, with the help of the Polish king, John III Sobieski, won a decisive victory. Subsequently, the Austrian armies under the command of Prince Eugene pushed deep into the Balkans. In the Peace of Karlowitz (1699), Austria regained long-occupied Hungary from the Ottoman Turks.

At home, the arts of the Baroque flourished. Vienna became a foremost cultural center, excelling in music, architecture, philosophy, and court poetry. There was a great religious revival. The Austrian population increased substantially.

## Brandenburg

Among the other German states, the most significant developments occurred in Brandenburg. This state, with Berlin as its capital, soon became Austria's rival for the leadership position in Germany. Several factors contributed to its rise. Its territory was greatly expanded after the Treaty of Westphalia. It was centrally located and had an industrious population. In the age of absolutism, it was fortunate enough to be governed by a succession of able rulers.

The most famous was Frederick William of the House of Hohenzollern, the so-called "Great Elector" (d. 1688), whose measures during his long regime made it possible for the country to recover from the devastations of war.

Mercantilist policies were pursued. Subsidies, tariffs, and monopolies were arranged in order to promote industries, such as glass-making and textiles. Land was reclaimed, and new agricultural products were sponsored. There were even some attempts at colonization. A decline in population was counteracted by the welcoming of immigrants. In particular, the Edict of Potsdam (1685) encouraged exiled French Huguenots to immigrate. They were generously endowed with land, houses, schools, churches, and the means to establish themselves successfully in agriculture and industry.

At the same time, a strong army was organized. There, the nobility, deprived of its old feudal privileges and prestige, found a new and special field of activity within the framework of the centralized state. The bureaucracy was inspired by concepts of duty and honesty. Wars were avoided as far as possible, and those that were unavoidable, such as wars against the Swedes, Poles, and Austrians, which were sometimes waged with the help of French subsidies, were essentially victorious. The success of the Great Elector's policies was made clear when, after his death, his successor, who inherited the Hohenzollern possessions on the Rhine and in Prussia in addition to Brandenburg, acquired the status of king.

## Eastern and Northern Europe

Eastern European developments followed patterns different from those of either the West or the North, except for one aspect: constant warfare.

### Poland

Poland's bid to subjugate Russia, attempted during the Times of Trouble in Russia, failed. Thereafter, the country became increasingly disorganized. Luxury-loving aristocrats and greedy, poorly educated nobles of lower status, the *slachta,* pursued private ambitions, nationalistic aims, and aggressive Catholic policies. Unwilling to subordinate their desires and aims to a strong monarchy, the nobility did not try to create a functioning parliament or *sejm*.

As a result, the state, which appeared strong, was undermined from within. Life in the towns, which had flourished in the 16th century, stagnated. The changes that should have been made to adapt to new conditions were neglected. This hindered the rise of a middle class as in Germany, France, or Italy. Consequently, the peasantry suffered, and the position of the many Jews in the country deteriorated. Enjoying certain tax privileges and allowed to govern their own communities, the Jews were both envied and disliked by their Polish neighbors and often maltreated.

Industrial production, which grew in neighboring countries, including Russia, did not advance. Agricultural activity was lively. Considerable income was derived from grain exports via Riga and especially Danzig, but the export trade remained mostly in the hands of German merchants and Dutch and English shippers.

Arrogance and ambition on the part of the upper classes, internal disorder, and lack of economic development brought external losses. The parts of Livonia which Poland-Lithuania had seized in the previous century were lost to the Swedes (1621). The eastern regions of the Ukraine fell to Russia in the Peace of Andrusovo (1667). The Cossacks—the freedom-loving, roaming inhabitants of the region who, although unreliable, had constituted a buffer against the Turks—were increasingly alienated. Through the "Union of Brest" (1595), the Poles had attempted to force the Cossacks to accept the Catholic Church and acknowledge the pope's authority. This would have given them nothing more than the right to retain some of the observances of their traditional Orthodox Church. As a result, part of the Ukraine joined with Russia. Ultimately, both Kiev and Smolensk were taken by Russia.

### Sweden

In contrast to Poland, Sweden experienced a *stormaktstid* (great power stage). Capable rulers, such as Gustavus II Adolphus, Charles X and Charles XI, and the great chancellor Axel Oxenstierna, understood how to ensure collaboration between Crown, nobles, and a diet in which other sectors of the population also participated. With the help of the resources of Finland, which formed part of the Swedish Empire, a strong economy was maintained. Timber, iron, and copper furnished valuable export goods. Shipping flourished thanks to Sweden's domination of the Livonian ports and Baltic Sea lanes. Despite Catholic counter-reformatory efforts, Lutheranism provided a strong bond between the peoples of the country. Schools were founded. Sweden's leading thinkers adopted the tenets of rationalism, notwithstanding the survival of myths and heathen beliefs among the peasant population. Descartes came to Sweden, sponsored by Queen Christina, the daughter of Gustavus Adolphus. He died there. The famous German jurist Pufendorf became a professor at the University of Lund.

However, the wars that Sweden waged against Denmark, Russia, Poland, and Germany exhausted the country, given its small population and limited resources. Successes could not be turned into permanent gains.

### *Russia*

Like most Continental nations, Sweden and Poland were heirs of the Renaissance. Russia traveled a different path. Few political and cultural concepts of the West were introduced there, despite the stream of English, Dutch, and German immigrants that began to arrive. They brought their ideas along with their skills. The immigrants' main effect was felt in the field of industry. They founded new industries, and they directed salt works, mines, glass factories, and more. A foreign, so-called German, suburb was founded in Moscow. This, and steadily increasing trade by way of Archangel over the free northern seaways, increased contact with the West. So, too, did the acquisition of Western territories that the Poles had previously annexed. However, it was chiefly in the 18th century that such contacts and acquisitions would become significant for the development of Russian civilization.

The gap that existed between Russia and the West in regard to social, legal, and political institutions was demonstrated by two important events. One was the introduction of a new code of law that was adopted in 1649. At the very time serfdom declined in the West, Russia introduced it. For more than a century, the Russian peasantry steadily lost their right to free movement. Now, the code of 1649 ensured their full attachment to the soil and confirmed the full rights of their landlords. Numerous revolts resulted. The climax was a large-scale revolution led by a peasant, Stenka Razin. The rebellion failed, however, and power remained in the hands of the absolute "autocratic" *tsar*. While reducing the influence of the old aristocracy, he strengthened the role of his own appointees as the backbone of his bureaucracy. These were largely petty nobles committed to service obligations. Their compensation consisted in landed estates or appointments to high administrative posts.

The other important event was the introduction of church reform. This bore little similarity to the Reformation in Western Europe and concerned mainly the elimination of errors that had, in the course of centuries, crept into the liturgical texts. Tsar Alexis I eventually supported the reformers, but thousands of believers refused to accept the changes to their hallowed traditions. They were outlawed and persecuted as schismatics ("Old Believers" or *Raskolniki*) who refused to recognize the creed of the official church, and thousands perished.

Thus, a split in the church occurred which was to last for centuries. The Old Believers held firm, even though the survivors of the persecutions were deprived of many of their civil rights. Not until the revolution in 1917 were they granted full citizenship rights. Unable to get administrative posts or land to work on, they turned, like other repressed minorities, to trading and other economic pursuits. They, thereby, contributed much to the growth of Russia as an economic power.

Still another development of major consequence marks Russian history during the 17th century: the extension of its territories. Borders were extended to China and the shores of the Pacific Ocean. Settlements were established in Siberia. Russia gained considerable wealth thanks to Siberia's richness in fur-bearing animals. These provided the country's most valuable export furs. In fact, the natives were required to provide the tax collectors with prescribed amounts of furs instead of money.

### **Colonies**

During the second half of the 17th century, European colonies overseas experienced changes that reflected the shift of power among the parent countries. Spain found itself exposed to continued hardships, especially in the Caribbean, because of incessant attacks by squadrons of English, Dutch, and

French fighters, pirates, and smugglers. In 1655, Jamaica, which was regarded as one of the most valuable assets of the Spanish Empire because of its sugar production, passed into the hands of England. Moreover, with all its wealth now part the English economy, Jamaica, like other conquered areas, became another outpost for English commercial and cultural penetration.

Similarly, Portuguese domination in the East weakened as the Dutch and other antagonists seized one territory after another. Other than a few ports in Asia and Africa, it was only in Brazil that Portugal, albeit with difficulty, succeeded in maintaining an important position. The resources of Brazil helped to compensate Portugal for many of the losses suffered in the East. Newly discovered diamond mines, combined with Brazilian gold and agricultural products, were sources of steady income. The Dutch, in turn, gained colonies in Asia and Africa, only to lose their holdings on the Hudson and Delaware Rivers in America. Last, all Europeans lost their rights and privileges in Japan when foreign traders were expelled. Japan permitted only a small, narrowly confined, and closely supervised group of Dutch to retain a tenuous foothold in the country.

Wherever changes in ownership occurred, corresponding changes in colonial life developed. These were especially pronounced in English North America. An ever-increasing stream of immigrants came to American shores. By 1732, all the original thirteen colonies of North America had been established. One of these was the prosperous Quaker colony of Pennsylvania, which devised a pattern of colonization based on their religious convictions and the democratic concepts of sharing, mutual helpfulness, and hard work.

The French in America could not match the English development of their colonies, although the mercantilistic mindset of officials such as Colbert sought to promote exploration and settlement. Most of the French people were very reluctant to leave their beautiful and prosperous homeland. Despite the potential wealth in furs, timber, spices, fish, and sugar, their colonies held little attraction for them.

The three large colonizing powers developed three different systems of colonial organization. The French set up few institutions and left it to the traders to win the cooperation of the native peoples and secure profits for the homeland. The Spanish settlers remained under close supervision by their home country. The English colonists were given a large measure of self-government.

During the Cromwellian revolution, the English colonists took advantage of the troubles at home to strengthen their position. During the Restoration and the revolution of 1688, they further expanded their liberties. Although the home country regained much of its lost authority when the revolutionary period was over, the attitude of the English colonists remained strongly independent and self-reliant. Their primary attachment was to the land on which they lived, and they felt far removed from the scene of the wars against Louis XIV into which they were drawn. The colonists referred to them as "King William's" or "Queen Anne's" wars, as if they were private undertakings of their rulers.

## ■THE CULTURAL SCENE

The great amount of attention paid by historians of the time to the political events of the later 17th century bears witness to the growing influence that political institutions, political thinking, social relationships, and national aspirations exercised in the life of modern peoples. In the Age of Louis XIV, the modern European state system was completed, and modern diplomacy was developed. Simultaneously, the tenets of the age found expression in many theoretical political writings.

### Political Thought

The protagonists of absolutism included the Frenchman Bossuet (d. 1704) and the Englishman Hobbes (d. 1679). These thinkers defended the prevailing concept of the divine right of kings, although they did not identify absolutism with arbitrary rule. Bossuet insisted that the royal will must be permeated with Christian doctrine. Hobbes, famous for his study of society and politics *(Leviathan,* 1651), thought that the royal will must be administered in accordance with the principles of a "natural" right to self-preservation. As Grotius had done, both demanded morality in international relations.

Their views were soon challenged by John Locke (d. 1704), who, in his *Treatises on Government* and *Letter on Toleration*, defended the idea that the relationship between ruler and subject is based upon a social order that binds both parties and not upon divine right. In this view, all subjects have a right to liberty and property and may justly revolt if their rights are violated.

## Philosophy

Locke, who was a man of affairs as well as a philosopher, derived his views from logic and observation, as his *Essay concerning Human Understanding* (1690) shows. Though he accepted the existence of God, he was an empiricist who relied on practical experience. Empiricist trends were the foundation for the work of most other philosophers of the age, notwithstanding Hobbes's criticism of Descarte's "mechanistic" approach and Pascal's attempts to harmonize Christian thought with that of his own age.

Besides Locke, other leading philosophers were the Dutchman Spinoza and the German Leibnitz. Spinoza (d. 1677), like Locke, defended the individual's right to political liberty. He is most famous for his "pantheism," which implied that everything is a part, an evidence, of the divine and that "God" works as a mathematical law permeating the universe. Leibnitz (d. 1716) emphasized mathematically ascertainable laws of nature. He relegated God to the position of an initial cause and saw the world filled with innumerable individual units of differing complexity, all independent of one another, following their own laws, yet in harmony with the world, the "best of all possible worlds," as made by God.

## Science

An age so devoted to logical thinking, mathematics, and experimentation necessarily produced remarkable scientific results. Numerous instruments (e.g., the telescope, microscope, air pump, and pendulum clock) were invented or improved. Statistical systems were devised. Technical methods in industry and mining were improved.

The Frenchman Pascal (d. 1662), inventor of the barometer, developed a mathematical theory of probability. The Englishman Boyle (d. 1691) laid the foundations for modern chemistry by investigating the pressure properties of gases. Another Englishman, Halley (d. 1742), observed and described the comets. The Dutchman Huyghens (d. 1695) investigated theories of light, and his countrymen Swammerdam (d. 1680) and Leeuwenhoek (d. 1723) studied microscopic organisms. Botanical works appeared in great numbers. In 1684, Leibnitz published his system of the calculus, a monumental achievement.

### *Newton*

The greatest scientist of the age, and one of the greatest of all time, was the Englishman Isaac Newton (d. 1727). This many-faceted genius, who was active in politics, independently devised a system of calculus (1687). Yet, he carried on so many studies in physics, optics, and astronomy that he laid the foundation for many areas of modern science. Occupying himself with the laws of mass and motion, he disclosed his greatest single discovery, the law of gravitation, in his great work *Principia Mathematica*, published in 1687. In all his work, Newton rejected transcendental speculation or hypothetical reasoning. He insisted that the prime goal of the scientist should be to describe accurately natural occurrences and their ascertainable causes.

### *Academy of Science*

A special place in the history of this age belongs to the Academy of Science. The first academy was founded in London in 1662. It was followed in 1666 by an academy in Paris and, later, by others in

Prussia, Austria, Russia, and elsewhere on the Continent. Their activities included philosophical discussions about nature and its laws, as well as the presentation of scientific papers on mathematical, biological, and physical problems. Many of the greatest minds of the age participated in their work and found in them the best forum for new ideas, testing them, and publicizing their conclusions. Men such as Leibnitz considered the academies so vital to the development of the intellectual forces of a nation that he championed the founding of an academy of science to the Russian emperor as the tsar's foremost task.

### Literature

From today's perspective, the advances in the sciences overshadow the late 17th-century accomplishments in literature and art. Yet, these achievements were by no means negligible. In France, creative writers included the celebrated dramatists Corneille *(Le Cid)* and Racine *(Britannicus, Athalie),* and the sharp, satirical critic of society, Moliere *(Bourgeois Gentilhomme, Tartuffe).* La Fontaine is famous for his *Fables.* At this time, the trend toward classical literary tradition reached its height. The tradition demanded adherence to normalized rules and conventions, to precepts of "good taste," and respect for the rational patterns of the day.

This trend also imparted certain sterility to some literature of the Age of Louis XIV that not only deterred later generations, but as early as 1680, brought about a "Battle of the Ancients and the Moderns." Against the normal demands of the "Ancients," there arose a cry for freedom of expression by the "Moderns." Nevertheless, throughout Europe the classical French literature of the 17th century, as represented by the "Ancients," had a decisive influence. Everywhere, it was imitated and praised as the perfection of taste and the model for values. Only in England did writers of genius build or preserve a different tradition. There, Milton (d. 1674; *Paradise Lost),* Bunyan (d.1688; *Pilgrim's Progress),* and Dryden (d. 1700; poems, satires) stand out. Germany contributed too. Grimmelshausen's *Simplicissimus* represents a lasting and potent literary contribution, but only the beginnings of a national literature emancipated from the French model can be traced.

### History

France made an important contribution in still another field. Mabillon (d. 1707), who undertook a methodological investigation of medieval documents, laid a foundation for systematic procedures and standards in history. The discipline of history thereby became an art and a science, and it has since served as a source of basic information concerning social conditions and human behavior, as well as a record of human fate and aspirations.

### Architecture

In the arts, the Baroque style dominated. It was superbly expressed in numerous palaces for which Versailles, elegant and grandiose in concept and clear in line, served as model. The buildings, fountains, statues, and specially designed shrubberies and flower beds, all geometrically arranged to satisfy the taste of the age, were imitated everywhere. The graceful Baroque style was well adapted to church construction, and some of its finest examples are found in southern Germany, Switzerland, and Austria.

In England, on the other hand, eminent architects continued resolutely in the classical, medieval, and Renaissance traditions. Christopher Wren designed St. Paul's Cathedral in London. The international influence of such architecture was slight. However, another side of the architectural arts in England made a real contribution to the stylistic concepts of all Western countries. This was the English garden. In contrast to the art of France, it emphasized naturalness. Lovely groups of trees or shrubbery, carefully and yet naturally arranged on wide lawns, appealed deeply to those who were unsatisfied with the formal ornamental style of the Age of Louis XIV.

## Painting

In painting, the French could pride themselves on the landscapes of Poussin (d. 1665) and Lorrain (d. 1682). A more lasting impression however, was left by artists in other nations. Catholic Spain contributed one great painter, Murillo (d. 1682), but it was the Protestant, secularly oriented Dutch painters who excelled—masters such as Frans Hals (d. 1666), Vermeer (d. 1675), and the landscape painter, Ruisdael (d. 1682). Their achievements may have been outstanding for any age, but these artists were overshadowed by the genius of Rembrandt (d. 1669). His luminous portraits and moving biblical scenes have a power, depth, and human significance equaling the best ever created.

## Perspective

*After the end of the Thirty Years' War, the persecution and expulsion of the Huguenots by the French, and the "Glorious Revolution" in England, religious issues ceased to dominate the political scene. Wealth, industry, banking, and shipping received ever-increasing attention. Peasant revolts and "cabinet wars" continued without bringing about major changes.*

*Spain and Portugal lost their prominent places; Sweden and, later, Brandenburg-Prussia emerged as major powers. The threat of Turkish invasions was put to an end. In the East, Poland was reduced in importance, while Russia emerged as a factor on the European political stage.*

*The principle of absolute monarchy was perfected everywhere except in England, where a parliamentary system took firm hold. In America, colonial rule persisted under Spanish and Portuguese viceroys and British governors. In steadily growing numbers, European immigrants entered the New World. A development took place that was to have grave consequences: black Africans were bought, sold, and sent as slaves into the British colonies.*

*In contrast to the misery that such trade brought and to the wretched situation of the lower classes, the court of Louis XIV and its imitators all over Europe indulged in luxury. Versailles set the example for style in building, dress, and manners. The age was also marked by works of fundamental importance, particularly in science, where logical, rational inquiry led to outstanding results.*

## Selected Readings

Beloff, Max. *The Age of Absolutism, 1660–1815* (New York: Harper, 1962).

Ashley, Maurice. *The Age of Absolutism, 1648–1775* (Springfield, Mass.: G. & C. Merriam Co., 1974).

Dukes, Paul. *The Making of Russian Absolutism 1613–1801* (London: Longman, 1990).

Okey, Robin. *The Habsburg Monarchy: From Enlightenment to Eclipse* (New York: St. Martin's Press, 2001).

Treasure, G. R. R. *Louis XIV* (New York: Longman, 2001).

Birn, Raymond. *Crisis, Absolutism, Revolution: Europe and the World, 1648-1789* (Orchard Park, New York: Broadview Press, 2005).

McKay, Derek, et al. *The Rise of the Great Powers, 1648–1815* (New York: Longman, 1983).

Slicher van Barth, B. H. *The Agrarian History of Western Europe* (New York: St. Martin's Press1983).

Trevelyan, George M. *England Under the Stuarts* (London: Metheun, 1930).

## Test Yourself

1. During the first 18 years of King Louis XIV's reign, the direction of French Affairs was entrusted to_____.
   A. Cardinal Wolsey
   B. Cardinal Mazerin
   C. Cardinal Richelieu
   D. Cardinal Colbert

2. Under Colbert, Louis XIV's capable minister, Marquette, Jolliet, and Robert de La Salle explored_____.
   A. The Ohio River Valley
   B. The Mississippi River region
   C. The Missouri River region
   D. None of the above

3. The English Revolution of 1688 was also known as _____.
   A. The Great Rebellion
   B. The Peaceful Revolution
   C. The Bloody Revolution
   D. The Glorious Revolution

4. The enormous castle of Versailles with its fabulous gardens was built during the reign of_____.
   A. Henry VIII
   B. Louis XIV
   C. Louis XVI
   D. James II

5. In 1699, Austria regained long-occupied Hungary from the Ottoman Turks after signing the _____.
   A. Peace of Augsburg
   B. Peace of Paris
   C. Peace of Karlowitz
   D. Peace of Vienna

6. The author of the work titled "Essay concerning Human Understanding" was_____.
   A. Descartes
   B. Spinoza
   C. Locke
   D. Hobbes

7. The Englishman Issac Newton is noted for his development of the Law of Gravity, but he was also pivotal in devising a system of _____.
   A. Calculus
   B. Geometry
   C. Algebra
   D. Theology

8. St Paul's Cathedral in London was designed by_____.
   A. James Rivers
   B. Isaac Newton
   C. Christopher Wren
   D. Jacques Cartier

## Answers and Explanations

1. **B.** During the first eighteen years of Louis XIV's reign, the direction of French affairs was entrusted to Cardinal Mazarin. It was Mazarin, a shrewd diplomat, who concluded the Peace of Westphalia, whereby France was raised to preeminence in Europe. It was also Mazarin who sealed the fate of the French nobility. Seeking to profit from the financial straits in which the young king found himself, the nobility staged, in 1648, a rebellion, the so-called "Fronde."

2. **B.** Colbert promoted colonizing activities during his period as minister. In his time, Marquette, Joliet, and La Salle explored the Mississippi region, resulting in the development of a substantial fur trade.

3. **D.** James II, who was a Catholic, showed greater tolerance to Catholics. They had been barred from public office by the Test Act of 1673. Intolerance toward Catholics remained undiminished in Parliament and in the community at large. James encouraged the return of absolutist trends. He also entered into close, economically undesirable political alliances with Spain, France, and other Catholic nations. The English consoled themselves with the hope that, since the old king had no sons, these trends would constitute no more than a brief setback. However, the king ultimately did beget a son, giving rise to new fears about Catholic influence. In 1688, a revolt, known as the "Glorious Revolution," began. Before blood was shed, James fled.

4. **B.** The arts and sciences found in Louis XIV a liberal and understanding patron, as long as they glorified him. Architectural projects, in particular, were greatly encouraged by Louis, although at excessive cost to the country. One prime example is the enormous castle of Versailles and its famous gardens, which was built during his reign.

5. **C.** In 1683, the Austrians' most dangerous enemy, the Ottoman Turks, who had regained their strength under the able leadership of the vizier Ahmed Kuprili, once more reached the gates of Vienna. The Austrians, with the help of the Polish king, John III Sobieski, won a decisive victory. Subsequently, the Austrian armies under the command of Prince Eugene pushed deep into the Balkans. In the Peace of Karlowitz (1699), Austria regained long-occupied Hungary from the Ottoman Turks.

6. **C.** Locke, who was a man of affairs as well as a philosopher, derived his views from logic and observation, as his *Essay concerning Human Understanding* (1690) shows. Though he accepted the existence of God, he was an empiricist who relied on practical experience.

7. **A.** The greatest scientist of the age, and one of the greatest of all time, was the Englishman Isaac Newton (d. 1727). This many-faceted genius, who was active in politics, independently devised a system of calculus (1687). Yet, he was involved with so many studies in physics, optics, and astronomy that he laid the foundation for many areas of modern science. Occupying himself with the laws of mass and motion, he disclosed his greatest single discovery, the law of gravitation, in his great work *Principia Mathematica,* which was published in 1687.

8. **C.** In England, eminent architects continued resolutely in the classical, medieval, and Renaissance traditions. Christopher Wren designed St. Paul's Cathedral in London.

# CHAPTER 9
# The Age of Enlightenment (1715-1774)

**1719** Defoe, *Robinson Crusoe*
**1720** "South Sea Bubble" in England
John Law in Paris
**1721** Peace of Nystad
Montesquieu, *Lettres Persanes (Persian Letters)*
**1729** Bach, *St. Matthew Passion*
**1733** Beginning of War of the Polish Succession
**1735** Linnaeus, *Systema Natura*
**1738** Invention of flying shuttle by Kay
**1739** Hume, *Treatise of Human Nature*
**1740** Maria Theresa becomes empress (Pragmatic Sanction)
Outbreak of First Silesian War (Frederick the Great)
**1741** Dupleix French governor general in India
Handel, *The Messiah*
**1742** Thermometer of Celsius
**1744** Second Silesian War
**1745** Louisbourg conquered by British
**1748** Peace of Aix-la-Chapelle
Montesquieu, *L'Esprit des Lois (Spirit of Laws)*
**1748** Bach, *Art of the Fugue*
**1752** Franklin's experiments on lightning and electricity
**1754** Beginning of French and Indian War
**1755** Lisbon earthquake
**1756** Outbreak of Seven Years' War
**1758** Quesnay, *Tableau economique*
**1759** Conquest of Quebec
Voltaire, Candide
**1760** Battle of Wandiwash
**1762** Rousseau, *Contrat Social (Social Contract)*
Gluck, *Orfeo*

**1763** End of Seven Years' War, Peace of Paris
**1765** Stamp Act for American colonies
**1768** Watt's steam engine
**1770** Cook returns from trip around world
**1771** Arkwright's spinning mill in England
**1772** First partition of Poland
**1773** Reorganization of English administration in India
Beginning of Pugachev Revolt in Russia
**1774** Turgot becomes controller-general
Goethe, *Sorrows of Young Werther*

*The 18th century is known as the "Age of Enlightenment." To a degree, the Age of Enlightenment was a conscious reaction to the artificiality of the times of Louis XIV, but in essence, it continued the trends of that period. It spread the light of reason among more widely and issued calls for action on the basis of rational thought. It emphasized science over religion, thought over faith, doubt over traditional authority.*

*Thinkers in the Age of Enlightenment believed that if scientific investigation were applied not only to inanimate nature, but to all aspects of human life, natural laws could be discovered which, like Newton's law of gravitation, would explain human actions. Human actions could then be so directed as to bring continuous progress to nations. Thus, attention was focused upon investigations of phenomena in the natural sciences, as well as investigations of social conditions, politics, and ethics.*

## ■ POLITICAL ENLIGHTENMENT

The practical application of enlightened theories in the political and economic life of Europe was promoted by the appearance of "enlightened monarchs" or "enlightened despots." As the term "despot" indicates, the concept of the "divine right of kings" or of "absolute monarchy" was retained. Enlightened monarchs were, indeed, far from accepting ideas, such as those of Locke concerning the natural rights of the governed in relation to their rulers, but they did show an affinity with the enlightened thought of their age. They did not claim that they and their states were one and the same, which is what Louis XIV expressed in his arrogant statement, "*L'Etat, c'est moi*," which implied that the welfare of the individual would be sacrificed to the glory of the king. Instead, they accepted ideals of tolerance, humanitarianism, equal justice, and other ideals that the Age of Reason brought. Frederick the Great's enlightened dictum, "I am the first servant of the state," reflected the new thinking about the proper role and function of a ruler.

### The National Scene

With the exception of England, whose parliamentary system, despite its many weaknesses, did not necessitate paternalistic guidance by a monarch; Poland, which was in the throes of anarchy; and France, which remained too much under the spell of Louis XIV, almost all European countries had their "enlightened" rulers. In Prussia, there was Frederick the Great, while Austria had Joseph II. Spain was ruled by Charles III, and in Sweden, Gustavus III was king. Russia had Catherine the Great. Denmark, Portugal, and Spain had ministers such as Struensee, Pombal, and Aranda, respectively. Frederick the Great of Prussia was the most representative example of enlightened despotism.

### Prussia

Prussia developed rapidly in the 18th century. In the time of Frederick's father, the efficiency of the government and the army had been greatly improved. Under this deeply religious, despotic, and extremely parsimonious ruler, the administration of the government had an honesty that was rare in the

18th-century. Serfdom was reduced. The judicial system was improved. Prussia's rank in Europe was firmly established.

### *External Policies*

When Frederick II, "the Great" (d. 1786), came to the throne in 1740, he inherited an extremely efficient governmental machinery. Making prompt use of his excellent army in three Silesian Wars, Frederick succeeded in doubling his realms, enlarging his economic resources, and raising Prussia to the status of a first-class power.

Frederick II, the son of Frederick William I, was born in Berlin. His childhood was spent in rigorous military training and education. As an adult, he studied music and French literature. As king, he guided the growth of the provincial kingdom he inherited to its place at the head of the German nations.

### *Internal Policies*

His fame, however, rests not only on his generalship in war, but also on his enlightened rule during 36 years of peace. While he, himself, was an irreligious man, he became a model of religious tolerance. Jesuits, Jews, and Protestants alike found refuge in his lands. Justice was dealt out speedily, humanely, and with great efforts at impartiality. Often, the poor were favored. Promotion for ability was common, although Frederick reserved the top posts in the army for the aristocracy and retained many class distinctions as well. Agriculture was the king's chief concern. Immigrants were welcomed, wastelands recovered, and modern technical improvements introduced. Serfdom was practiced only in its mildest form. Housing was provided for workers. The cultivation of new crops, including the potato, was encouraged, and the king supervised these matters personally. He also resettled the veterans of war, to whom he distributed land, seed, and horses.

### *Economic Policies*

In his policy toward industry, Frederick was essentially a mercantilist. He passed measures to stimulate production and trade and subsidized both the silk industry and the new porcelain industry. He founded a state bank and stabilized prices through state purchases in times of plenty and sales in times of distress. He developed mines in newly conquered Silesia. He prohibited the importation of luxury goods (e.g., tobacco and coffee) because payments for them would diminish his bullion.

## Austria

In Austria, Joseph II (d. 1790) was Frederick's great admirer and imitator. Austria was on the road to a steep decline. Prussia challenged Austria's leading position in Germany, and the Hapsburg princes proved incapable of modernizing their multinational state. They were chiefly interested in the preservation of their *Hausmacht*. Austria could no longer maintain its standing. Joseph's mother, Empress Maria Theresa, who was a kind and conscientious ruler, had pursued an overly conservative policy.

When he came to power, Joseph introduced new, enlightened policies. However, he pushed his reforms forward at such a pace that the disturbances, revolts, and setbacks he caused were equal to the progress he made. Yet, Joseph did make improvements in administration and education. He introduced civil marriage, abolished serfdom, and encouraged toleration and equality for all, including Jews.

## Russia

The remarkable improvements that enlightened despotism brought to many nations should not blind us as to its inherent weakness, however. As its very nature required the continued use of arbitrary and absolute rule, its advantages were dependent upon whether or not the government was in the hands of a conscientious and progressive monarch. If such a monarch were followed by a less progressive successor, society could suffer. This aspect of enlightened despotism was demonstrated by events in Russia.

### Peter the Great

Enlightenment came to Russia in the early 18th century, largely because of the personal influence of Peter I, "the Great" (d. 1725). Peter was a man of inexhaustible energy. He personally and conscientiously attended to innumerable duties and supervised an incredible amount of detail. He reformed the administration, removed clerical influences from state affairs, built a civil service based on ability, and reduced class discrimination in the courts. He improved the economy of his state by adhering to the principles of mercantilism. In his time, the production of iron in Russia surpassed that of England. He reformed the army and expanded the national domain through successful wars.

Peter gave special attention to the Westernization of his country—a trend that had begun under his father, Alexis. He sought to improve educational standards and to introduce the teaching of foreign languages. He founded an academy of sciences. He obtained teachers from foreign lands, especially Germany, and brought technicians from Holland, and traders from England. He sponsored explorations in Siberia and in the Pacific and Bering Sea regions.

Peter tried to transform the manners, appearance, and clothing of his countrymen in imitation of Western models. He founded St. Petersburg to provide a permanent link with the West in 1703. Some of Peter's successors sought to eliminate the political and intellectual guidance of foreigners, however, and almost destroyed Peter's legacy. Only when Catherine II, "the Great" (d. 1796), came to the throne were enlightened policies renewed.

### Catherine the Great

This German princess led a dissipated life, but she excelled in intelligence, devotion to duty, administrative ability, and artistic and literary taste. Under Catherine's direction, the influence of France instead of Germany was strengthened. Plans for enlightened legislation were developed. Hospitals were improved, and she introduced the prophylactic measure of inoculation to Russia.

However, the two fundamental weaknesses in the Russian system, autocracy and serfdom, prevented the development of a healthy peasant class, progressive industry, or a strong middle class. Many peasant

*Figure 9–1 Peter the Great, 1672–1725*

revolts occurred, including the protracted and dangerous rebellion of Pugachev. Toward the end of the century, the nation faced greater social problems than at the beginning, in spite of its territorial expansion, improved education, and increased production.

## Poland

The rapid progress of Russia brought an end to the political prestige enjoyed by its smaller neighbors. In particular, Russian progress brought about the collapse of Poland. The collapse was hastened by the deplorable situation within the country—anarchical conditions, the arrogance and luxury of a small upper class, and the miserable status of the masses. Disunity in the aristocratic hierarchy made it impossible for any individual or group to govern efficiently. This situation invited foreign interference and soon proved detrimental to Polish interests.

Moreover, an arbitrary policy in favor of Catholicism alienated the Orthodox and Protestant sectors. The policy was doubly dangerous because the majority of Poland's inhabitants were not Polish, but Lithuanian, German, or Russian. In 1772, these conditions created a division of the country among the nations of Russia, Prussia, and Austria, the so-called "first partition," which restored most of the non-Polish territories to the neighbors from whom they had been alienated.

## Sweden

Sweden narrowly escaped the same fate. Its period of greatness under Gustavus Adolphus had been short. Not long after the death of Gustavus Adolphus, Brandenburg began to regain some of the annexed German lands. By 1721, Sweden's Livonian possessions had all been lost to Russia. The rest of its German territories had been relinquished to the German states.

With their territory thus reduced, the Swedes prudently took the necessary steps of adjustment. Absolutism was followed by enlightened despotism. Industry and trade prospered. The condition of the peasants—serfdom had never been widely practiced—improved substantially with the end of Poland's military adventures. A measure of popular representation by means of a national diet helped to stabilize the government on a sound basis.

## Spain and Portugal

Enlightened despotism brought revival even to Spain and Portugal. Through numerous wars, Spain lost much of its territory in the Pyrenees region and in the colonies, as well as much of its population. Still, Spain gradually regained strength. Its recovery began in 1713, when the succession to the throne was settled. England had gained a stake in Spain's lucrative slave trade, but Spain adjusted itself to the new conditions. Trade restrictions were relaxed, and new industries were established. The schools and the army were modernized. The downward trend of population was reversed.

Under Charles III (d. 1788) and his minister, Aranda, the government functioned more efficiently. It reduced taxes to encourage private enterprise. In line with the trend toward a more centralized administration, it abolished the internal customs barriers that had obstructed trade. In the colonies, the regime gave up the system of *encomienda*. It appointed able administrative officers and restructured the gradually expanding territory into appropriate administrative units. The pervasive influence of the Jesuits in state affairs was eliminated. Simultaneously, neighboring Portugal carried out similar reforms, both in Portugal and in Brazil.

## France

Unlike other European countries, France, which was the home of enlightened philosophy, did not adopt progressive ideas in its own political system. Whether under the dissipated, but capable and intelligent regent, the Duke of Orleans (d. 1723), or under lazy, luxury-loving Louis XV (d. 1774), France retained the outmoded institutions of the previous century. Only in religious affairs was a more liberal policy instituted. The nobility retained its economic advantages. The administrative service and tax system were left unaltered. Colonization was but halfheartedly supported. The wasteful court continued to drain the treasury.

A crushing debt had accumulated as a result of Louis XIV's ambitions and extravagance, and the Scottish financier, John Law, attempted to reestablish French credit in 1720. He organized a state bank, stabilized the currency, and took over tax collection. Law founded the Mississippi Company, a large colonial enterprise, but his fundamentally sound efforts to expand production and trade were misdirected because of his personal ambitions. His efforts led to mad speculation and economic collapse. French credit fell to a new low. Under the circumstances, the peaceful policies of two able ministers, Dubois and Fleury, could not forestall the rapid political deterioration of the French administrative apparatus, nor could the essential prosperity of individual merchants and peasants and the natural wealth of the most populous and productive country in Europe at the time prevent the decline of French power.

## England

The evolution of the English government in the 18th century followed neither the pattern of French absolutism nor that of enlightened despotism. England's past political experiences, its social conditions, its technological and industrial advances, and its overseas commitments favored neither such path. Instead, Parliament extended the scope of its political leadership. During the early 18th century, the Stuarts failed in their attempts to regain the throne, which, after the death of Queen Anne, was handed over to Germans from Hanover.

The first two Hanoverian kings were chiefly concerned with their Continental possessions, and they paid scant attention to English affairs. Consequently, Parliament was able to exercise its powers without hindrance. A financial storm arose because of speculation and the collapse of the South Sea Company, an enterprise similar to what John Law had done in France, but it was weathered without undermining the credit of the country. Commerce flourished after the wars of the 17th century eliminated Dutch competition, and with successes in international diplomacy, the authority of parliamentary government increased. A strong national bank, sound monetary policy, and an adequate and broadly based system of taxation—which, unlike the French system, did not exempt the nobility—supported a healthy treasury.

### Parliament and Parties

Peace was maintained under the cautious and efficient administration of Sir Robert Walpole (d. 1745). Through Walpole's influence, enduring precedents for the conduct of government were established. As a "prime minister," the first in English history, Walpole surrounded himself with advisers who could count upon the support of their parties—Whig or Tory—in Parliament. He thus secured the backing of Parliament, especially of the House of Commons, to which, in a sense, he then became responsible. The advisers themselves became the king's ministers. The group, the "cabinet," became the executive organ of the state. Bribery, dishonesty, and a tendency to cater to the interests of minorities and favored individuals may have continued, and Parliament, whose members represented only a small fraction of the population—mainly the privileged, wealthy landowning group—may not have represented the nation at large, but the basic interests of the nation as a whole were safeguarded.

### Reign of George III

The effective functioning of these developing institutions was undermined when the third Hanoverian, George III (d. 1820), came to the throne in 1760. Opposed to the Whigs who had been in power for decades, George III chose his ministers not according to party affiliation, but according to his personal preference. He held them accountable to himself alone. However, his policies—often opposed by men like the elder Pitt (d. 1778)—were not successful. During George's reign, England lost its 13 colonies in North America.

Internal affairs unfolded differently than he expected. In spite of his attempts to increase his royal prerogatives and in spite of the widespread corruption, the parliamentary system continued to develop. In the economic sphere, mercantilist views were increasingly replaced by laissez-faire theories. With the introduction of steam power, industrialism and modern capitalism established the pattern for future production methods and for relations between government and business.

## ■ THE INTERNATIONAL SCENE

The direction that the internal developments in the individual national states had taken in the second half of the 17th century, as well as the path on which they proceeded during the following fifty years, required new international relationships. By 1700, a system of government had gradually and naturally developed, and it became the conscious property of European diplomats. It even provided a basis for a theory of international relations by appealing to the rational attitude of the age and to its sense of order. This theory is known as the "balance of power." On the Continent such a balance was not really new. It constituted a normal aim within the European community, and it had existed within many earlier state systems, including that of 16th-century Italy. At the beginning of the 18th century, however, it gained in importance because the danger represented by the French hegemony under Louis XIV had again focused attention upon the problem. The "balance of power" meant that no single power or group of powers should be permitted to develop enough strength to dominate the others.

The policy of upholding this balance served Britain well. Since Britain stayed outside the system, it could use the policy to prevent the emergence of any overwhelmingly strong European competitor. Whenever the balance was upset, Britain would throw its weight to the weaker side, and by assuming the role of protector of the weak, it would try to reestablish the balance.

The advantage of the system was that the independence of the various states, especially the smaller ones, could thereby be safeguarded. The disadvantage was that it hampered European cooperation and led to incessant wars, which arose because changes in the balance of power were unavoidable under the pressure of economic developments and the emergence of strong-minded personalities in positions of authority.

### International Objectives

Within the framework of the balance of power, many old and long-standing trends in European policies persisted. France's objectives were to expand to the Rhine and to prevent a renewed collaboration of the German Empire and Spain as had existed when both were under Hapsburg rule. England's policy was to keep European attention focused on European problems, rather than on overseas acquisitions, and to prevent the conquest of the coast of the English Channel by any strong power. Hapsburg Austria's aspirations were to increase the *Hausmacht* and retain ascendancy over the Turks. Spain's ambitions were to preserve its Italian possessions and keep its overseas trade routes open. Prussia's goals were to reduce Hapsburg influence in the German Empire and secure the territories separating its outlying possessions on the Rhine and in East Prussia from Brandenburg at its center. Finally, Russia maintained an expansionist zeal, and wanted to gain access to the Baltic and Black seas.

### Balance of Power and the European States

These aims and aspirations led to numerous entanglements. Within the concept of "balance of power," they usually defied resolution except by resorting to war. Diplomacy, despite the assumed rationality of human beings, failed.

However, the wars were largely "cabinet wars," fought with small armies in restricted areas. They aroused little passion and affected the general populations of the countries involved much less than earlier religious wars or the later extensive national wars. The destructive power of weapons was limited. National and religious hatreds were absent. As if by convention, mutual respect and consideration among the warring yet interdependent princes prevented excesses in the conduct of war or the annihilation of states in the making of peace.

### The Great Northern War (1700-1721)

Before Louis XIV's last war (the War of the Spanish Succession) had begun, another war broke out: the Great Northern War between Russia and Sweden. After some brilliant initial victories, the Swedish king, Charles XII, who is considered one of history's great military geniuses, was decisively beaten at Poltava (1709). However, it took the Russians another 12 years to evict the Swedes from all of Livonia, to secure in the Peace of Nystad (1721) the long-coveted harbors on the Baltic Sea. This achievement so enhanced the prestige of Russia that, henceforth, all the European nations had to take Russia's views into consideration when creating diplomatic initiatives.

### War of the Polish Succession (1733-1735)

A new war broke out in 1733. Dubois and Fleury tried to keep France from getting involved while it was trying to recover from the wars of Louis XIV. Nevertheless, the minor question of the succession to the Polish throne brought France into the new entanglement, and Hapsburg and Bourbon vied with each other for control of the succession. The war ended with the failure of the Bourbons to secure the throne for their candidate.

### War of the Austrian Succession (1740-1748)

The Hapsburg success was short-lived, however. Soon, Austria found itself threatened from another side. Upon the accession of Maria Theresa to the imperial throne—her father had sacrificed numerous Hapsburg interests to secure her right of succession—a series of other wars broke out. On one hand, Prussia attacked Austria. Ignoring Prussia's promise to respect a "Pragmatic Sanction," by which most European powers had consented to Maria Theresa's succession, Frederick II of Prussia invaded and conquered Silesia (1741). On the other hand, France, which also went against Austria, became involved in a new war with England.

This seemed to offer an opportunity for Maria Theresa to try to recover Silesia, but in 1745, her armies were again defeated by Frederick. France, her other enemy, was defeated by England. Not until 1748 was peace restored (Peace of Aix-la-Chapelle). This prepared the ground for a revolution in the balance-of-power system. Both France and Austria, traditional rivals, were so weakened that neither had to fear the hegemony of the other. They, therefore, settled their age-old differences, came to an understanding, and allied themselves against the victors, Prussia and England.

### Seven Years' War (1756-1763)

Consequently, in 1756, a new war broke out, the Seven Years' War. This took on global dimensions. Russia joined the Franco-Austrian alliance against Prussia, while outside of Europe, Spain became involved in the conflict against England. Thus wars were fought on three continents—Europe, Asia, and America.

In Europe, the war centered again on Prussia's struggle for the possession of Silesia. Despite a series of brilliant victories, Frederick soon found himself in grave difficulties. Only the death of Russia's empress, Elizabeth, solved his predicament. Elizabeth's successor, Peter III, was an admirer of Frederick,

*Figure 9–2  The Seven Years' War, 1756–1763*

and he withdrew the Russian armies. France and Austria were compelled to make peace on the basis of the status quo, and Frederick kept Silesia.

In Asia and in America, where the war became known as the "French and Indian War," England, which contributed little but money to the European phase, gained the upper hand. The peace, which was concluded at Paris in 1763, cost France a large part of her overseas possessions.

### Russo-Turkish War (1768-1774)

Once the Seven Years' War was over, Russia turned its attention to the Black Sea region, which Peter the Great had tried to dominate. Russia defeated the Ottoman Turks and finally gained access to the Black Sea (1774). Having achieved this long-coveted aim, Russia began to push on relentlessly, seeking to secure the entire Black Sea coast. Russia's aim was to eliminate Turkish influence in Europe and the Turkish domination of the Bosporus and the Dardanelles. It also wanted to gain direct and free access to the Mediterranean.

## Balance of Power and Overseas Expansion

Despite changing alignments among the European nations, the long series of wars that mark the 18th century brought shifts in the balance of power. The wars were fought to preserve existing power relationships rather than to upset them. They increased the international prestige of Prussia and Russia without putting either of them in a position to attain continental hegemony.

Overseas, however, no balance of power was preserved. On the contrary, in all the wars that paralleled the European conflicts and were fought in colonial areas—in particular, the War of Jenkins's Ear (1739–1741), King George's War (1743-48), and the French and Indian War (1754–1763)—Britain expanded its power and empire at the cost of France and Spain, particularly in both the East and the West (East India and America), where Britain gained predominance.

### East India

At the time, East India seemed to be the most important colonial holding. It appeared that France would be able to secure this prize because, beginning with its settlement at Pondichery, France had vigorously expanded its Indian possessions in mid-century. A competent agent, Dupleix, knew how to gain the good will of important local princes. In 1746, he annexed the large trading town of Madras. When, owing to French weakness at home, the town had to be ceded back to England (by the terms of the Peace of Aix-la-Chapelle in 1748), Dupleix concentrated on other areas and won domination over most of southern India.

However, the English were determined to drive the French out. In Robert Clive, England found a leader equal in ability to Dupleix. Like the Frenchman, Clive sought the support of native princes. He impressed them as a man of action when he avenged the capture of Calcutta by a native prince. He wooed their services through generous gifts, and then he turned against the French.

Unfortunately for France, Dupleix, accused of dishonesty, had been recalled in 1754. His able successor, Lally Tollendal, obtained no help from the home government. Consequently, the British, who dominated the sea lanes and were willing to invest the necessary funds, defeated the French in the decisive Battle of Wandiwash (1760). Tollendal was recalled and put to death by an ungrateful government. Peace was concluded in Paris in 1763. Notwithstanding all the efforts and sacrifices of the French agents, and notwithstanding the economic importance of the colony, France had to surrender most of its holdings in India to the British.

Promptly, the British set about reorganizing the administration of their colony and exploiting its wealth. After recalling Clive without rewarding him for his services in the struggle against France, they deprived the East India Company of its control over the country. They subjected the government to strict supervision from London. Warren Hastings was sent to India as governor in 1773. With his regime, a new chapter in Anglo-Indian history began.

### North America

At the Peace of Paris in 1763, France lost not only India, but also most of its North American holdings. In the course of the 18th century, the French had tried to turn the colonial empire, which mercantilist theory and thirst for glory had driven them to acquire, into a possession that would yield practical returns. Their colonies in Canada, the Mississippi Valley, and the Caribbean islands showed considerable promise. Trading in commodities, such as sugar, timber, fish, and furs, and slaves, to and from the homeland and among the colonies increased.

However, competition with Britain and the pressure of British colonists in North America hindered peaceful progress among the thinly settled French dominions. As in India, the British home government backed the commercial interests, "the flag following the trade." In 1745, the colonists in America attacked and conquered the French fortress of Louisbourg. The terms of the Peace of Aix-la-Chapelle required the British to return the fort to France, but ill feeling between the British colonists and their French neighbors led to continual, localized encounters, especially in Acadia (Nova Scotia) and in the Ohio Valley.

By 1754, these local conflicts had developed into a general war. Britain sent expeditionary forces to America, but these forces, as well as the American colonists themselves, were defeated. The resulting danger to the colonies brought more concentrated efforts, especially when the energetic and able William

*Figure 9–3  The Seven Years' War in North America*

Pitt assumed the direction of affairs in England. Naval forces were sent to America and destroyed the French fleet. On land, British troops conquered Quebec and Montreal in 1759 and 1760, respectively.

Disaster now threatened the French. Belated Spanish intervention on the French side failed to reestablish a balance of power against England. Unable to continue the war, France and Spain had to submit to British demands. In the Peace of Paris, Spain gave up Florida. The French, choosing to retain the commercially profitable islands in the West Indies, ceded Canada and the Mississippi region.

## The Thirteen Colonies

At the time of the Peace of Paris, the British people could hardly foresee that the most valuable part of their American possessions would be lost, at least politically, within little more than a dozen years. During the Seven Years' War (the French and Indian War), the colonists had cooperated, if reluctantly, with the home country. Whether the colonists had originally come from England, Scotland, and Ireland or from Switzerland, Germany, and Holland, and whether they had emigrated for political, economic, or religious reasons, they were generally animated by a thirst for liberty.

They had moved to a new land not only for material gain, but also for independence and for freedom from compulsion. They objected to all exploitation of their land by the home country, and they objected to British mercantilist tactics. Moreover, they pressed steadily westward from the seaboard and were angered at the interference of European issues and diplomacy with their own expansionist objectives. They had already secured a large measure of self-government, a prosperous economic condition, and, as leaders like Benjamin Franklin demonstrated, a considerable amount of intellectual stature. In turn, they were unwilling to take upon themselves the burdens that the British, who had incurred large expenditures in the wars against France, tried to impose upon them without their consent.

Furthermore, they denounced a Stamp Act (1765), which Parliament devised as a source of revenue from the colonies. They forced its repeal in the following year, but Parliament, insisting upon its right to tax the colonies for revenue, imposed other burdens. The Declaratory Act, Townshend Act, Quebec Act, and so-called "Intolerable" Acts succeeded one another quickly, and provided either for new taxes, customs duties, or fines. The situation was further aggravated because these impositions coincided with the absolutist tendencies of George III.

A violent propaganda campaign began, supported by leaders brought up in the spirit of enlightenment. One of these was Thomas Paine, who demanded a radical break with Britain. The discontented colonists finally assembled a Continental Congress, which at first prescribed a boycott of British goods. Later, in 1775, it raised an army. This was followed, in July 1776, by the assembling of representatives from the various colonies, who took the decisive step and declared the independence of the American colonies from Britain.

## ■ CULTURAL ENLIGHTENMENT

No matter how important the changes were that occurred on the political scene of England and the enlightened countries of the Continent, the social and intellectual pattern of the West was even more deeply affected by the economic evolution of the 18th century. Mercantilist practices were modified as the modern capitalistic system, which was based on new production methods, got under way. Agriculture and industry adapted to the new technical knowledge and scientific spirit.

### Industry, Trade, and Society

The changes were less noticeable in central and Eastern Europe, which lacked colonial possessions and had only limited access to raw materials and markets. In the Western countries, however, the changes were very evident. Private enterprises benefited from colonial supplies, technical advances and—especially in England—political conditions.

### *Trade and Industry*

Everywhere, the coal and iron industries expanded. Serfdom, which had limited the industrial labor supply, steadily weakened or disappeared. Forced labor obligations were transformed into monetary obligations. This shift allowed greater mobility for the peasants and a broader labor market for the entrepreneur. An educated bourgeoisie aimed for higher material living standards and became increasingly influential.

The Western countries steadily enhanced their trade relations with America, the Near East, and India. In order to maintain this prospering trade, they promoted domestic industries and were quick to introduce technical improvements. Spinning and weaving machines, invented by Hargreaves, Arkwright, and Whitney, were brought into use. Large organizations developed and introduced well-planned methods of production and distribution.

### *Society*

The costs for the introduction of labor-saving industries had to be borne by the free artisans and workers who lost their jobs and independence. As Hogarth's pictures from England show, they lived in hopeless misery. The burden was also carried by the inhabitants of the overseas possessions of the Western countries. Thus, England, besides exploiting the resources of India, sought to derive the greatest possible profit from its 13 colonies in North America and from its Caribbean possessions. Its exports included Eastern products, iron, and finished goods; its imports from the Caribbean—in a triangular trade

*Figure 9–4 The Industrial Revolution in Europe.*

(Liverpool-Boston-Havana)—sugar, molasses, and rum. Britain also monopolized the slave trade to the New World and derived a large income from this source.

## Population

The industrial products created in Europe and the resources derived from the colonies contributed to the food supply, and, thereby, to population growth. Advances in medicine added to this trend. Microbes were discovered. The people benefited from a better understanding of physiology and from some of the initial improvements made in gynecology. Principles of hygiene were published and applied. Early in the century, families were very large, often with ten to twenty children, but the majority of these children died in infancy. Families were smaller in the second half of the century, but more of the children survived.

On the Continent, women began to play a larger role in the world outside the household. Advanced education was made available to greater numbers of women. They organized *salons* where the ideas of the day were discussed, and they participated in important and learned gatherings. Women did not yet excel in creating major works in art, philosophy, literature, or science, however.

### Economic and Legal Thought: Humanitarianism

In line with these changing economic conditions and the philosophical views that emphasized natural laws, the existing social organization was challenged. Economic thinking changed. Mercantilism, with its many regulations, appeared to interfere with the free play of "natural" forces. The freedom of the individual to pursue the activities for which he or she felt best suited was advocated as the basis of prosperity. Some economists, like the "physiocrats," led by Quesnay (d. 1774) in France, held that it was not money or bullion that constituted wealth, but rather a country's total national product. This, in turn, was said to result from exploiting the resources of soil and subsoil and the labor invested in producing goods. Others applied the theory of freedom to a broader arena, focusing on trade and industry. They advocated the adoption of the doctrine of *laissez-faire*, believing that noninterference in the free and natural play of economic forces would work to the benefit of the nation. The most famous advocate of *laissez-faire* was Adam Smith (d. 1790). Smith's 1776 groundwork study, *The Wealth of Nations,* established the foundation for the field of modern economics.

Underlying the thought of these economists was the twofold goal of finding natural laws and contributing to the progress, the "happiness," of the human race. With this aim in view, the economists exercised a profound influence on law. Quesnay, for instance, advocated that governments confine themselves to restraining evildoers and not interfere with the citizen's legitimate activities. In the view of Quesnay and his fellow economists, all people have a right to work as they please as long as they do not hurt others. Adam Smith similarly favored the unimpeded right to work. Wealth, he argued, is the result of labor.

In the same spirit of promoting freedom and humanitarian aims, various reformers denounced restrictive laws. Beccaria, about 1764, objected to the use of torture. Prison for debtors was assailed as useless and inhumane. Serfdom was condemned. Superstitions, such as those responsible for the persecution of "witches," were ridiculed.

### Science

The practical economic effect of rational thought and scientific orientation was clearly visible to the economists and scientists of the 18th century. They were, therefore, in favor of further efforts to expand scientific knowledge. Academies of science, like those of England, France, Prussia, and Russia, played a leading role in these efforts.

Expeditions for geographical discovery were sponsored. Descriptions of foreign lands—of their fauna, flora, rivers, mountains, and populations—were published. Vitus Bering, a Danish explorer in Russian service, found the straits separating Asia and America. The Germans Gmelin, Steller, and Pallas, also in Russian service, explored Siberia from the Urals to China and the Pacific. Other explorations were undertaken by the English and French in the New World. Almost automatically, European ideas were spread to many parts of the globe. Conversely, considerable influence was exerted by newly discovered areas upon the economics, politics, manners, and thoughts of the European nations.

The discoveries abroad contributed much to the imposing works of Buffon (d. 1788) and the Swede Linnaeus (d. 1778). Buffon described the animal world. Linnaeus undertook the fundamental task of not only describing plants, but also classifying them on the basis of their reproductive organs. In physiology,

Haller investigated respiration and the development of the embryo. Spallanzani (d. 1799) rejected the view that living matter can be generated by nonliving matter and proved that "spontaneous generation" does not occur in nature.

To the already flourishing fields of mathematics and astronomy, geniuses such as the Swiss mathematician Euler (d. 1783) and the philosopher Kant (d. 1804) made notable contributions.

Many discoveries were made in chemistry and physics. Boerhaave (d. 1738) and Priestley, whose work on oxygen, published in 1774, was fundamental, paved the way for scientific chemistry, which was soon developed by Lavoisier. Benjamin Franklin (d. 1790) occupied part of his time with scientific problems. His contemporaries owed to him a broad understanding of electrical forces, the significance of positive and negative electrical charges, and the conservation of electrical energy. In medicine, immunization against smallpox was achieved.

## Technology

Theoretical knowledge was soon applied to practical problems. Reaumur's work on the analysis of steel was published in 1722. Reliable measurements for longitude and latitude aided navigation. A steam engine was invented in 1705 by Newcomen and later modernized by Polzunov (1764) and Watt (1768). Technology even had an effect on the world of art, as shown by improvements in musical instruments.

## Social Sciences

Developments in social science were as significant as those in the natural sciences. Three Frenchmen—Montesquieu (d. 1755), Voltaire (d. 1778), and Rousseau (d. 1778)—may have added little to the insights already gained by such English social thinkers as Locke and his successor, Hume (d. 1776), but their practical influence as propagandists for the new social ideas far surpassed that of their English counterparts. In his *Persian Letters,* Montesquieu derided contemporary conditions in France; in his *Spirit of Laws* (1748), he emphasized the importance of the material basis of all social institutions and the influence of climate on the laws and character of a nation. He advocated a type of government limited by checks and balances. Voltaire, poet and historian, directed his wit against prejudice, unreasoning tradition, intolerance, and injustice. He firmly believed in the perfectibility of mankind.

Rousseau was the most sensitive of these three great Frenchmen, and the only political radical. In his *Nouvelle Heloise* and his educational treatise *Emile,* he defended a new, utopian way of life that, he thought, would result from turning away from civilization and back to nature. Thereby, he hoped the people of the West would be led to virtue and happiness. In his *Social Contract,* Rousseau set forth his thoughts on the inalienable rights of all human beings and on popular government.

Rousseau's ideas were spread further by the so-called "Encyclopedists," such men as Diderot (d. 1784) and d'Alembert (d. 1783), who, like Voltaire and Rousseau, faced censorship, exile, and imprisonment, yet pursued their work of propagating "enlightened" thought. They published a comprehensive alphabetical dictionary in which they used entries for political, religious, and other important terms to discuss enlightened ideas. It was writings such as these that provided the subject matter in the numerous salons, in pamphlets and newspapers. The increase in literacy increased their impact.

## Religion

The entire movement of the Enlightenment appealed to the human conscience and humanitarian feelings. Yet, people's overconfidence in progress, their neglect of metaphysical urges, and their materialism were bound to lead to criticism and reaction.

### Atheism and Deism

Only a few of the enlightened thinkers altogether rejected the idea of God and religion. Hume, who saw religion as an outmoded state of human evolution, and d'Holbach (d. 1789), a determined atheist, were among them. There was also a strong trend toward skepticism and atheism. This trend was attributable, on one hand, to the conventionalism and rigidity within traditional churches, and, on the other, to the failure to find a faith that would reconcile traditional religious beliefs with new scientific insights.

A vague middle position was provided by "deism." The deists rejected traditional revelation, and with it, the dogma of the existing Christian churches. While accepting a God as a first cause and as a source for the good, they built their views of the universe on the basis of rationalistic thought and mathematical laws.

### Pietism and Methodism

Deism lacked deep emotional appeal. It was soon surpassed in importance by a countermovement, antagonistic to rationalism, which had been established during the 17th century. This countermovement originated with the German pastors Spener and Francke. Their initiative developed into the Pietist trend. "Pietism" now brought to Christian communities a new devotion, spirituality, charity, and a revived mysticism and missionary fervor. Emphasis was placed not on reason, but on the attributes of the heart. The movement satisfied the longings of many who were seeking a truly Christian life.

Its individualistic tendencies also led to conflicts with state authority, however. Pietist groups, such as the Moravians under the leadership of Count Zinzendorf, were forced to emigrate. Many went to the New World, where they eventually exercised a certain distinct cultural influence. Likewise, many adherents of Wesley (d. 1791), who had sponsored a similar revolt in England against a natural religion emptied of Christian content, came to America. Everywhere, the Age of Enlightenment saw two conflicting trends: the one toward rejection of the Christian doctrine, the other toward reaffirmation of it.

### Literature

The interests of the age and its preoccupations with societal structure and with laws of nature left a definite mark on literature. In France, the outstanding writers were Voltaire and Rousseau. Two works of special interest, the Abbe Prevost's *Manon Lescaut* and Bernardin de Saint-Pierre's *Paul et Virginie*, stirred the hearts of 18th-century readers even more deeply, and they deserve mention as permanent treasures of world literature.

England contributed notable works, such as *Robinson Crusoe* by Defoe (d. 1731), *Gulliver's Travels* by Swift (d. 1745), and satirical writings with their implied criticism of existing prejudices. A number of authors of wide renown appeared, including Pope (d. 1744; *Essays on Thais*), Fielding (d. 1754; *Tom Jones*), Samuel Richardson *(Pamela)*, Sterne (d. 1768; *Tristam Shandy)*, Oliver Goldsmith (d. 1774; *Vicar of Wakefield)*, and Samuel Johnson and his biographer, Boswell (d. 1795).

Germany witnessed, with Klopstock (d. 1803) and Lessing (d. 1781), the beginnings of one of its greatest periods in literature. Lessing, in particular, helped free 18th-century literature from the artistic structure of the classical French tradition. He recalled the great and free heritage of Shakespeare to a public that had been inclined to forget or belittle the great English dramatist. Russia, too, began to produce significant literature; Lomonosov, and after him, the future historian Karamsin, laid foundations for the literary and scientific evolution of their country.

A number of historians of lasting importance appeared in the mid-18th century. Besides those who, in the tradition of Mabillon, investigated and edited sources, Voltaire and Gibbon *(Decline and Fall of the Roman Empire)* combined artistic style with sound scholarship. Historical interest was, thereafter, steadily heightened. Classical studies increased rapidly. Because of his studies in the excavations of Pompeii and Greece, the German archaeologist Winckelmann revealed to the world the beauty and meaning of the classical heritage.

## Art

With the growth of a reading public, the visual arts declined in significance. Few artists stand out. There were the three Italian Baroque painters, Antonio Canaletto, Francesco Guardi, and Giovanni Tiepolo, the latter famous for his great wall and ceiling paintings, and there were three English painters: Gainsborough (d. 1788), Joshua Reynolds (d. 1792), and the engraver Hogarth (d. 1764). All three were interested in social matters. Gainsborough and Reynolds made portraits of the high nobility, while Hogarth depicted the vices and misery of the poor. The Baroque style turned into "Rococo." Rococo possessed charm and intimacy. Its stunning buildings (palaces, theaters, and churches), staircases, and furniture, with shell-like structures and curved windows to let in light, adorned the countries of Italy, Spain, France, and southern Germany. Rococo also increased the trend toward sentimentality and affectation.

## Music

Simultaneous with the playfulness in the Rococo arts, we witness some of the grandest, most meaningful works of music ever created. During the second half of the 17th century, the innovations of the preceding period had already borne many fruits. The violin and the violoncello had been brought to perfection. Composers of the stature of Corelli (d. 1713) and Alessandro Scarlatti (d. 1725) in Italy, and Purcell (d. 1695) in England had promoted the art of the contrapuntal style and created instrumental music of rare beauty. Reflecting both a rational trend and sincere emotion, they added purity, simplicity, and strictness of form to a content rich in thought and feeling.

They prepared the way for the great masters who were to dominate the first half of the 18th century. It was then that Johann Sebastian Bach (d. 1750) and George Frideric Handel (d. 1759) composed their works. Handel *(The Messiah)*, besides writing numerous other works of the highest achievement, also excelled in the oratorio and opera. Bach did not publish any opera. It was in his compositions for orchestra, organ, and harpsichord; his church cantatas, chorales, and sonatas; his *St. John Passion* and *St. Matthew Passion;* and his *Art of the Fugue* that Bach embodied profound Christian inspiration and a human sense of beauty, grace, and compassion.

## Perspective

*On the political stage, the ideas of the Enlightenment were spread widely through the writings of the prominent thinkers of the age, many of whom were French. They animated rulers, "penlightened despots," who, in contrast to the style of Louis XIV, considered service to their states and their subjects as their foremost duty. Under these rulers, and under England's parliamentary system, an outdated aristocracy found new tasks. It filled the middle and high ranks of administration, the army, and navy. The commercial classes, bankers, and financiers benefited from the growing trade and, because of numerous mechanical inventions, from rapid industrial expansion.*

*In the cultural field, the Enlightenment strengthened the scientific approach to the study of nature and human life. Plants, animals, and natural surroundings were described, illustrated, and classified. Biology and medicine profited from scientific methods. Studies of electrical forces led to major discoveries. The scientific trends caused many philosophers to question the value of religious beliefs and religious institutions. Some rejected all belief in an all-embracing God. In reaction to such tendencies, there emerged also an opposite trend toward renewed faith and strict interpretation of the Bible, toward pietism and mysticism. Still others sought to reconcile conflicting ideas by accepting deist or pantheist views.*

*One area of the cultural life of the West reached a turning point during the Enlightenment, and that was music. A number of great German composers stood at the beginning of a full century of outstanding musical achievements.*

**Selected Readings**

Gay, Peter, comp., *The Enlightenment: A Comprehensive Anthology* (New York: Simon and Schuster, 1973).

Gipson, Laurence H. *The British Empire before the American Revolution* (New York: Knopf, 1939-1970).

MacDonogh, Giles. *Frederick the Great: A Life in Deed and Letters* (London: Weidenfeld & Nicolson, 1999).

Gooch, George O. *Frederick the Great* (New York: A. A. Knopf, 1947).

Jones, J. R. *Britain and the World, 1649-1815* (Brighton, Sussex: Harvester Press, 1980).

Kluchevsky, Vasily O. *Peter the Great* (New York: St. Martin's Press, 1958).

Krieger, Leonard. *Kings and Philosophers, 1689–1789* (New York: W. W. Norton, 1970).

Brinton, Crane. *The Portable Age of Reason Reader* (New York: Viking Press, 1956).

McKay, Derek, and Scott, H. M. *The Rise of the Great Powers, 1648–1815* (1983).

Raeff, Marc. *The Well-Ordered Police State, Social and Institutional Change Through Law in the Germanies and Russia, 1600–1800* (New Haven: Yale University Press, 1983).

Williams, Glyndwin. *The Expansion of Europe in the Eighteenth Century* (London: Blandford, 1966).

## Test Yourself

1. Frederick II, "The Great," came to the throne in_____.
   A. 1700
   B. 1740
   C. 1750
   D. 1710

2. The Enlightenment came to Russia in the early 18th century, largely owing to the personal influence of_____.
   A. Ivan IV
   B. Peter I
   C. Alexander I
   D. Nicholas II

3. The two fundamental weaknesses in the Russian system that prevented the development of a healthy society were_____.
   A. Militarism and religion
   B. The Ottoman Turkish threat and famine
   C. Autocracy and serfdom
   D. All of the above

4. Under the Spanish monarch, Charles III, and his minister Aranda, the government functioned efficiently by_____.
   A. Enforcing old tax laws
   B. Abandoning the *encomienda* system in Spanish colonies
   C. Reducing taxes to encourage private enterprise
   D. B and C

5. At the Peace of Paris in 1763,_____.
   A. France lost India
   B. France lost most of its North American colonies
   C. France lost Egypt
   D. A and B

6. Montesquieu's 1748 *Spirit of the Laws* advocated a government _____.
   A. based on monarchy
   B. limited by checks and balances
   C. controlled by the clergy
   D. all of the above

7. Jean Jacques Rousseau set forth his thoughts on the inalienable rights of all human beings in 1762 in his great work titled_____.
   A. *The Rights of Man*
   B. *The Social Contract*
   C. *The Leviathan*
   D. *The Persian Letters*

8. The Deists _____
   A. rejected traditional revelation
   B. rejected existing Christian church dogma
   C. accepted God as the first cause and course of all good
   D. all of the above

## Answers and Explanations

1. **B.** When Frederick II, "the Great" (d. 1786), came to the throne in 1740, he inherited very efficient governmental machinery. Making prompt use of his excellent army in three Silesian Wars, Frederick succeeded in doubling his realms and economic resources and in raising Prussia to the status of a first-class power.

2. **B.** Enlightenment came to Russia in the early 18th century, largely owing to the personal influence of Peter I, "the Great" (d. 1725). Peter was a man of inexhaustible energy; he personally and conscientiously attended to innumerable duties and supervised an almost incredible amount of detail. He reformed the administration, removed clerical influences from state affairs, built a civil service based on ability, and reduced class discrimination in law courts. He improved the economy of his state by adhering to the principles of mercantilism. In his time, iron production in Russia surpassed that of England. He reformed the army, and through successful wars, expanded the national domain.

3. **C.** Under Catherine the Great, the two fundamental weaknesses in the Russian system, autocracy and serfdom, prevented the development of a healthy peasant class, progressive industry, and a strong middle class. Many revolts of the peasants occurred (including the protracted and dangerous rebellion of Pugachev). Toward the end of the century, the nation, notwithstanding its territorial expansion, improved education, and increased production, faced greater social problems than at the beginning.

4. **D.** Under King Charles III (d. 1788) and his minister, Aranda, the Spanish government functioned more efficiently. It reduced taxes to encourage private enterprise. In line with the trend toward a more centralized administration, it abolished the internal customs barriers that obstructed trade. In the colonies, the regime gave up the system of *encomienda*.

5. **D.** At the Peace of Paris in 1763, France lost not only India, but also most of its North American holdings. In the course of the 18th century, the French had tried to turn the colonial empire, which mercantilist theory and thirst for glory had driven them to acquire, into a possession that would yield practical returns. Their colonies in Canada, the Mississippi Valley, and the Caribbean islands showed considerable promise. Trading in commodities (sugar, timber, fish, and furs) and in slaves increased, both to and from the homeland and among the colonies.

6. **B.** In Montesquieu's *Spirit of Laws* (1748), he emphasized the importance of the material basis of all social institutions and the influence of climate on the laws and character of a nation. He advocated a type of government limited by checks and balances.

7. **B.** In his *Social Contract,* Rousseau set forth his thoughts on the inalienable rights of all human beings and on popular government.

8. **D.** The deists rejected traditional revelation, and with it, the dogma of the existing Christian churches. While accepting a God as a first cause and as a source for good, they built their views of the universe on the basis of rationalistic thought and mathematical laws.

**CHAPTER 10**

# The Age of Revolution (1775-1795)

**1776** American Declaration of Independence
Adam Smith, *Wealth of Nations*
**1781** Kant, *Kritik der reinen Vernunft (Critique of Pure Reason)*
**1782** Watt's steam engine
**1783** Second Peace of Paris
**1787** Mozart, *Don Giovanni*
**1789** U.S. Constitution in force
Beginning of great French Revolution
Fall of the Bastille
**1792** War against France
Russian-Turkish Peace of Jassy
**1793** Louis XVI guillotined
**1794** Robespierre guillotined
**1795** Peace of Basle
Third partition of Poland

*The ferment created by the ideas of the Enlightenment spread rapidly among forward-thinking people in all Western countries. Progress made possible by new methods of production added to the unrest. Impatience grew despite reforms introduced by enlightened governments. With a firm belief in the perfectibility of mankind, individuals belonging to the most diverse social strata demanded far-reaching changes in the organization of society.*

*In the face of this trend toward social evolution, many who held economic and political power stood firm. Instead of seeking ways to adapt themselves to the new situation, they rejected any idea of a retreat from their privileged positions. They hoped, in the spirit of Louis XV's "Apres moi le deluge," to be able at least to postpone the Day of Judgment.*

*Nevertheless, the ideology of freedom and equality, and the fervor engendered by it, irrevocably undermined the faith in the old order, even for those who had a material interest in it. Thus, without a serious economic crisis, the ground was prepared for a quick, violent transformation of social and political institutions.*

## ■ REVOLUTIONARY MOVEMENTS IN THE COLONIES

The first great assault upon the traditional social system occurred in England's thirteen American colonies. They were comparatively free and prosperous and subject to a rather generous, progressive government. The assault was led not by the oppressed, but by those who had little to gain except the fulfillment of certain ideals rooted in the spirit of the Enlightenment.

## Birth of the United States

After the thirteen English colonies had declared their independence in 1776, they faced the task of making their new social construct a reality. The struggle encompassed two phases: first, liberation from foreign domination, and second, establishment of a working government in line with the most progressive ideology of the age. Notwithstanding vigorous opposition by conservative forces, both tasks were successfully accomplished.

The American Declaration of Independence was carefully drafted under the guidance of Thomas Jefferson. Aside from enumerating the grievances against the British, it stated that man possesses "natural rights," that it is self-evident that "all men are created equal," that they have the right to "Life, Liberty, and the Pursuit of Happiness," and that government derives its power from the consent of the governed. It thus gave expression to the enlightened views of the century and sought to transform theory into practice. In this way, it set a model for the organization of democratic governments in many countries.

### American War of Independence

In order to achieve their goal of self-determination, the colonists undertook armed resistance against the most formidable power of the time, Great Britain. The war lasted seven years. But it was won, despite many setbacks and internal dissensions, by American colonial troops under the inspired leadership of George Washington (d. 1799). The English had the advantage of overwhelming naval superiority, but they conducted the war halfheartedly. The British troops and generals sent to America were mostly ill equipped.

The Americans, on the other hand, had concluded alliances with France and Spain in 1778; they had received decisive support from them. American leaders, George Washington in particular, performed their duties with great devotion and perseverance. In 1781, General Cornwallis and his English troops were forced to surrender at Yorktown (with formal surrender in 1783), whereupon the British home government acknowledged American independence. The peace treaty, concluded in the same year at Paris, sealed Britain's loss of all thirteen colonies. Moreover, it forced Britain to hand back Florida and the Mediterranean island of Minorca to Spain. France gained nothing except acknowledgment of its claims to French settlements in America.

### The Constitution of the United States

Even before the end of the war, the colonists had provided for postwar cooperation among themselves. They drew up the "Articles of Confederation." The articles vested most legislative and executive powers in the representative houses of the individual states; they limited the powers of the central government. This first attempt provided so weak a link among the various states that the formation of a healthy nation became a dubious prospect.

Moreover, economic conditions after the war were unsatisfactory. A number of revolts occurred, and bitterness between factions persisted; efficient tax collection for the government was impossible for lack of a central enforcing agency. Issues such as westward expansion and the problem of slavery divided the states. During this period, the eastern seaboard states voluntarily surrendered their claims to western lands they could have acquired. This willingness also indicated some possibility of future cooperation. However, the leading figures in the colonies, Benjamin Franklin, George Washington, John Adams, Thomas Jefferson, and Alexander Hamilton, were concerned with the newly independent country's prospects of survival in view of the dissensions within.

In 1787, several of them met with like-minded leaders in a new Constitutional Convention. With seven states represented, the Convention, which was led by George Washington, agreed upon a constitution, whose drafting was largely the work of James Madison. It provided for a national government with three separate branches—legislative, executive, and judicial. These were intended to provide checks and balances, thereby preventing the exercise of arbitrary power. Among other stipulations, it also provided for the separation of church and state. Although full of compromises, it constituted a workable frame of government. Although being very concerned with property rights, it lacked an overall statement about civil rights. Amendments specifically addressing civil rights had to be subsequently added.

With acceptance of the Constitution by the legislatures of all thirteen colonies (ratification by nine was required), the "United States" came into being. George Washington was elected the first president in 1789, with his duties under the Constitution including those of enforcing the law, appointing judges, and acting as military commander-in-chief. The new nation began to function as a republic, and in a way very different from that of the European models. Through its progressive Constitution, the United States was to later exercise considerable influence on political and social thought and organization in Europe. Yet, the new nation was also a true child of Europe, especially of the French enlightenment and the Anglo-Saxon legal traditions.

### Unrest in South America

The example set by the United States could not be followed in other colonial areas. In Spanish and Portuguese South America, training in self-government was lacking. A gulf existed between the Europeans, who included many wealthy and well-educated people, and the Indians, blacks, and mixed races that were in the majority in South America. The European settlers feared that if they lost home support, then the lower classes would rise in revolt and overwhelm them.

Moreover, the economic situation did not favor independence. Despite the abolition of the *encomienda* system, agriculture was still backward; mining depended on the markets in the home countries; and business organization was weak. Uprisings against Spain and Portugal took place between 1780 and 1784. However, since allegiance was stronger than the spirit of revolt, the winning of independence was long deferred.

### Activity in Asia and Africa

No revolutionary outbreaks occurred in other continents where independence movements would have had to originate with native (non-European) populations. The latter, notwithstanding their great numbers, never developed military power to equal that of the Europeans, who could therefore not only maintain their position but also extend their territorial holdings. Consequently, Europeans seized additional colonies in Africa and India. During Warren Hastings's administration, India came almost completely under English rule. Furthermore, a whole new continent was opened for colonization when, in 1797, a penal settlement was established in Australia, which eventually developed into a prosperous commonwealth.

## ■ REVOLUTION IN EUROPE

Shortly after Europe witnessed the startling innovation of a republic in America, it was shocked by a major revolution against the "Old Regime" in France. This appeared to be another result of the philosophy of enlightenment. Revolts also occurred in Belgium, Italy, and Poland. But it was the French Revolution that would have the greatest dramatic and lasting impact upon most of Europe.

### Conditions Before the Revolution

French institutions were not altogether backward. French rulers had not been entirely lacking in political enlightenment. After the death of Louis XV in 1774, attempts had been made under weak-spirited Louis XVI and his capable minister, Turgot (d. 1781), to improve agriculture. By abolishing numerous internal customs' barriers and improving the roads, Turgot provided greater freedom for trade. The privileges of the nobility were reduced, and the remnants of serfdom dissolved. Special efforts were made to end the abuses of an inequitable tax system and check the system of buying offices. Also, the highest court of law, the Parlement de Paris, was given increased authority. The Parlement, however, was inclined to abuse its position of power in favor of the privileged classes.

The reactionary forces everywhere were still strong. Turgot was dismissed in 1776. The divisions among the French people in regard to laws, customs' barriers, tax systems, and the different weights and measures, all of which favored the traditional distribution of power, continued to exist. Social distinctions were upheld in favor of the first two estates (the clergy and the nobility). The third estate (the middle class and the peasantry, the latter alone accounting for four-fifths of the population) had no political rights, and its members were discriminated against when seeking high positions and economic advancement. Overland traffic was unsafe, and vagabondage was commonplace. Moreover, each social stratum was divided within itself. Each of the three estates had its wealthy and its poor constituents; often the wealthy individuals belonging to one estate cooperated with those in another, rather than with members of their own estate.

## Path to Revolution

Under such conditions, the incentives to revolt were many:

(1) There were the ideologies of the age: the philosophy of enlightenment, freedom, equality, and political rights for the bourgeoisie; the ideas of free enterprise, free development of trade, and free access to all positions in state and army according to ability instead of birth; the rejection of the corrupted morals of court and nobility; and the opposition to existing types of censorship. Actually, many members of the nobility had themselves accepted these ideas. They gathered in fashionable *salons* frequented also by the intellectuals (the *philosophes*) of the time, and these *salons* became centers for the dissemination of the new concepts.

(2) There were political incentives, the example of the American colonies, and the dissatisfaction with foreign policies and with the military defeats of France at a time when a nationalistic spirit was spreading everywhere. Furthermore, there were the corrupt law courts and the still existing, though seldom employed, *lettres de cachet,* which meant arbitrary arrest at the king's pleasure. The entire system was out of tune with contemporary conditions under enlightened monarchies or parliamentary regimes.

(3) Many had personal grievances against the weakness of an otherwise well-meaning king, the haughtiness, interference, and extravagance of the queen, Marie Antoinette, and the influence of favorites, whose abilities contrasted sadly with those of the leaders of discontented groups.

(4) Most important, however, were the economic motives for dissatisfaction. Although poverty was not exceptionally widespread in France and conditions in France among the lower classes compared rather favorably with those in England and other countries, confidence in the government's ability was lacking. The people had to contend with a steady rise in prices, intermittent food shortages—partly owing to bad harvests in 1788 and 1789—and recurrent periods of unemployment.

Moreover, many among the privileged were determined to preserve the inequalities of the tax system. The land tax, or *taille,* continued to be levied only upon the property of the third estate. The nobles, on the other hand, paid an amount that they themselves regarded as appropriate; the clergy confined itself to a voluntary "gift." The salt tax, or *gabelle,* was imposed upon everyone, but the tax on this indispensable commodity was burdensome primarily to the poor. The *cot-Me,* a tax in the form of compulsory work for the lords by those peasants who had not yet become free, was levied exclusively on the lower classes. In addition, the landed nobility enjoyed certain exclusive privileges, such as special-milling and hunting rights. Then there were tithes, and extra tithes *(vingtieme),* a wine tax *(trop bu),* and other levies. Nor could the peasants lighten their burdens through purchase of additional land as this was prohibited.

**Outbreak of the Revolution**

The foregoing difficulties might have been overcome had the public treasury not been depleted and had the Parlement not opposed legislation that would have made necessary funds available through taxation of the privileged groups. The financial credit of the government was soon exhausted. The king appointed as his chief minister Jacques Necker, who was popular but whom he dismissed in 1789. Eventually, Louis XVI was persuaded to call a meeting of the long-abandoned Estates-General. Elections were held. The people gave their representatives written instructions in so-called *cahiers* enumerating their grievances. In May 1789, the Estates-General assembled. It broke up in June over the question of voting because the third estate, composed of the middle classes and peasants, feared that the combined clergy and nobles would always outvote them. Their representatives, many of them young people and among these numerous lawyers, therefore convened on a nearby tennis court, where under the inspired leadership of the noted orator Mirabeau, an oath was taken not to disband until voting by head was introduced and a constitution for all of France was drafted.

The king capitulated. But this political victory by the third estate did not solve its economic difficulties. Instead, it brought further unemployment and, finally, the first violent uprisings. On July 14, 1789, the Bastille, where the assumedly innocent political victims of absolutism were confined, was stormed by a mob. This event was a foreshadowing of the revolution to come. Unrest spread throughout France. Necker had to be recalled. Some of the nobility hastily fled the country. Ordinary citizens armed themselves, and the people adopted a new, revolutionary flag.

**The Constitution**

In response, a memorable night session of the Estates-General was held on August 4, 1789. The privileged classes divested themselves of most of their prerogatives: serfdom was abolished; equality of taxation was introduced; eligibility for governmental jobs was extended to every qualified citizen, irrespective of class or wealth; and all internal customs' barriers were abolished. This was followed on August 26, 1789 by the Declaration of the Rights of Man, proclaiming equality, liberty, and justice for all, as well as guaranteeing property rights to all classes.

In the face of these events, the king proved himself unequal to his task. He weakly submitted to a mob's demands and moved his court back from Versailles to Paris, so he could be "closer to his people." Revolutionaries formed "clubs" (Jacobins, Cordeliers, Feuillants, and others), and enthusiastic leaders (e.g., Marat, Danton, and Robespierre) took over their direction.

Thereupon, the Estates-General took another momentous step. In order to avoid imminent state bankruptcy, it decreed the confiscation of all Church lands. A new currency (the *assignat),* based on land, was issued. During the next year, 1790, a constitution was drafted, with the abbot Sieyes playing a leading role as constitution maker. This new constitution established a limited monarchy. The country was reorganized into eighty-three "departments," each administered by elective officers. Religious freedom was proclaimed. A jury system was introduced.

Voting rights were granted to the male taxpaying segment of the population, whether nobility or burghers. A representative assembly was given legislative powers and control of finances. It was largely composed of people influenced by the ideas of the enlightened philosophers. Furthermore, a "civil organization of the clergy" was introduced. Monasteries were abolished; clerical offices were to be filled by electoral vote of the communities; and papal power was confined to the right of consecration. The clergy, having lost their lands, were to have their salaries paid by the state and, in exchange, were to take an oath to uphold the constitution.

*Figure 10–1 Revolutionary France, 1789–1793*

## Repercussions Abroad

The new institutions meant a move toward radicalism. This, combined with the agitation of French *émigrés* (nobles who had left revolutionary France and were organizing a counterrevolutionary army), led to repercussions abroad. Foreign monarchs began to fear for their own safety and for the political systems on which their authority rested. The situation worsened when Louis XVI was persuaded in 1791 to seek refuge abroad but, together with his entire family, was intercepted at the Belgian border. Strikes were called and bloody new riots occurred, whereupon the Austrian emperor decided to come to the aid of his French sister, Marie Antoinette; other monarchs joined him in organizing an army to invade France.

The Russian empress, Catherine, now old, conservative, and thoroughly afraid of any revolutionary movement, used the opportunity to act upon a scheme of her own. Fearing similar disturbances in anarchical Poland, she proposed and, together with the Prussian king, carried out a second partition of Poland. The Poles had begun too late to undertake long-overdue internal reforms. Patriots, such as Kosciusko, had begun too late to direct their efforts toward modernization of Polish institutions. Even a reformed Poland was no longer acceptable to its neighbors. The second partition was followed in 1795 by a third one, whereby Russia, Austria, and Prussia abolished the Polish state.

## War

Meanwhile, in 1792, revolutionary France had answered the threats of the European powers with a declaration of war. A leftist party, the Girondins, had taken over the government; it began to confiscate the property of the *émigrés* and to deport any priest who refused to take the prescribed oath in support of the constitution. When Louis XVI opposed these measures, another move toward radicalism—typical of all revolutions in progress—occurred. His palace, the Tuileries, was invaded. The king and his family were subjected to numerous indignities.

Just then, an arrogant and ill-timed manifesto by the commander of the allies, who was leading a victorious army into France, contributed to the furor of the revolutionaries. Again, they invaded the palace, massacred the guards, and forced the royal family to seek refuge in the hall of the assembly. The assembly decided to jail the king and arrange for new elections on the basis of an equal, general franchise. Under the pressure of the Jacobins, who formed a more extreme left wing than the Girondins, the new assembly, known as the Convention, proclaimed a republic. Meanwhile at Valmy, the French troops gained their first decisive victory over the foreign invaders. This helped to strengthen the position of the Convention.

## Terror

The Convention proceeded promptly to depose the king, introduce a new calendar that would date from the revolution instead of the birth of Christ, and abolish all remaining tax burdens on the peasants. It also brought the king to trial and had him executed in January 1793. Thereafter the guillotine worked constantly in what has come to be known as the "Reign of Terror." This, in turn, led to a series of revolts in western and southern France against the revolutionary government and to an even more dangerous consequence—an all-European war. Spain, England, and Holland joined Austria and Prussia in an alliance against France.

Revolutionary France met the danger with resolute action. A general draft was ordered. A large army was promptly organized, and a Committee of Public Safety was appointed. Composed largely of Jacobins, this Committee soon dominated both in the Convention and in the Girondist government; the latter was forced to resign. Centralizing all power, the Committee then pushed through legislation that actually abolished the very freedoms it advocated. When one of the most radical leaders, Marat, was murdered, Danton and Robespierre continued the revolutionary program. A new constitution was drafted. Laws were passed against speculators and against anyone suspected of disloyalty (Law of Suspects). Social legislation was broadened, though property rights were still respected. To supplant religion, a "Cult of Reason" was introduced, followed by a "Cult of the Supreme Being," which reflected vague deistic concepts.

In 1794, Robespierre seized complete control; he even had Danton arrested and guillotined. Robespierre was a fanatical devotee of Rousseau's utopian teachings, untiring and incorruptible. But suspicious of everyone, he promoted the "Great Terror" whereby he intended to cleanse the nation and introduce the new age—that of universal brotherhood. He advocated equal rights for all, including women and Jews, and opposed the luxuries and manners of the former privileged classes; he insisted on simplicity in lifestyle.

## Reaction

After five years of stirring events, insecurity, and disruption of traditional ties, a point was reached when the reestablishment of security and order seemed more desirable than liberty and utopia. A reactionary party emerged that succeeded in July 1794 (9th of Thermidor) in overthrowing Robespierre's regime and sending him to the guillotine. The powers of the Committee of Public Safety were abolished, restrictive laws revoked, revolutionary clubs closed, and some priests were allowed to return. In 1795—a year that brought an exceptionally bad harvest and a sharp depreciation of the paper money, the assignat—a new constitution was instituted that provided for a "Directory" of five men and for two representative houses elected by people of property.

The revolution had no socialistic content; indeed, throughout the upheaval, property rights were regarded as inalienable. The small and weak working class, whose belated separate uprising under Babeuf was readily suppressed, gained nothing further for the peasantry. Nor did it bring political liberty, equality, or brotherhood, or solve France's financial problems. But it did end absolutism, feudal privileges, arbitrary arrest, the mercantilist economy, and Church predominance. It brought France glory by formulating the Rights of Man, fighting for them, and setting an example for other nations. It gained for the peasants full possession of their lands and freedom from feudal burdens, and it brought success to the middle class, which through its wealth became the dominating factor in the state.

## Perspective

*The Age of Enlightenment ended, as far as Western civilization's political evolution was concerned, with revolutions in America and Europe. In some regions, they failed. In Britain's American colonies, a war of independence brought into being, however, a state with a government that, under a Constitution, attained many of the ideals with regard to freedom, government, and individual rights that the Enlightenment had cherished.*

*In Europe, revolution in France put an end to the numerous surviving remnants of feudalism. Recently, a French historian wrote: "The revolution is over." What he meant was that now, after two hundred years, the debate over its significance for Western civilization is exhausted. Perhaps the revolution was the most important specific event in European civilization since the Reformation. Its course from mild to radical reform, with accompanying internal and foreign war, and terror, all ending in reaction, has been considered a model for all revolutions.*

*Many of the hopes for "progress" voiced during the revolution were, as in its American counterpart, realized, even though some of the idealistic aims were lost. Neither the French nor the American Revolution gave consideration to economic equality.*

## Selected Readings

Brinton, Crane. *Anatomy of Revolution* (New York: Vintage Books, 1965).
Cohn, Hans. *Nationalism: Its Meaning and History* (Princeton: Princeton University Press, 1965).
Doyle, W. *Origins of the French Revolution* (Oxford: Oxford University Press, 1980).
_____. *The Oxford History of the French Revolution* (Oxford: Oxford University Press, 1990).
Hampson, Norman. *The Life and Opinions of Maximilien Robespierre* (1974).
Hobshawn, E. J. *The Age of Revolution: Europe 1789-1848* (Cleveland: World Pub. Co., 1970).
Lefebvre, Georges. *The French Revolution*, 2 vols. (London: Routledge, 1962).
Palmer, Robert R. *Age of the Democratic Revolution: A Political History of Europe and America, 1760-1800*, 2 vols. (Princeton: Princeton University Press, 1964).
Morton, Joseph. *The American Revolution* (London: Greenwood Press, 2003).
Spaeth, Harold J. and Smith, Edward C. *The Constitution of the United States* (New York: Harper Perennial, 1991).

## Test Yourself

1. In 1787, a convention led by George Washington agreed upon the constitution whose drafting was largely the work of_____.
   A. James Madison
   B. Thomas Jefferson
   C. George Washington
   D. Benjamin Franklin

2. George Washington was elected the first president of the United States in _____.
   A. 1776
   B. 1789
   C. 1791
   D. 1790

3. A turning point in the French Revolution was marked by_____.
   A. The execution of Robespierre
   B. The execution of Louis XVI
   C. The execution of the peasants
   D. The storming of the Bastille on July 14, 1789

4. Under the "Declaration of the Rights of Man," the French were granted_____.
   A. Equality, liberty and justice
   B. Property rights for all
   C. The end of monarchy
   D. A and B

5. The key features during the Reign of Terror included_____.
   A. Introduction of a new calendar
   B. Abolition of all tax burdens on the peasants
   C. Trial and execution of Louis XVI
   D. All of the above

6. Not included among the French radicals during the Reign of Terror were_____.
   A. Marat
   B. Colbert
   C. Robespierre
   D. All of the above

## Answers and Explanations

1. **A.** In 1787, several men met with like-minded leaders in a new Constitutional Convention. With seven states represented, the Convention under Washington's presidency agreed upon a constitution, whose drafting was largely the work of James Madison. It provided for a national government with three separate branches—legislative, executive, and judicial. These were intended to provide checks and balances and thereby prevent the exercise of arbitrary power.

2. **B.** With acceptance of the Constitution by the legislatures of all thirteen colonies (ratification by nine was required), the "United States" came into being. George Washington was elected the first president (in 1789), with his duties under the Constitution including those of enforcing the law, appointing judges, and acting as military commander-in-chief.

3. **D.** On July 14, the Bastille, where assumedly innocent political victims of absolutism were confined, was stormed by a mob. This event was a foreshadowing of the revolution to come. Unrest spread throughout France. Necker had to be recalled. Some of the nobility hastily fled the country. Ordinary citizens armed themselves and the people adopted a new, revolutionary flag.

4. **D.** In the "Declaration of the Rights of Man" (August 26, 1789), its framers proclaimed equality, liberty, and justice, and guaranteed property rights to all.

5. **D.** The Reign of Terror proceeded promptly to depose the king, introduce a new calendar that would date from the revolution instead of the birth of Christ, and abolish all remaining tax burdens on the peasants. It also brought the king to trial and (in January 1793) had him executed. Thereafter the guillotine worked constantly in a "Reign of Terror." This, in turn, led to a series of revolts in western and southern France against the revolutionary government and to an even more dangerous consequence—an all-European war. Spain, England, and Holland joined Austria and Prussia in an alliance against France.

6. **B.** Colbert was a minister under Louis XIV and not one of the French radicals. Robespierre, one of the major French radicals, seized complete control; he even had Danton arrested and guillotined. Robespierre was a fanatical devotee of Rousseau's utopian teachings, untiring and incorruptible. But, suspicious of everyone, he promoted the "Great Terror" whereby he intended to cleanse the nation and introduce the new age—that of universal brotherhood. He advocated equal rights for all, including women and Jews, and opposed the luxuries and manners of the former privileged classes; he insisted on simplicity in lifestyle.

# CHAPTER 11
# The Napoleonic Era (1795-1815)

**1796** Napoleon's Italian campaign
**1797** Haydn, *Emperor Quartet*
**1798** Napoleon's Egyptian campaign
Wordsworth and Coleridge, *Lyrical Ballads*
Malthus, *Essay on the Principle of Population*
**1799** Napoleon becomes First Consul
**1803** Purchase of Louisiana Territory by United States of America
**1804** Schiller, *Wilhelm Tell*
Napoleon becomes emperor
**1805** Battle of Trafalgar
Battle of Austerlitz
**1806** End of Holy Roman Empire
**1807** Reforms in Prussia (vom Stein)
Fulton's steamship on the Hudson
Introduction of Continental System
**1808** Goethe, *Faust* (first part)
**1812** Napoleon's Russian campaign
War between England and U.S.A.
Byron, *Childe Harold's Pilgrimage*
**1813** Wars of Liberation against Napoleon
**1814** Stephenson's steam locomotive built
**1815** Battle of Waterloo: Napoleon exiled to St. Helena
Congress of Vienna concluded
Holy Alliance founded

*As often happens with revolutions, the French Revolution ended in dictatorship. A "gilded youth," which sought to "enjoy" life after the great issues demanding unselfish devotion had been settled, engaged in numerous follies in dress, manners, and behavior, and neglected the tasks that the newly gained liberty necessitated. But the man to direct France's destiny for the next two decades was already on hand: Napoleon Bonaparte (1769-1821). His role during the period 1795-1815 was pivotal in the context of France and its relations with the rest of Europe.*

*The name reflects the predominantly political preoccupations of past historians but does not do justice to a period that belonged, culturally, among the greatest in Western civilization. And while it was*

*France that excelled in the sciences, it was Germany that contributed most to the greatness of the age in other cultural areas. Three names suffice to indicate achievements in that country: Kant, Goethe, and Beethoven.*

## ■ POLITICAL STRUGGLES IN EUROPE

The counterrevolutionaries of 1795 were disappointed in their hopes, which the end of the revolution had aroused. Terror was ended; internal order was restored; and a measure of security was again provided for the average citizen. The fears of France's neighbors were alleviated. But the revolutionary and nationalistic elements in France were not satisfied with the results; they helped to pave the way for the rise of Napoleon. Obsessed with dictatorial ambitions, he gave Europe two decades of even more dangerous and destructive upheavals.

### Rise of Napoleon

Napoleon, born in the French-purchased island of Corsica, had studied military science in France and had been a member of Robespierre's party. He excelled as artillery general in the war against the English. His exceptional ability, friendly relations with one of the members of the Directory, and advantageous marriage with an influential widow, Josephine Beauharnais, brought this capable young general the command of an army.

At his own suggestion, he was sent into Italy to terminate the war by attacking the Austrian possessions there. Although Prussia and Spain had signed a peace treaty at Basel in 1795, renouncing the entire

*Figure 11–1 Napoleon Bonaparte, 1769–1821*

left bank of the Rhine in favor of France, and although Holland had been defeated and had become a "Batavian Republic" under a French protectorate, Austria and England had continued the war. The Italian campaign, conducted brilliantly by Napoleon, brought a string of victories and military glory to France. It made plunder available to fill France's empty treasury; it spread revolutionary ideas abroad. It ended not only with Austria's withdrawal from the war, but also with France's acquisition of extensive territory gained in the Peace of Campoformio (1797).

After he defeated Austria, Napoleon prepared to attack England. He contemplated an assault across the English Channel, but instead chose to break England's "lifeline" to India through the conquest of Egypt in 1798. Napoleon conducted another brilliant campaign, winning a great victory at the Pyramids. After a British sea victory at Abu Kir, however, he was unable to reach his objective because the French lost control of the Mediterranean supply lines. He was fortunate to escape with his life. He fled to Paris, leaving his army to perish in Egypt.

### The Consulate (1799-1804)

Meanwhile, the Directory had squandered the spoils of the Italian campaign and had forfeited the confidence of the nation. Its foreign policy had by 1799 provoked a new anti-French coalition, this time joined by Russia. Russian and Austrian troops, under the command of Suvorov, had driven the French out of most of the Po Valley. At home, inflation raged; corruption made orderly government impossible; and new revolts staged chiefly by reactionary forces were underway. Napoleon regarded this as the opportune moment to carry out his own ambitious plans. In October 1799, he overthrew the government and dictated a new constitution, which provided for a consulate in which he, himself, took first place as the executive power. He saw to it that his action was confirmed by a plebiscite.

Napoleon's next step was to reconquer Austrian Italy. After another brilliant victory at Marengo, and after defeating the Austrians again at Hohenlinden, he induced the latter to make peace at Luneville (1801). He then turned his attention to England and successfully pressed the British to sign a peace treaty at Amiens in 1802 that restored to France all colonies seized by England since the beginning of the war.

Napoleon then set to work on internal reforms, initiating a dictatorial but highly beneficial regime. The revolutionary era was declared at an end. The normal calendar was reinstated. A concordat was concluded with the pope. Although it did not return Church lands, it restored the prestige of Catholicism; dissatisfied priests, peasants, and burghers were pacified. Religious tolerance was extended to Jews. Government finances were systematized; a central bank was founded; and a new currency (the franc, backed by a sound tax system) was introduced.

Agriculture was promoted. The raising of new crops, such as sugar beets, was encouraged in order to make Europe independent of imports from British colonies. Roads, tunnels, harbors, and canals were built. The school system was expanded, higher education supported, and the French Academy reorganized. But censorship was strict, and the propaganda apparatus worked to personally benefit Napoleon. By his appointments to local administrative posts and by dispensing honors, he secured supporters and faithful service to himself. Highly beneficial legal reforms were initiated under the *Code Napoleon*. Based on Roman law, the *Code* embodied many of the liberal, equalitarian, and humanitarian concepts for which the revolution had been fought. It became a model for the Western world. It provided for equality before the law and confirmed the inviolability of property rights. However, it deprived women of the gains secured by them during the revolution.

### Napoleon's European Conquests

Personal ambitions and the very nature of his regime impelled Napoleon, however, to initiate dangerous foreign enterprises. Aspiring to become a "new Charlemagne," he had himself crowned emperor in 1804, and he then engaged in further wars. In 1805, he defeated Austria and Russia in his most famous victory, at Austerlitz, gained through tactics based on the great mobility of his forces. In 1806, he destroyed the Prussian army and conquered nearly all of Prussia. Numerous smaller German states were abolished; many were transferred to French jurisdiction. The Holy Roman Empire, which had endured nearly a millennium, declared itself dissolved, and the Hapsburgs kept only the emperorship of Austria.

Another attack on England was contemplated, but invasion plans were abandoned after Admiral Lord Nelson's fleet destroyed the French naval forces in 1805 at the Battle of Trafalgar. Nevertheless, Napoleon set up a barrier against England by prohibiting the importation of British goods on the Continent, thus establishing the "Continental System." Moreover, his troops invaded and occupied most of Spain and Portugal, and even ventured to attack the Papal States. Russia, defeated in East Prussia when coming to the aid of the Prussians, was forced to make peace and conclude an alliance with France (Tilsit, 1807). Napoleon then arranged a spectacular congress at Erfurt attended by kings, princes, and a host of famous people. It marked the apex of Napoleon's career.

## Decline of Napoleon's Empire

Napoleon's conquests created a problem of overexpansion; he lacked the resources needed in order to protect and administer his acquisitions. The halfhearted, mutually distrustful alliance with Russia, providing for a division of European hegemony between the two partners, gave little assurance of safety.

Furthermore, Napoleon had to contend with serious new difficulties. His treatment of the papacy, culminating in the annexation of the Papal States (1809) and the arrest of the pope had alienated the

*Figure 11–2 Napoleon's Empire, around 1812*

Catholics and their sympathizers. Censorship and arbitrary restrictions had infuriated the liberals. The military campaigns had exhausted French manpower and had intensified the popular discontent within France. Most ominous was Napoleon's failure to subdue Spain, which with English help resisted the invader. The revolutionary ideal of liberty seemed lost. A new nobility had supplanted the old. People were weary of war, but peace did not come.

Moreover, Napoleon's intellectual power and military genius seemed to be declining at the same time that his enemies were learning to overcome his strategy. His megalomania—reinforcing his habitual distrust of others and his steadfast loyalty to his family—had caused him to place his brothers and sisters on various European thrones. Their overall lack of capability soon showed this move to have been ill advised. Under their rule, the vast array of satellite states did not form a reliable foundation for the empire.

Nationalistic fervor now aided the cause of his opponents. In Spain, continued guerrilla warfare resulted in a constant drain on French strength. England gave no indications of wanting to make peace. Revolts occurred in Holland, Switzerland, Italy, and the Tyrol. Since the Continental System could not be enforced along all the coasts of Europe (enforcement would have been contrary to the interests of the various nations), it actually worked to the advantage of England, rather than of France. Smuggling increased, bringing with it more discontent and greater disregard of law and order. In 1809, Austria risked a new war against France. Although defeated once again, and forced to allow the Austrian emperor's daughter to marry Napoleon after his divorce from Josephine, the Hapsburgs demonstrated the possibility of continued resistance. Finally, a rising anti-Napoleon tide arose in Prussia, where owing to statesmen such as vom Stein and Hardenberg, as well as General Scharnhorst, comprehensive reforms were undertaken. Planning a war of liberation, the Prussians adopted many practices from the French Revolution. They modernized and centralized the administrative system, abolished old-fashioned guilds, and eradicated serfdom. They extended the scope of religious freedom, and they founded new schools and universities. While the government adopted many of the liberal concepts of the Napoleonic law code, poets and educators stirred up a widespread feeling of national pride.

### Russian Campaign (1812)

In order to meet the danger, Napoleon should have strengthened his alliance with Russia. Instead, he antagonized it by insisting on the enforcement of the Continental System. Finally, he decided to break up the alliance. Aware of his aggressive intentions, Russia brought an end to two wars in which it was engaged: one with Sweden over the possession of Finland and another with Ottoman Turkey over territory along the Black Sea coast.

In June 1812, Napoleon ordered a French invasion of Russia. The dramatic war (described in Tolstoy's *War and Peace*) began. The Russians were forced to retreat; after a terrible, but indecisive battle near Borodino, Napoleon entered Moscow. By that time, however, Russia had collected its strength, whereas Napoleon had lost half his army. Beleaguered in the capital city, where shortly after his entry a terrible fire deprived his troops of supplies and shelter, and with winter approaching, Napoleon in vain tendered peace offers to the tsar. A Russian army under the command of General Kutuzov cut off his escape to southern Russia, where he had planned to spend the cold season, and the French were forced to retreat. As a result of severe weather conditions, the disorganization of the French, and the Russian attacks, the retreat became one of the worst military disasters in history.

### Wars of Liberation

Under Prussian leadership, a widespread revolt against the French began almost as soon as the remnants of Napoleon's army reached German soil. Many of the conscripted foreign troops deserted. After numerous defeats and victories, an alliance of Prussian, Austrian, Russian, and Swedish troops defeated

Napoleon decisively in the Battle of Leipzig in October 1813. The French troops were forced to flee back to France.

In the meantime, the combined forces of England, Holland, and Spain had attacked from north and south. In March 1814, an allied army marched triumphantly into Paris. Napoleon abdicated and upon the advice of the wily minister Talleyrand—a man who had already served the Catholic Church, then the revolutionary regime, then the Directorate, then Napoleon, and now his enemies the victors—reinstated the Bourbons. Louis XVI's brother, Louis XVIII, was called back from exile in England; he began to rule as a constitutional monarch under a "Charter." A "Peace of Paris" reestablished France's borders as they had existed in 1792.

### Waterloo (1815)

A reorganization of the European political framework was undertaken in a congress convened in Vienna. Prince Metternich, first minister of Austria, presided; Alexander I of Russia, the Duke of Wellington from England, and Hardenberg of Prussia were the chief figures. Almost all the nations of Europe participated in the splendid meetings. Eventually even Talleyrand, representing the new Bourbon France, was admitted.

Relations among the allies were tense. Austria and England wanted to reduce Russia's commanding power and prestige, whereas Prussia sought the backing of Russia for its numerous territorial wishes. France attempted to divide the victors by promoting the demands of various small nations.

Advised of these dissensions, Napoleon returned to France from exile on the island of Elba. But despite his enthusiastic reception in many places, his arrival was premature. Faced with this renewed threat, the allies composed their differences. At Waterloo (1815), Anglo-Prussian forces under Wellington and Blucher decisively defeated the hastily raised army of Napoleon. Again compelled to abdicate, he was now sent to the lonely, arid island of St. Helena, where he died in 1821.

### Congress of Vienna (1815)

The Congress of Vienna concluded its proceedings in June 1815 with statesmanlike wisdom; the diplomats did not crush defeated France, but reestablished it within the borders it had possessed in 1792. Colonial issues had already been resolved by the two peace treaties in Paris (1814 and 1815). They had given England all it had demanded by way of colonies, including the island of Malta, and had made it heir to the profitable French slave trade. Germany was reconstituted as a loose federation of 38 states with an Austrian as president. Austria, itself, regained and extended its Italian holdings. Prussia annexed large areas in central Germany. Russia seized most of Poland (which was made a kingdom under the tsar) and obtained recognition of its domination over Finland. Sweden, in exchange for Finland, took over Norway, which Denmark, Napoleon's longtime ally, had to relinquish. Holland and Belgium were united into one new state. In general, the congress aimed to restore the old domains to the legitimate rulers of the prewar period or to give them due compensation. A belt of sufficiently powerful nations was drawn around France to deter it from future aggression.

National aspirations, which had been strengthened by the revolutionary spirit, were ignored in favor of an effective balance of power in Europe. At the insistence of Alexander I, the treaties were supplemented by a "Holy Alliance," an international organization intended to guarantee cooperation among the rulers and benevolent treatment of their subjects. This alliance was designed to safeguard both the international arrangements made at Vienna and the existing internal status of the various countries.

## ■ POLITICAL DEVELOPMENTS IN THE AMERICAS

Significantly, before the Napoleonic era had ended, America had begun to play an important part in Western affairs. Napoleon's wars did not involve the Western Hemisphere in the same way as the Seven

Years' War had. Yet, the French revolutionary spirit and Napoleon's conquests had a radical effect on South and Central America. The conquest of Spain and Portugal by Napoleon removed the ruling dynasties, forcing the American colonies to search for a new governmental authority. The Napoleonic wars had an indirect effect on the United States, as Britain was forced to concentrate its attention upon Europe. This gave the United States an opportunity to build its new nation without interference from England.

### North America

At the time the French Revolution began, Washington had just become president of the United States. During his two administrations, steps were undertaken to perfect the system devised by the Constitution. These steps were of considerable importance for all of Western civilization because they dealt with the issue of federalism versus a highly centralized union, state, or empire.

In the United States, a Bill of Rights was introduced into the Constitution by amendment, and a Supreme Court and a national bank were created; these developments involved intense controversies over the desirability of interpreting the Constitution broadly or of adhering to it strictly. The division of opinion divided the country, resulting in the formation of political parties. Despite bitterness and strife under Washington's successors, Adams (elected 1796) and Jefferson (elected 1800), the struggle proved advantageous insofar as the issue of the interpretation of the Constitution was decided. Those who advocated the broader view prevailed, and a tradition of a legal opposition was established. Continued criticism led to progressive improvements.

In its external policy, the United States avoided European entanglements, but it could not escape them entirely. In 1803, the United States of America accepted Napoleon's offer to sell French Louisiana. It thereby not only protected itself against Spain, but also enlarged its territory enormously. It defended its right to unimpeded overseas trade. When forced to it by English blockades and embargo acts, the U.S.A. reasserted its position by entering into a new war against Britain in 1812.

After victories and defeats (the English burned the newly built capital of Washington), a treaty was signed at Ghent in 1814. The peace treaty gave little to either side, but it reaffirmed America's independent statehood. Henceforth, the United States had an opportunity to develop its own resources further and turn its attention to westward expansion. It continued its march across the North American continent and attracted vast numbers of immigrants from European countries in search of economic advancement. It entered a period of "good feeling."

### South America

In South America, the independence movement received new impetus when Napoleon's occupation of Spain and Portugal interrupted their exercise of legal authority over their American colonies. Revolts under inspiring leaders, such as Bolivar, Miranda, Morelos, and San Martin, occurred. By 1811, Venezuela and Paraguay had achieved independence. Mexico followed in 1813, the La Plata region (Argentina, Uruguay, and Paraguay) in 1816, Chile in 1818, and Peru in 1821. Subsequent attempts by the Spanish and Portuguese kings to regain their authority failed, but so did all efforts of the South American nations to form a federation. The individual nations, however, were soon able to influence, first, the economic life and, later, the cultural and political life, of the Western world. Brazil, which also separated from its parent country, played a special role. Brazil, alone, did not become a republic, but in 1822 made Pedro, the son of the last Portuguese regent, an emperor.

## ■ CULTURAL TRENDS

While Napoleon's wars left hatred, destruction, and death in their wake, in other respects they had a permanent and beneficial influence on the progress of civilization. They engendered, especially among France's adversaries, enthusiasm, devotion, and idealism; they also disseminated many of the French *philosophes'* ideas and encouraged people abroad to build institutions promoting concepts of liberty and equality. The introduction of the *Napoleonic Code* in many parts of the Western world is but one example of this fact. The impact of the entire movement of revolution and war was so much deeper since it came at a time when the old political and social order was crumbling and the bourgeoisie, with its economic and progressive attitudes, gained predominance. People's minds were open to new and different ideas concerning politics, society, art, and science.

## Advancements in Pure Science

During the forty years from 1775 to 1815, logical thought and the investigation of nature added many fundamental scientific insights to those gained earlier. These were embodied in a wealth of scholarly treatises of revolutionary character.

### *Chemistry*

In the field of chemistry, the pioneer work of Priestley and Cavendish (d. 1810; studies of hydrogen, ca. 1766) was continued by these same men and by others—Gay-Lussac, Avogadro, and most notably Lavoisier (guillotined 1794). Lavoisier carried on the investigation of oxygen and hydrogen, established the fact that matter may alter its "state" but not its "quantity," studied the connection between oxidation and respiration, and placed chemical nomenclature on a scientific basis. He enunciated the principle of the conservation of mass.

### *Other Sciences*

In biology, the works of the Swiss von Haller and the Frenchman Lamarck (d. 1829) were outstanding. In astronomy, new insights into the structure of the cosmos were introduced. For example, Laplace's (d. 1827) conception of the origin of the planets opened new vistas for the study of the universe. In geology, Saussure (d. 1799) excelled, investigating rivers, mountains, and glaciers. In mathematics, besides Laplace—famous for his development of the calculus—Lagrange (d. 1813) was a leading figure. His special contribution lay in his investigation of geometrical problems.

### *Medicine and Engineering*

In medicine, therapeutic studies were greatly advanced; tissue physiology was investigated; and vaccination was introduced by Jenner (1796). The danger of scurvy was reduced after experience with fresh fruits and vegetables had been gained during Captain Cook's trip around the world. In electricity, Galvani's discovery of animal electricity led to Volta's work (1800) on electrical currents and on the storing of electricity in batteries.

### *Archaeology and History*

In archaeology and history, a new stage was entered with Winckelmann's discoveries and Herder's philosophy of the history of mankind. As for philology, Napoleon's Egyptian campaign had brought the discovery of the so-called "Rosetta stone," which made possible the deciphering of the ancient Egyptian Hieroglyphic language.

## Advancements in Technology

Technological innovations made possible the rapid transition to an industrial society. In 1807, a successful steamship was operated in America. In 1814, Stephenson's locomotive was constructed in England. Balloons to carry human beings aloft were designed and used. Numerous improvements were introduced in two basic industries: mining and textiles. The use of interchangeable machine parts spread and made possible cheaper, more efficient production. Agricultural yields rose with growing understanding of nature and with the use of machinery. The production of iron and steel increased in importance.

Britain took the lead in technological advancement. Its colonial empire, greatly expanded by new territories in South Africa and India, not only made industries possible, but also necessitated their expansion and modernization. This growth of industrial capacity enabled Britain to export goods to independent states as well as its possessions. Both European and American nations came to depend upon British machinery.

The English working population endured numerous adverse consequences of these technical advances, suffering grievously through unemployment and low wages. The government was slow to extend protection to the workers. The "classical" economists of the age, in line with Adam Smith's laissez-faire policies, believed that through free play of economic forces, adjustments would come by themselves; and they hoped with Jeremy Bentham (d. 1832), who adhered to "Utilitarianism," with its accent on practical aims, that the "greatest good for the greatest number" would eventually result.

### Religious Liberalism and Mysticism
The utilitarian spirit, prevailing in economic thoughts and mechanistic trends, generated a reaction that was strengthened by the miseries accompanying revolution, war, and industrialization. This reaction expressed itself in a religious revival that took two different directions. On one hand, it led to a liberal interpretation of Christian doctrine, with emphasis on love for all and tolerance. (Schleiermacher [d. 1834] in Berlin was to lead this movement toward religious liberalism.) On the other hand, a revival of mysticism took place, an inner rejection of the evils of the world and its self-assured knowledge. With this revival came a search for direct communion with God. Numerous groups expressed such feelings; typical was the Russian Baroness Krüdener, who sponsored a revivalist movement; her influence helped bring about the formation of the Holy Alliance by Alexander I. Simultaneously, there was a renaissance within traditional churches. In their search for guidance away from the materialistic path on which scientific knowledge seemed to lead, many people turned to Catholicism.

### Philosophy
Philosophy was another field upon which the growing scientific and utilitarian spirit continued to leave a deep impression. Toward the end of the eighteenth century, belief in the unlimited possibilities of human understanding was badly shaken; so also was belief in the perfectibility of the human race. Philosophers came to recognize that there are limits to human knowledge and that scientific laws are inadequate to explain our ethical and spiritual nature.

### *Kant*
It was the achievement of Kant (d. 1804; *Critique of Pure Reason*) to propose a philosophical system that embraced both an understanding of physical science and a recognition of the human moral instinct. Kant held that physical science gives a dependable knowledge of nature and its workings, but that moral law—an inner voice of duty—gives the human race a unique role in the material universe. This moral law, like that of nature, touches our rational nature, leading us to a sense of fellowship with all others. "Freedom," he insisted, "is a condition necessary for the full development of human rationality and ethical behavior."

At least three great compatriots of Kant built on similar foundations: Fichte (d. 1814), Schelling (d. 1854), and Hegel (d. 1831). Like Kant, all three were heirs of the Enlightenment; all emphasized the need for freedom. Hegel postulated freedom as the ultimate aim of history, in the pursuit of which God's will expresses itself.

## Music

The powerful forces of rational investigation did not dim the love of beauty and the spirit of imagination, fantasy, and vision that mark so many of the greatest achievements in art. Especially in music, some of the most beautiful works in world history were created. Germany continued, after the death of Bach, to be the center of European musical life. The great musicians of the time overcame the conventions, routine, artificiality, and constraints that the taste of the aristocrats, who sponsored many of the composers, required. For these patrons, music, to the extent to which it was not Church music, was often no more than an ornament at their social gatherings—and mere virtuosity was much applauded. But though abandoning to a certain extent the contrapuntal style of Bach, the good composers continued his work and gave expression to the deepest emotions and human feelings. Building on precedents that can be traced through the earlier baroque period, they devoted themselves to creating masterpieces for the piano (which thus gained new importance) and to producing symphonies and string quartets that stirred a new generation while retaining their appeal for all future ages. Haydn (d. 1809) was not only one of the most famous composers *(Creation, Te Deum),* but also a gifted teacher. He and his somewhat older contemporary, Gluck (d. 1787; *Alceste, Iphigenie en Tauride),* were in fact the most outstanding teachers since Bach and Handel. Gluck emphasized that "music is not just an art that pleases the ear, but one of the greatest means to touch the heart and arouse passion." The era's musical apex was reached with Mozart and Beethoven and their sonatas, symphonies, quartets and quintets, and requiem masses—and their operas: Mozart's (d. 1791) *Don Giovanni, Magic Flute,* and *Marriage of Figaro,* and Beethoven's (d. 1827) *Fidelio*.

Thus, the musical world entered its own "Classical Age." Verbal descriptions cannot convey a sense of the inspired works of these great composers or even those of the many lesser ones. With the death of Beethoven, the last of the group, the Classical Age came to an end. In his later years, indeed, Beethoven himself introduced a new period—that of Romanticism.

## Painting, Architecture, and Sculpture

Far less meaningful for future generations were the works in the fine arts created during the Revolutionary and Napoleonic periods. Perhaps there was an absence of artists of true genius, or perhaps painting, architecture, and sculpture were not so well suited to express the spirit of the age; in any case, little of great renown was brought forth in these areas. The Frenchman David (d. 1825) is practically the only painter worth mentioning—aside from the strange and very modern genius of the Spaniard Goya (d. 1828). Goya's portrayals of the Spanish war against France endure as a realistic and gripping monument to the horrors of a time that prided itself on its idealism.

Nor was any high achievement shown in architecture and sculpture; these arts were rather influenced by neoclassicism, i.e., an imitation of classical models. With its simple, restrained lines and its clarity and dignity of style, neoclassicism was received as a welcome relief from baroque and rococo, even if its design lacked original, creative thought.

## Literature

In contrast to the fine arts, literature provided an adequate and influential means of expression for the age. It came to a particularly high development in Germany. While Germany was politically and industrially backward, it produced in the late eighteenth and early nineteenth centuries some of the greatest writers of the modern age in literature—to complement its leaders in music and philosophy. The period from 1760 to 1800 is regarded as Germany's "Classical Age of Literature," which then was followed by Germany's "Romantic Age."

### Classicism

The two great figures in Germany's Classical Age, following Lessing, were Goethe (1749–1832) and Schiller (1759–1805). They expressed in classical form the eternal human longings for freedom and self-expression. Their works (Goethe's lyrics, *Sorrows of Werther, Goetz, Wilhelm Meister,* and *Faust* and Schiller's ballads, *The Robbers, Wallenstein,* and *Wilhelm Tell*) have been translated into many languages and have remained a source of inspiration.

### Romanticism

Goethe and Schiller were followed by a long line of Romantic poets. "Romanticism" represents one aspect of the reaction against the artificiality and rationalism of earlier ages. The word is a much-abused term for one of the most meaningful developments in Western culture. Although Romanticism's sentimentality and vagueness were to antagonize later generations, its love of nature and of human beings in their noble aspirations, its search for inwardness, its sensitivity to beauty, and its youthful ardor and imagination were to remain ever-inspiring. It placed the accent of life on the worth of the individual.

The English Romantic movement was highlighted by the poems of Wordsworth, Coleridge, Byron, Shelley, and Keats. Of these English poets, Byron was probably the most widely read, even in Russia. His reputation was enhanced by his devotion to the cause of Greek liberty and by his early death.

German Romanticism inherited artistic restraint and clarity of expression from the preceding Classical Age. Among its most famous representatives were Kleist, Eichendorff, Morike, who wrote beautiful lyrics and short stories, and E. T. A. Hoffmann, famous for his tales. Italy, France, and Russia, too, had their periods of Romanticism, the Frenchman Chateaubriand being regarded as one of the founders of the Romantic Movement.

The ideal of freedom was extolled everywhere; imagination and sentiment, sometimes pervaded by mystic beliefs, fired poetic fantasy. The Romantic writers found a special source to draw upon, little considered in the past, in the stories and folk tales that had lived on in the oral traditions of the various nations and to which Herder, in particular, had drawn attention—calling to mind the long-buried treasures of the Slavic world. Folklore thus became one of the chief fountains of inspiration, not only for poets, but also for philologists, historians, social critics, and educators. Similarly, the Roman Catholic world of the Middle Ages captivated the emotions of many and, in turn, affected the religious trends of the age.

## ■ CULTURAL CROSSROADS: GOETHE'S FAUST

At this turning point in the history of modern times—a point when Western civilization appeared to stand on the threshold of change toward new horizons—stands Goethe's majestic two-part dramatic poem, *Faust*. Just as Dante's *Divina Commedia* came at the highest point of the Middle Ages and on the eve of the Renaissance, Goethe's *Faust* was written at a time of cultural transition. Goethe was a man of action, as well as of thought, a scientist and philosopher, a statesman and prime minister, an artist and a poet. In *Faust,* he sums up the spirit of the Modern Age and expresses its aspirations. The protagonist, Faust does not adhere to formulated human or divine creed, but is an eternal seeker of truth. Disappointed by years of study, including the black art of magic, Faust makes a compact with Mephistopheles that stipulates that he must surrender his soul to the devil if ever he becomes satisfied—if ever he becomes ready to confess that he has achieved what he has been striving after. Mephistopheles tries Faust with pleasures, carnal love, wealth, classical perfection, and worldly power. But not until Faust is old and blind does he discern his goal: creative work, the winning of new life for a new and free people. This goal, of course, will never really be attained; it remains an ideal for which to strive. Thus in *Faust* is summarized the spirit of the modern world—eternally dissatisfied, eternally seeking, eternally striving, and through creative endeavor, eternally aspiring toward new horizons.

## Perspective

The Napoleonic Era was one of incessant warfare. Having risen through military exploits to a virtual dictatorship as emperor of the French, Napoleon made an attempt at dominating all of Europe. In the process, the European state system was altered and many of the ideas of the French Revolution gained wide acceptance. But Napoleon's attempt at domination failed when his invasion of Russia ended in disaster. He was ultimately banished to a small Atlantic island, St. Helena, where he died.

The American countries stayed out of the European wars, and ultimately benefited from them. In South America, the colonies seized the opportunity to begin wars of independence. In North America, the newly independent United States completed its liberation from Britain. It also began to build its own republican institutions, many of which were in harmony with the ideals of the French Revolution.

Some of the greatest accomplishments of the Napoleonic Era took place in cultural fields such as science, mathematics, archaeology, philosophy, music, and literature.

## Selected Readings

Hudson, Pat. *The Industrial Revolution* (London: E. Arnold, 1992).

Stearns, Peter and Hinshaw, John. *The ABC-CLIO World History Companion to the Industrial Revolution.* (St. Barbara, CA: ABC-CLIO, 1996).

Johnston, R. M., ed., *The Corsican: A Diary of Napoleon's Life in His Own Words* (Boston: Houghton Mifflin, 1910).

Dukes, Paul. *A History of Europe, 1648–1948* (1985).

Grout, Donald J., and Palisca, Claude V. *A History of Western Music* (New York: Norton, 1988).

Lefebvre, Georges. *Napoleon.* 2 vols. (New York: Routledge and K. Paul, 1969).

Cronin, Vincent. *Napoleon Bonaparte* (New York: Morrow, 1972).

Morison, Samuel E. *The Oxford History of the American People*. 3 vols. (Oxford: Oxford University Press, 1972).

### Test Yourself

1. Based on Roman law, the Code Napoleon featured _____.
   A. Equality before the law
   B. The right to own property
   C. Advance in women's rights
   D. Both A and B

2. The French naval force was destroyed in 1805 by Admiral Nelson's fleet at the battle of_____.
   A. Tordesillas
   B. The Nile
   C. Trafalgar
   D. Waterloo

3. In 1812, Napoleon ordered an invasion of Russia, a war best described in the novel *War and Peace* by the Russian writer _____.
   A. Chekov
   B. Godonev
   C. Voltaire
   D. Tolstoy

4. At the Battle of Waterloo in 1815, Napoleon was defeated and exiled to the island of_____.
   A. St. Helena
   B. Elba
   C. Corsica
   D. Sardinia

5. In 1803 the United States accepted Napoleon's offer to sell_____.
   A. Canada
   B. Florida
   C. Louisiana
   D. Haiti

6. Kant brilliantly proposed a philosophical system that embraced both an understanding of physical science and recognition of the human moral instinct in a work titled_____.
   A. *A Critique of Pure Reason*
   B. *The Natural Philosophy of Mathematics*
   C. *The Social Contract*
   D. *On the Origin of Species*

7. The two great figures in Germany's classical literature following Lessing were_____.
   A. Goethe and Schiller
   B. Faust and Stiller
   C. Schmidt and Kleist
   D. Morike and Kant

8. Napoleon's Egyptian campaign brought about a revolution in the deciphering of ancient Egyptian hieroglyphs by the discovery of the so-called_____.
   A. Napoleon's Code
   B. The Philosopher's Stone
   C. The Rosetta stone
   D. The Blarney Stone

## Answers and Explanations

1. **D.** Highly beneficial legal reforms were initiated under the *Code Napoleon*. Based on Roman law, the *Code* embodied many of the liberal, equalitarian, and humanitarian concepts for which the revolution had been fought. It became a model for the Western world. It provided for equality before the law and confirmed the inviolability of property rights. But it deprived women of the gains secured by them during the revolution.

2. **C.** An attack on England was contemplated, but invasion plans were abandoned after the French naval forces had been destroyed (in 1805) by Admiral Nelson's fleet at the Battle of Trafalgar.

3. **D.** In June 1812, Napoleon ordered a French invasion of Russia. The dramatic war (described in Tolstoy's *War and Peace*) began.

4. **A.** At Waterloo (1815), Anglo-Prussian forces under Wellington and Blucher decisively defeated the hastily raised army of Napoleon. Again compelled to abdicate, he was now sent to the lonely, arid island of St. Helena, where he died in 1821.

5. **C.** In its external policy, the United States avoided European entanglements, but it could not escape them entirely. In 1803, the United States of America accepted Napoleon's offer to sell French Louisiana. It thereby not only protected itself against Spain, but also enlarged its territory enormously. It defended its right to unimpeded overseas trade. When forced to it by English blockades and embargo acts, the U.S.A. reasserted its position by entering into a new war against Britain.

6. **A.** It was the achievement of Kant (d. 1804; *Critique of Pure Reason*) to propose a philosophical system that embraced both an understanding of physical science and a recognition of the human moral instinct. Kant held that physical science gives a dependable knowledge of nature and its workings, but that moral law—an inner voice of duty—gives the human race a unique role in the material universe. This moral law, like that of nature, touches our rational nature, leads us to a sense of fellowship with all others. "Freedom," he insisted, "is a condition necessary for the full development of human rationality and ethical behavior."

7. **A.** The two great figures in Germany's Classical Age, following Lessing, were Goethe (1749–1832) and Schiller (1759–1805). They expressed in classical form eternal human longings for freedom and self-expression. Their works (Goethe's lyrics, *Sorrows of Werther, Goetz, Wilhelm Meister,* and *Faust* and Schiller's ballads, *The Robbers, Wallenstein,* and *Wilhelm Tell*) have been translated into many languages and have remained a source of inspiration ever since.

8. **C.** In archaeology and history, a new stage was entered with Winckelmann's discoveries and Herder's philosophy of the history of mankind. As for philology, Napoleon's Egyptian campaign had brought the discovery of the so-called "Rosetta stone," which made possible the deciphering of the ancient Egyptian Hieroglyphic language.

# CHAPTER 12
# Nationalism, Liberalism, Industrialism (1815-1830)

**1818** Chile and La Plata region declare independence from Spain
Congress of Aachen
**1819** Carlsbad decrees
Bolivar founds Republic of Gran Columbia
**1820** Revolutions in Italy: Congress of Troppau
Scott, *Ivanhoe*
Missouri Compromise
**1821** Weber, *Freischutz*
**1822** Congress of Verona
Independence of Brazil
**1823** Monroe Doctrine
**1824** Beethoven, *Ninth Symphony*
Hegel, lectures on *Philosophy of History*
**1825** Robert Owen's establishment of New Harmony, Indiana
Dekabrist revolt in Russia
**1827** Battle of Navarino
Heine, *Book of Songs*
Schubert, *Trout Quintet*
**1829** Peace of Adrianople
Catholic Emancipation Act in England
**1830** Greek independence declared
France seizes Algeria
July Revolution in France
Victor Hugo, *Hernani* premier in Paris

*Wars may not alter the course of events, but often tend to slow or accelerate changes already in progress. Despite the reactionary tenor of the Congress of Vienna, the Napoleonic Wars accelerated certain Western trends. For centuries, steady advances had been made toward the formation of national states. Now, the process was speeded up. The "Age of Nationalism" was at hand, and with it an age of "Liberalism" and "Industrialism."*

*Nationalism had been gradually developing within Western civilization since the end of the Middle Ages. An otherworldly orientation and the concept of an all-controlling Church had been giving way to wider, worldly interests. Gradually, the ideal of a united Christendom had become subordinated to the particular needs and ambitions of individual nations. Nationalism was based on the conviction that peoples with a common language, history, tradition, and attitude toward life should be united into single independent states. To such a state, all members should show their supreme loyalty.*

*Liberalism, which was usually coupled with 19th-century nationalism, was not only reflected in an attitude toward life but in a political and economic program as well. It aspired to guarantee the personal and political freedom of individuals and protect their human rights. It envisioned equal justice for all, a constitutional government, and the free development of all members of society according to their natural gifts and education, regardless of birth. Its main creed was embodied in the "Rights of Man" of the French Revolution.*

*Industrialism was a correlative of liberal thought. The right to private property was one of liberalism's chief tenets. Therefore, liberalism favored the growth of capitalism. Capitalism, in turn, provided for the economic exploitation of the scientific discoveries of the past; it made possible the new production methods that eventually came to characterize all Western civilization. The machine replaced the work of the craftsman. An "Age of Industrialism" led to fundamental sociological changes, encompassing moral as well as material, and possibly even biological, aspects of Western civilization.*

*Nationalism, liberalism, and industrialism were viewed with disfavor by conservative groups of the populations: the royalty, many members of the clergy, and the landed aristocracy. National aspirations, liberal views, and industrial production methods were, however, promoted by a young generation—heirs to the Enlightenment, who believed in "progress." They comprised idealists from many camps, especially professors and students, men and women, professionals and businessmen who had steadily gained in economic weight and intellectual leadership without gaining proportionately in political influence.*

## ■ PERIOD OF CONGRESSES (1818-1823)

The leading statesmen of 1815 were mainly conservatives. Having rearranged the political world at Vienna, they now sought the preservation of their product. Afraid of further change, they devised at Vienna a system of international consultation that was to be used whenever a challenge arose.

### Congress of Aachen (1818)

The first opportunity to apply this system arose when France asked to be relieved of various burdens put upon it after its defeat in the Napoleonic Wars. This issue was successfully resolved because some of the victorious nations desired an early restitution of French power to balance that of Russia. The statesmen met in a congress at Aachen (Aix-la-Chapelle) and agreed to end the occupation of France and to reduce its war indemnity. They refused, however, to settle other issues ardently advocated by the liberal bourgeoisie, such as the abolition of the slave trade and the widening of international cooperation.

### Congress of Carlsbad (1819)

The following year witnessed a second occasion for international consultation. Liberal agitation increased, especially in the German states, where university students demanded constitutional government and longed for a united nation. In order to prevent the spread of such ideas, which would have undermined the domination of Austria, Metternich called a congress at Carlsbad. Suppressive measures were taken. Censorship of newspapers and books was established in many German states, and restrictions were imposed upon universities.

### Congress of Troppau-Laibach (1820–1821)

Repression could not stop the growth of national and liberal sentiments. They showed themselves everywhere—in Italy, Spain, Portugal, Greece, and Latin America. Particularly threatening to the existing system were rebellious outbreaks in Austria's Italian provinces. A new congress was held in Troppau, Austria, and later continued in Laibach. Metternich succeeded in winning Tsar Alexander's support; under the banner of the "sacredness and inviolability of treaties," the two insisted on strict maintenance of the status quo.

In the meantime however, differences of opinion and interests, both among nations and within each nation, had increased. Britain, in particular, saw its advantage in a relaxation of the Viennese system. It refused to cooperate in the planned military action. In consequence, it had to be undertaken by Austria alone. A second issue jeopardizing the peace settlements, the Greek struggle for independence from the Ottoman Turks, did not lead to better cooperation. (Condemned in principle, Grecian independence nevertheless found support from both Russia and England, who were eager to reduce Turkish power.) Similarly, an accord was not reached in matters regarding overseas revolts in Latin America.

### Congress of (1820–1821)

The next and last congress was held at Verona; it concerned the national Verona (1822) movements in Greece, Spain, and Latin America. The Greek issue led to the same dissensions as those of the previous year, and no international action was taken.

### Spain

As to Spain, the old monarchy, which had been reestablished after the war, was overthrown in a bitter rebellion; the liberal constitution of 1812 was reintroduced. Fearful for its own political system, France, which had been readmitted to the council of nations, protested and demanded armed intervention. Again, England refused to participate in a military venture. France was left to act alone. It proceeded to subdue the Spanish forces and to restore the reactionary government of the king.

### Latin America

With regard to Latin America, Britain continued to be at odds with the Continental powers. It saw an important prospective market in autonomous Latin American republics and wished to prevent the interference of other European powers. It therefore addressed itself to the United States. However, the United States independently issued the "Monroe Doctrine" in 1823. Thereby all attempts by the Congress of Verona to arrange matters in Spain's former colonies and to forestall the extension of the liberal-led national revolt there were blocked. European collaboration came to an end.

### Results

The Holy Alliance and the congresses constituted an attempt at international organization and cooperation in line with objectives largely generated by all-encompassing wars. The attempts of 1815 to 1823 generated little results; some of the victors used the new organization to prevent change. It is likely that the congresses were an offense to the moral conscience of Europe. England's foreign minister, George Canning, had already rejected the concepts of morality as an unfit guide for national policies, even if, as he cynically added, "they justly immortalize the hero." National self-interest was extolled everywhere. A measure of international anarchy came to prevail that had been unknown to past centuries, during which time it had been prevented by common dynastic principles, interests and connections.

## ■ CONSERVATISM VERSUS LIBERALISM (1815-1830)

Once the unrest of the postwar period had been calmed, conservatism triumphed in most parts of Europe. Not only in Russia, but also in Austria, Prussia, England, and Spain, movements were suppressed for extensions of civil rights and freedoms. France, for a time, followed a more moderate path, but eventually it too reverted to conservative views. The United States, alone among the Western countries, continued to build upon the foundation of liberal principles.

Yet, liberalism continued to gain ground among the educated classes in Europe. New disturbances affected the internal political conditions in the various European countries and upset the international order, which was now under the firm control of conservative statesmen. Within little more than a decade, liberal aspirations once again led to revolution.

### France

In France, King Louis XVIII ruled from 1815 to 1824. While holding extremists in check, he followed a conservative path in line with the Charter imposed on France. This Charter provided for monarchical rule, limited by certain legislative powers vested in an assembly. The assembly was elected by the landowners and upper-middle class, constituting about four percent of the population—the small well-to-do sector of the French people. The usefulness of such a system was extolled by writers like Joseph de Maistre in France and Edmund Burke in England. The very introduction of a Charter indicated a break with Bourbon absolutism and Napoleonic dictatorship. It permitted a beginning of popular participation in government. The Charter protected civil rights; the *Napoleonic Code* was retained along with other reforms.

The principles for which Charter and Code stood were, however, abandoned when Louis XVIII died and his brother, Charles X, succeeded him. Charles attempted to secure for his friends, the old *émigrés* of the revolution, an enormous sum to compensate them for the loss of lands. He sought to restore former Church privileges; he offended the spirit of the times by exacting the death penalty for thefts of sacred objects. He suppressed public opinion and imposed a stamp tax and other restrictive measures upon newspapers. In personal conduct, he displayed pre-Revolutionary royal splendor. Simultaneously, he tried to divert the attention of his people from his internal policies by catering to their longing for glory; he engaged in a new military venture—an expedition for the conquest of Algiers. His ill-conceived policies brought about the breakdown of his own regime.

### Central Europe

In Italy and most of the Germanic states, Metternich's conservatism dominated. However, in three German states—one of them the small principality of Saxe-Weimar, where Goethe had been prime minister—no constitution was developed. The *Code Napoleon,* with its liberal spirit, was not retained. In essence, government was administered in accordance with principles of enlightened despotism. This conservative trend brought conflict with the liberals. In Italy, a number of secret societies were founded, like the *Carbonari,* which supported the liberal cause. In Germany, a comparable liberal movement led to unrest among students and to the formation of *Burschenschaften* (fraternities) and other liberal societies. The Italian movement attracted some outstanding leaders; among them were the writers Manzoni and Gioberti, as well as the famous politician Mazzini. In Germany, idealistic thinkers joined the cause—the great scientist Humboldt, the philosopher Fichte, the statesman vom Stein, the poet Arndt, the Brothers Grimm, and many others.

However, liberal hopes in Italy were undermined when attempts at revolution failed in 1820 and 1821. Thereafter, justice favored the old privileged class once again. Clericalism was supported anew; scientific education was hindered; and censorship controlled public opinion. Foreign domination remained.

In Germany, also, the liberal forces proved too weak. In 1817, students organized a festival on the Wartburg, where revolutionary speeches were made. In 1819, a liberal murdered a poet, von Kotzebue, who was accused of spying for Russia. This event spurred Metternich to call the Congress of Carlsbad; its decrees and repressive police measures put a stop to the agitation and initiated a calm period of firm conservative rule.

## England

Similar conservatism marked English policies, with the leaders convinced that a small group of aristocrats should govern the ordinary people. The royal court system was outdated and dissolute. The office of prime minister from 1815 to 1830 was in the hands of the Tory party, which dominated in Parliament and passed little progressive legislation. The right to vote was even more restricted than in France. Modernization of agriculture was neglected; the common fields were almost entirely enclosed; and freeholders constantly diminished in number. Corn Laws were passed and provided for protective tariffs on grain imports; they benefited the few rich landlords.

Little was done for the impoverished. A severe business crisis, following the war period, brought unemployment. When worker uprisings occurred, the government resorted to suspension of the *habeas corpus* in 1817, and in one instance in 1819, to bloody suppression. A stamp tax and censorship were introduced. Public mass meetings were forbidden. Little understanding was shown for the fact that while Britain grew rich—London inherited the position of financial center of the world, formerly held by Amsterdam—and while the Midlands became "the workshop of the world," the workers and the lower bourgeoisie reaped meager benefits.

Only slowly, with improvement in business in the early 1820s, did a countermovement appear within the Tory party itself. So-called "liberal Tories," like Sir Robert Peel and George Canning, gained influence. Owing to their endeavors, penalties for political offenses were eased, and the police system made more lenient. Tariffs were reduced, and trade policies were liberalized. The currency was stabilized through the introduction of the gold standard. Attempts to pass labor legislation were initiated. In 1828 and 1829, laws were passed that accorded long-withheld political emancipation to dissenters and Catholics in England. But more far-reaching liberal legislation had to await, in England as elsewhere, the impetus of the French "July Revolution" of 1830.

## Russia

Despite the reputation for liberalism, which the Russian tsar, Alexander I, had acquired in his youth, reaction proved to be the strongest political force in Russia. Liberal tendencies, which could threaten existing autocratic institutions, were crushed. Nationalistic aspirations, which caused unrest among subjugated nationalities like the Poles, were forcefully combated.

Early in Alexander's rule, his confidant, the minister Speransky, had proposed a reform program: consultative assemblies on the national level, a measure of local self-government, gradual reduction of serfdom, and lessening of class distinctions. After the Napoleonic Wars, plans were made for modernization of agriculture and industry. But the lack of qualified administrators and increasing corruption, along with Alexander's conservative leaning, hindered this reform effort. Few improvements were undertaken in the educational system, the law courts, or the provincial administration. Serfs remained in bondage except on the estates of the German Balts, who were more progressive than the Russian landholders and who foresaw the economic advantage of emancipation. The constitution and autonomy granted to the Poles were often violated. Universities were founded, but their work was subjected to police supervision. Obscurantism prevailed.

Additional bondage was introduced through the establishment of military colonies. The unhappy inhabitants of areas set aside for these colonies became permanent soldiers. Together with their families, they were subjected, even during peacetime agricultural work, to the absolute command of the military authorities. They received material care throughout their lives, but they lost all individual rights.

As a result, when Alexander died in December (Russian *Dekabr*) 1825, a revolt broke out. This "Dekabrist" revolt, initiated to bring freedom and constitutional government to Russian lands and led by idealistic, liberal young officers (most of them from the nobility), was put down with extreme brutality. From then on, the new tsar, Nicholas I, combated all liberal leanings. Again, Russia was insulated from Western influences. The old autocracy imposed its despotism anew.

## The United States

While liberal political and economic ideas between 1815 and 1830 were largely rejected by the governments of Europe, and all but disappearing in Russia, they were gaining ground in the United States.

Democratic institutions were strengthened. Voting privileges were consistently extended; educational opportunities were broadened. Upon becoming president in 1829, Andrew Jackson declared that, unlike his predecessors, he would emphasize fulfillment of the needs of ordinary citizens. With this aim, he attacked the existing banking system, which he reformed; an independent treasury was created. He even opposed the courts. He surrounded himself with new men—political supporters who would replace political adversaries holding influential and lucrative offices. The resulting "spoils system" came into political practice.

Aside from these changes in political arrangements, a number of issues had to be dealt with which were unknown to other countries in the Western world. Some of them arose from the fact that in the United States (as in Russia), farmers had the opportunity to cultivate wide areas of sparsely settled territory, an opportunity not available to those living in narrowly confined European nations, where the peasants practiced intensive cultivation out of necessity. Westward expansion at the expense of the American Indians became one of the most pressing issues. The Eastern tribes, already decimated in battles they had waged to defend their lands, were deprived of their possessions, expelled from their territories, and driven mercilessly beyond the Mississippi River. Their lands were then cleared of forests and given to pioneers, who prepared them for agriculture. Cities were built and irrigation projects started. Canals were dug. Settlers continued westward migration, and resultant population shifts brought new political problems.

Just as agriculture and expansion multiplied problems, so did industrial growth. The United States government introduced protective tariffs—a measure that ran counter to liberal European economic theory. In addition, the government had to deal with the problem of immigration. This led to heated debates over preferential treatment and admittance of immigrants, who were expected to assimilate and integrate as Americans.

Furthermore, the question of slavery invited intense debates. It brought bitter strife and was settled only temporarily in 1820 by the Missouri Compromise, which delineated the areas in which it was legal to own slaves. Finally, there was the issue of the validity of federal legislation in states that objected to the laws. Many of these states assumed "nullification" rights upon federal acts. The struggle, which at the time involved preservation of the Union, centered on the imposition of tariffs. It was, likewise, only precariously settled in 1832.

The internal problems of the United States, exacerbated by its geography and political origin, forced it to follow a course in many respects radically different from that dominating the rest of Western civilization.

## ■ REVOLUTION

In 1830, whatever hopes conservatives may have entertained about preserving the status quo in the face of concessions which, especially in England, had been forced upon them was shattered when a new revolution broke out in France. It was at first feared that this would lead to an upheaval comparable to that of 1789; perhaps this fear contributed to the quick surrender of the French king. But in its course, the revolutionary movement did not again overturn society; instead, it was stopped in its early stages. Further, the instigators had never envisioned more than the restitution of those liberal principles on which the post-Napoleonic settlement had been based.

## July Revolution (1830)

The July Revolution was brought about by the shortsightedness of Charles X, who violated the Charter and ignored petitions asking him to respect it. Finally, he issued "four ordinances," whereby the electoral law was arbitrarily changed to the exclusive advantage of the landowners. New elections were decreed, and the freedom of the press was further curtailed. On July 27, 1830, the printers went on strike, and barricades were put up in the streets of Paris. King Charles X quickly fled. The moderate royalist forces, under the veteran leadership of Talleyrand and Lafayette, succeeded in preventing bloodshed. They deposed Charles and accepted his cousin, Louis Philippe, prince of Orleans, as a suitable successor to the throne.

Louis Philippe had always boasted of his liberalism; he was proud of his "bourgeois" ways; and he could be expected to respect the Charter. The "four ordinances" were revoked; censorship was abolished. By the lowering of voting qualifications, the electorate was approximately doubled. The citizens' National Guard, formed to counterbalance the regular armed forces controlled by the king, was reorganized to ensure the gains of the revolution. The reforms satisfied the upper bourgeoisie; sporadic further revolts by the lower classes (still poor and weak) were ruthlessly suppressed.

## Repercussions in Western Europe

The July outbreaks in Paris set off revolts in various parts of Europe. The neighboring Belgians, ever dissatisfied with the Vienna arrangement that had forced them into a union with Holland, rebelled. They clamored for constitutional government and national independence. Within a decade, Belgium was established as an independent state. Disturbances occurred in Switzerland and Italy, some of them successful in bringing about more liberal laws. In Germany, a number of princes hurried to grant their peoples long-promised constitutions. The German unification movement, advocated by liberal and national groups, made some progress, at least in the economic sphere. Under Prussian leadership, *a Zollverein,* a customs union that had been created earlier, was broadened to include almost all the states of northern Germany. It facilitated the extension of the railway system and greatly served industrialization. In Britain, after fifty years of Tory rule, a Whig cabinet took over in 1830. Under Earl Grey, energetic work was started to reform the electoral laws. In 1832, though not without meeting violent resistance, a first "Reform Bill" was passed. It abolished "rotten boroughs" (electoral districts which, though depopulated, had still enjoyed the traditional right of representation in Parliament) and created new electoral districts in urban areas. It thus broke the monopoly of the landowning nobility, with its medieval privileges, just as the Catholic Emancipation Act had broken that of the Anglican Church. It made room for broader representation of the bourgeoisie. While the industrial proletariat gained nothing, and the composition of Parliament was not promptly changed, the First Reform Bill paved the way for future reforms.

## Repercussions in Eastern Europe

The July Revolution indirectly helped the Greeks. Since 1819, they had struggled against the Turkish sultan. England and Russia had given them aid and in 1827 had destroyed the Ottoman Turkish fleet at Navarino. Russia had continued the war until it could impose the Peace of Adrianople. With the Ottoman Turks defeated and the liberal national movement invigorated by the July Revolution, Greece's claim to independent statehood was recognized. In 1832, the new nation was established.

In addition, it was only in Russia that the July Revolution failed to have a tangible effect. There, the bourgeois class was too weak; the universities were too small and too firmly controlled. Ever since the Dekabrist uprising, the autocratic government had been alert to any revolutionary action. The July

Figure 12–1 Post-Napoleon Europe, 1815

7. Under the reign of Tsar Nicolas I in Russia_____.
   A. Liberals lost ground
   B. Conservatives gained power
   C. The old autocracy imposed its despotism
   D. All of the above

8. The Independence of Greece from the grip of the Ottoman Empire was officially established in_____.
   A. 1830
   B. 1832
   C. 1864
   D. 1820

## Answers and Explanations

1. **D.** The first opportunity to apply this system arose when France asked to be relieved of various burdens put upon it after its defeat in the Napoleonic Wars. This issue was successfully resolved because some of the victorious nations desired an early restitution of French power to balance that of Russia. The statesmen met in a congress at Aachen (Aix-la-Chapelle) and agreed to end the occupation of France and to reduce its war indemnity. They refused, however, to settle other issues ardently advocated by the liberal bourgeoisie, such as the abolition of the slave trade and the widening of international cooperation.

2. **C.** The United States independently issued the "Monroe Doctrine," in 1823, which prohibited the interference of European Powers in the Americas. Thereby all attempts by the Congress of Verona to arrange matters in Spain's former colonies and to forestall the extension of the liberal-national revolt there were blocked. European collaboration came to an end.

3. **A.** In France, King Louis XVIII ruled from 1815 to 1824. While holding extremists in check, he followed a conservative path in line with the Charter imposed on France. This Charter provided for monarchical rule, limited by certain legislative powers vested in an assembly.

4. **B.** The office of prime minister from 1815 to 1830 was in the hands of the Tory party, which dominated in Parliament and passed little progressive legislation. The right to vote was even more restricted than in France.

5. **A.** Upon becoming president in 1829, Andrew Jackson declared that, unlike his predecessors, he would emphasize fulfillment of the needs of ordinary citizens. With this aim, he attacked the existing banking system, which he reformed; an independent Treasury was created. He even opposed the courts. He surrounded himself with new men—political supporters who would replace political adversaries holding influential and lucrative offices. The resulting "spoils system" came into political practice.

6. **B.** The question of slavery invited intense debates. It brought bitter strife and was settled only temporarily by the Missouri Compromise in 1820, which delineated the areas in which it was legal to own slaves. Finally, there was the issue of the validity of federal legislation in states that objected to the laws and therefore assumed "nullification" rights upon federal acts.

7. **D.** When Tsar Alexander died in December (Russian *Dekabr*) 1825, a revolt broke out. This "Dekabrist" revolt, initiated to bring freedom and constitutional government to Russian lands and led by idealistic, liberal young officers (most of them from the nobility), was put down with extreme brutality. From then on, the new tsar, Nicholas I, combated all liberal leanings. Again, Russia was insulated from Western influences. The old autocracy imposed its despotism anew.

8. **B.** The July Revolution indirectly helped the Greeks. Since 1819, they had struggled against the Turkish sultan. England and Russia had given them aid and had destroyed the Ottoman Turkish fleet at Navarino in 1827. Russia had continued the war until it could impose the Peace of Adrianople. With the Ottoman Turks defeated and the liberal national movement invigorated by the July Revolution, Greece's claim to independent statehood was recognized. In 1832, the new nation was established.

# CHAPTER 13

# Society, Arts, and Sciences (1815-1848)

**1819** Sir Walter Scott, *Ivanhoe*
**1831** Victor Hugo, *The Hunchback of Notre Dame*
**1833** Pushkin, *Eugene Onegin*
British Parliament prohibits children employment
**1845** Berlioz, *Symphonic Fantastique*

*The stirring events of the great French Revolution and the Napoleonic Age, despite the widespread suffering and sense of failure that ensued, did not destroy the idealism that had marked the preceding Age of Enlightenment. A strong element of unrest remained. Intellectual vigor was remarkable. Social questions and scientific problems were attacked with unequaled fervor. Yet, despite its efforts and enthusiasms, the generation that lived in the years following the Congress of Vienna experienced bitter disappointments.*

## ■ SOCIETY: PRACTICE AND THEORY

In a sense, the Revolution of 1830 accomplished what the great Revolution of 1789 had failed to achieve. Professional men and those who controlled finance, trade, and the growing industrial apparatus, gained almost everywhere a full share in the exercise of political power. "Bourgeois" views penetrated all facets of Western civilization.

In line with the trends of the times, social stratification was modified. The old nobility retained much of its landed wealth, as well as its role at the royal courts and in the administrations of many countries. However, it no longer set the pattern in manners, taste, and social attitudes. The proportion of peasants in the population declined, even though they still comprised the overwhelming majority. Yet, they achieved no active political role. Industrial workers increased in numbers, but owing to their economic weakness, were unable to influence either national or economic policies.

It was thus the middle class, the bourgeoisie, which most influenced the age. Within this group, it was the "captains of industry"—as the historian Carlyle called them—or successful self-made men who shaped the ways of modern society. Their specialized knowledge, ambition, and (in some cases) erudition and culture enabled them to challenge the old upper classes. They gained influence by means of hard work. They adopted or imitated many of the views and prejudices of the old society, but they were also receptive to modern ideologies.

As a whole, the middle class cherished liberal thought, to which it owed its rise. It generally advocated equality of opportunity, and favored the founding of schools and universities. It was interested in the progress of science. Although many of its members supported the religious institutions of the past, they now showed less religious fervor. They were tolerant in their treatment of minority groups, such as the Jews, who composed a significantly influential portion of their ranks. The latter were emancipated politically; many attained leading positions in science and trade. The middle class was devoted—though often more in theory than in practice—to "propriety," stability, and honesty; it served as a new patron of art and learning.

## Women

In view of the political organization of the country, women in England could not participate in the conduct of public affairs, nor did they have any political rights. In the building, mining, and textile industries, women's labor was exploited, as it had been throughout history everywhere. Long working hours at low wages and hard labor were demanded, not only in agriculture, but also in industry. Women of the well-to-do classes attended to their households, supported by maids; they occupied themselves with gardening, reading, writing (as did Jane Austen, d. 1817; *Pride and Prejudice),* and social gatherings. The political role of women in the United States was similar. But, as in other pioneering societies, the influence of women, especially in frontier regions, was considerable. Living conditions were largely determined by their activities and decisions.

In Continental Europe, conditions were different. Since industry was not as advanced as in Britain, there was less exploitation through industrial labor. Then, too, the women in Germany and France held a higher place in public affairs. Mme. de Stael, Mme. Roland and, later, George Sand in France and Bettina von Amim, Rahel von Varnhagen, Caroline Schlegel, and Henrietta Herz in Germany exercised far-reaching influence. Their writings were of no less importance than their *salons.* In these salons, philosophers and generals, theologians and princes, historians and literary figures, gathered. Their discussions of existing views and problems led to action in various political arenas. Moreover, especially in Germany, women often took charge of businesses when their husbands had died early, and directed them, as did, for instance, Therese Krupp, the widow of the founder of the famous steel works. To the numbers of active and influential women should also be added Baroness de Krüdener of Holy Alliance fame and others, such as the traveler Alexandra Gripenberg from Scandinavia.

## Mechanization of Industry

The "prise of the bourgeoisie" owed most of its impetus to the mechanization of production methods. Mechanization brought changes so profound that later the expression "Industrial Revolution" was coined to describe the era—a misleading term, for no revolution took place, but rather a series of economic changes drawn out over a long period of time. These changes came first and proceeded most rapidly in Britain. Its insular position, fast-growing population, insufficiency of foodstuffs but control of raw materials at home and in its colonies, and —most of all—enterprising commercial spirit favored early adoption of new production methods. Mechanization of the textile industry started the spiral of general industrialization; it led to the growth of machine industry, which, in turn, stimulated coal and iron mining, shipbuilding, and, after 1825, railroad construction.

Railway construction—challenged in Russia, as well as in the United States, by canal building—thereafter became the chief motor force in the industrialization process. It demanded vast amounts of supply in coal and steel—for a century the standard measurement of a country's industrial progress. It gave jobs to large numbers of workers, stimulated the machine industry serving numerous branches of the economy, and opened the path for additional research and technical progress. Railways alone could provide the new needs for transportation; they made it possible to reach the wider markets that developed with population growth and the demands of industrial workers, who were not as self-sustaining as their

Society, Arts, and Sciences (1815-1848) **169**

Figure 13-1 *Revolutions of 1830 and 1848 across Europe*

peasant counterparts. They opened up possibilities for passenger services that changed the living habits of millions of people. As large enterprises, they were in need of large amounts of financing, and this demand, in turn, contributed to the growth of banking.

Trade increased, prices rose, a boom resulted, and new industries came into being. European countries followed the British lead, albeit at a slower pace. In France, where coal and iron were scarce and agriculture flourishing, and where cheap labor was neither as abundant nor concentrated as in urban areas, industrialization was delayed. Spain, Italy, the Netherlands, and the Scandinavian countries lagged still further behind. However, Germany's rise to prominence in industry, though later than Britain's and France's, was rapid when it came in the 1830s.

## Social Conditions

The mass poverty resulting from industrialization was most observed in Britain, which became both the industrial and social workshop of the world. It was there that theorists occupied themselves most intensely with new economic and social problems.

### Social Theories

Medieval thinkers had condemned covetousness, ambition, competition, and economic exploitation. Though not overly concerned with poverty, which was considered inevitable in human society, they had demanded Christian charity. They had insisted on a "just" price and had opposed interest-taking. They had approved regulation of trade and enforcement of quality standards through the formation of guilds and monopolies.

Most of these fundamental views had been reversed by the classical economic theory of 18th and early 19th-century Britain. Ambition was no longer considered a vice. Price determination by the laws of supply and demand, without reference to ethical principles, was regarded as natural and proper. Interest-taking was accepted as a normal function of the money market. Monopolies were condemned, and regulation of trade and production as to quality and quantity was left to "natural" forces.

In line with liberal trends, and inspired by Adam Smith's laissez-faire views, economists defended modern capitalism and private property. They extolled the division of labor and investigated the economics of money, rent, labor, and value. Most of them held to the liberal proposition that the free play of economic activities would bring the most favorable general conditions. They also believed that individuals are the best judges of their own interests, and that individuals serve society best when they promote their own interests.

But an increasingly pessimistic strain can be noticed even among these economists. David Ricardo felt that the various social interests could never be harmonized. Sismondi doubted that new production possibilities could improve the situation of the masses; he prophesied a succession of crises that would forever disturb social relationships. Malthus, following in this liberal path, insisted that population will always tend to outrun the means of subsistence; he therefore considered economic planning and artificial relief measures to be senseless.

### Social Reality

Evidence seemed to support such pessimistic views. Industrialization brought unforeseen results. The personal relationship between employer and employee was lost in the conduct of the new large-scale enterprises; individual workers became mere units in a chain of production. Their employment and wages came to depend less upon personal achievement than upon impersonal trends and business cycles. They no longer took pride in, or gained satisfaction and a comfortable living from, craftsmanship and skill. Low-paid, unskilled workers (often women and children) sufficed to attend to machinery; family incomes declined.

Many farm laborers were cruelly uprooted and separated from the soil from which they had drawn strength and a measure of security. They had to perform monotonous tasks as a result of the widespread division of labor. They were exhausted by excessive working hours and long trips to and from their work. Living in dismal slums, they no longer had the solace of the quiet and beauty of the countryside.

Scientific progress, however, did open up new vistas. It was now possible to prolong the average life span, to introduce new comforts of life, and to reduce manual labor through machinery that performed miracles of strength, speed, and precision. At first these benefits were only for the few, however, and were paid for by both worker and peasant, whose lives were spent in toil. People's ruthless competitive instincts were stimulated; wealth was increasingly concentrated in the hands of entrepreneurs. The gulf between rich and poor continued to widen. Large fortunes were made, not only through the production of goods but also by finance. Even on the land, the newly gained freedom from serfdom was of little benefit to the peasant. The need for scientific farming methods, for fertilizer, for the planting of new mass crops such as potatoes and sugar beets, and, consequently, for financial means forced many to quit farming and leave their homes. A smaller number of farmers could feed the increasing populations.

### *Population*

There was a change in the population ratio of town and country, as there was in the average life span. Medicine and hygiene helped to prolong life, and more people survived infancy. Around 1800, Spain and Britain counted about ten million inhabitants each; France and Germany almost three times as many, and Russia still more. The bourgeoisie and the working class (the "proletariat") grew fastest.

## Challenging Economic Thought

In view of such conditions, many leading thinkers in the second quarter of the 19th century began to occupy themselves with a revision of economic theories.

### *Modified Laissez-Faire*

Jean Baptiste Say abandoned many of the positions of the classical economists; he taught that utility is the measure of value and that labor must be judged by utilitarian standards. Friedrich List advocated a certain amount of state direction and a protective tariff. John Stuart Mill, a foe of intolerance *(On Liberty, Essay on the Subjection of Women),* somewhat later insisted, like List, that a measure of regulation and social reform directed by the state was necessary to guarantee the freedom of the individual. Most of them recognized that the availability of industrial goods created "needs" that had not been felt before, and that consumption would rapidly increase.

### *Utopianism and Anarchism*

A more radical departure from the laissez-faire theory can be traced to various idealistic groups of the first half of the 19th century. Of special importance were the "utopians," who, believing in the goodness of people if wisely led, expected a better future from the full development of their rational and moral qualities. Robert Owen, an English textile worker who had become owner of a mill, best represented their views and aims. Starting with social improvements in his own factory, where he limited the working hours of children, paid wages during periods of unemployment, and instituted schools for workers and looked after their health, he then turned his attention to British national problems. He moved temporarily to America and, in 1825, founded in New Harmony, Indiana, a community for people who would renounce private property. Those who lived there adopted uniform housing, clothing, and education. They worked as a community and received credit for their labor in accordance with the extent of their participation in the activities of the community. The project collapsed, however, because the participants lacked the devotion and individual initiative Owen had expected.

A more scientific approach than Owen's can be ascribed to Saint-Simon. This noted Frenchman, a wealthy count and devoted Christian who sacrificed all his possessions for his ideals, taught that society must be scientifically planned, that true freedom consists in serving the community, and that spiritual values depend upon economic conditions. He held that property corrupts people. In this, his compatriots, Fourier and Proudhon, agreed with him. But not from society, church, or state—agents of law, protectors of property, and therefore vicious—did the latter two expect salvation. They expected salvation from the individual's rationality. Reason, they thought, would induce people to enter freely into contracts with fellows. On such a basis, a healthy, moral, and stateless (anarchical) society could be built.

In opposition, Louis Blanc extended Saint-Simon's views, insisting that, at least for the time being, the state alone could guarantee a fair distribution of wealth. He therefore demanded that governments attend to the task of organizing work. In many respects, Blanc represented the view of the modern socialist camp.

## Socialism

Socialism, which in its early stages was indistinguishable from communism, was not a 19th-century invention. It had antecedents in some of Plato's teachings, as well as in the Gospels, Thomas More's writings, and certain Egyptian and Aztec institutions. Nineteenth-century socialism differed, however, from earlier movements in that it addressed itself mainly to the new industrial worker and only indirectly to the peasant. It concerned itself largely with the relationship between entrepreneur and laborer and with questions of profit. Socialism embraced a great variety of views. Some socialists based their precepts on moral grounds, others on materialistic concepts. But all shared the fundamental principle that private property is evil and that the means of production, and possibly even those of distribution, should be in the hands of the community. They demanded an equal distribution of the national wealth, with remuneration for all according to their work or according to their needs. Traditional concepts, including inherited religious views, were rejected by most of them; socialists tried to be "scientific."

## Social Legislation

Under the impact of utopianism, anarchism, and scientific socialism, both workers and governments acted to cope with the problems of the new industrial age. Workers and craftsmen who at the beginning of mechanization saw their livelihood threatened and had resorted to destruction of machinery gave up such desperate measures. Instead, they began to form associations and unions, which were to give strength to their cause. They organized the first trade union, an illegal enterprise, in 1824. They also began to organize producers' and consumers' cooperatives in agriculture, industry, and trade. Thus they planned to bring a sector of the national economy under their own control and to share in the profits made possible by the new production methods.

Governments reacted by passing factory legislation reforms, beginning with provisions for sanitation and the whitewashing of buildings, and continuing with regulations against the exploitation of children. In 1819, Britain forbade the employment of children less than nine years of age in the cotton mills. Factory codes (1833) and other laws for the protection of women and children followed, even though enforcement was slack. By 1847, a maximum working day of ten hours had been established for women and minors in certain trades. All European governments, however, held out against recognition of the workers' right to form associations or to resort to strikes. Nor did they propose unemployment-relief measures. They attributed poverty and hardships to the assumed laziness of the individual. In fact, especially in Britain, attempts were made to meet the problem of poverty by making governmental "poor relief" worse than poverty itself.

# ■ LITERATURE, SCIENCE, AND ARTS

Preoccupation of thinkers with societal changes did not hinder a vigorous literary and artistic life after the Napoleonic Wars were over.

## Literature

Goethe died in 1832, one year after finishing *Faust*. Germany continued to create beautiful lyrical poetry (Heinrich Heine, d. 1856) and some of the most enchanting tales of fantasy (E. T. A. Hoffmann, d. 1822). Moreover, in a period when drama was neglected and "became divorced from popular stage production," Germany contributed two eminent playwrights: Grillparzer and Hebbel. With penetrating psychological insight into the problems arising from the human situation, Hebbel paved the way for the modern drama. In France, the age of the novelist *(romancier)* dawned. Stendhal (d. 1842; *The Red and the Black),* Balzac (d. 1850; *The Human Comedy),* and Flaubert (d. 1880; *Madame Bovary)* wrote their great novels, and the elder Dumas composed his famous stories (d. 1870; *The Three Musketeers).* Perhaps the most important of these writers was Victor Hugo *(The Hunchback of Notre Dame),* who lived until 1885, and whose historical novels have continued to enjoy wide popularity.

In Britain, as in Germany, the Romantic Movement continued. Keats (d. 1821; "Ode to a Nightingale"), Shelley (d. 1822; "Ode to the West Wind"), and Byron (d. 1824; *Childe Harold)* died too young to reach their full potential, but Wordsworth lived until 1850. He had won fame before 1800 with his poetry and essays, marked by rejection of classicist trends and by emphasis on a direct and warm relationship to nature. He continued to create similar works that served as models for many of his contemporaries. Romanticism lived on also in the historical novels of Walter Scott *(Ivanhoe),* in the writings of Thackeray *(The Vicar of Wakefield),* to a certain extent even in the social novels of Charles Dickens, who documented the underside of the Industrial Age, and in the writings of the Bronte sisters (Emily's *Wuthering Heights).* Literature in the English language was enriched by American writers, among whom Edgar Allan Poe (d. 1849; mysteries and poetry) and James Fenimore Cooper (d. 1851; *Leatherstocking Tales)* gained international renown.

Like the United States, Russia entered the world's literary stage as a newcomer. Its writers displayed unique artistic gifts. Pushkin (d. 1837; *Eugene Onegin,* "Queen of Spades") with his exquisite lyrics, powerful dramas, and enchanting stories stands at the beginning of a long list of Russian artists of outstanding genius. The novels of Gogol *(Dead Souls)* and Goncharov *(Oblomov)* depict the strange atmosphere of the Russian landscape, consciousness, and way of life; they have captured the imagination of readers everywhere. Writers of accomplishment also included Mickiewicz in Poland and Manzoni *(Promised Bride)* in Italy.

## Philosophy and History

Except in Germany, the first half of the 19th century did not produce any lasting philosophical works. In Britain, a shallow utilitarianism was expounded. Even Jeremy Bentham, with his sober studies of human nature and love of liberty and his desire for progress, showed in his search for the "greatest happiness for the greatest number" little insight into the human condition. But in Germany, Hegel, Fichte, and Schelling kept alive the traditions of the great thinkers: In the search for freedom, they saw the goal of history and the workings of Providence. Their idealism was opposed by a fourth eminent philosopher, Schopenhauer (d. 1860; *The World As Will and Idea),* who expressed deep pessimism. Not in moral attitudes, but in the will to live, he saw the driving force of human action; ideas were but reflections of that will and of human selfishness.

Philosophical thought, which had been so closely connected with religion and with the rational attitudes of the Enlightenment, came to be increasingly interwoven with historical studies. Out of combined progress in these fields came a new understanding of human attitudes and aspirations, as well as an account on environmental conditions. A great collection of historical sources was started in Germany, *the*

*Monumenta Germaniae Historica.* B. G. Niebuhr wrote his fundamental work on Roman law; the famous modern historian Leopold von Ranke began his long and fruitful career.

## Science

A major influence on 19th-century thinking was exercised by the physical sciences. The fundamental work of the 18th century was broadened and applied. Faraday discovered electromagnetic induction. Gauss, Helmholtz, Maxwell, and many others studied light, electricity, heat and energy, laying a basis from which successors could carry on. They investigated electromagnetic waves and electrochemistry. Fraunhofer discovered the method of spectrum analysis. The field of thermodynamics was studied. New machinery, appliances, and lighting systems were invented. The most varied kinds of power-driven apparatus (for steamships, locomotives, and motors in factories) were created. Coal mining and steel manufacturing became the most important industries. Likewise, the fields of geography and geology were scientifically developed (e.g., by Alexander von Humboldt and Sir Charles Lyell).

## Art

While literature and science flourished, the fine arts produced less of lasting merit. Two painters of note appeared in Britain: Turner and Constable, the one famous for his paintings of Venice, the other for his landscapes. France took pride in Delacroix and Ingres. Among the best in other countries were Bocklin of Switzerland, and Caspar David Friedrich of Germany, both with their romantic landscapes. In architecture and sculpture, the neoclassical style of the early 19th century, represented by artists such as the Danish sculptor Thorwaldsen, gave way to another imitative art form, the neo-Gothic. Cities, which grew rapidly, showed an increasingly dismal picture: somber and pretentious dwellings and, often, graceless villas and public buildings began to mar town and countryside, especially in newly industrialized regions.

## Music

Romanticism, which embraced many areas of human endeavor, became dominant in the field of music during the first half of the 19th century. The Romantic composers sought freedom of self-expression, delved into the mysteries of human life, and, above all, tried to depict emotion. Inspired by folk traditions, as well as by patriotic movements, they created some of the most beautiful works ever written. One of the most famous Romantics was Franz Schubert (d. 1828). In addition to chamber music and symphonies, he composed *Lieder* (songs), which have become a permanent treasure of the musical world.

His tradition was carried on by composers like Schumann and Mendelssohn, and later, Brahms. Outside of Germany, Berlioz *(Symphonic fantastique)* and the Polish exile Chopin in France excelled—Chopin equally great as pianist and as composer of nocturnes, dance works, and preludes. In German opera, the chief Romantic work was *Der Freischutz* by Weber, while in Italy Donizetti and Rossini *(Barber of Seville)* stand out. The Italian composers adhered rather firmly to traditional forms and lacked some of the depth of feeling evinced by the Romantics. They often catered to the demands of a public that wanted to be entertained and amused and that was fascinated by such virtuosity as was displayed by the Italian composer and violinist Paganini *(Carnival of Venice),* and by the Hungarian composer and pianist Franz Liszt. Immensely admired by his contemporaries, Liszt's work enriched harmonic expression and greatly enhanced Church music. He became teacher to many excellent performers.

## Perspective

*During the times of reaction and conservatism, industrialism advanced, and with it, the role that the middle class could play. Industrialists accumulated wealth. Laissez-faire views supported such development, but it resulted in the deterioration of living standards among craftsmen, small businessmen, and workers. Voices calling for alleviation of suffering among the lower classes became stronger. New theories were developed, and some legislation, though inadequate, was passed to limit laissez-faire practices.*

*Music continued to flourish. Intellectual works in philosophy and history retained and even strengthened their place on the cultural stage of the European countries. In literature, new forms evolved and were accepted. The novel, in particular, emerged as a major force. Many works of considerable merit appeared in France, England, and Italy, and for the first time, Russian authors made significant literary contributions.*

## Selected Readings

Bruun, Geoffrey. *Nineteenth-Century European Civilization* (New York: Oxford University Press, 1960).

Cairns, John C., ed. *The Nineteenth Century* (New York: Free Press, 1965).

Landes, David S. *The Unbound Prometheus: Technological Change and Industrial Development in Western Europe from 1750 to the Present* (London: Cambridge University Press, 1969).

*The Cambridge Economic History of Europe.* 6 vols. (Cambridge: Cambridge University Press, 1966).

Trebilcock, C. *The Industrialization of the Continental Powers, 1780–1914* (London: Longman, 1981).

Newman, Michael. *Socialism: A Very Short Introduction* (Oxford: Oxford University Press, 2005).

Venturi, F. *Roots of Revolution* (New York: Knopf, 1960).

Miller, David. *Anarchism* (London: J. M. Dent, 1984).

Snyder, Paula. *The European Women's Almanac* (New York: Columbia University Press, 1992).

Woodward, Ernest L. *The Age of Reform, 1815-1870* (Oxford: Clarendon Press, 1962).

## Test Yourself

1. The novel *Pride and Prejudice* is one of the most celebrated works of_____.
   A. Jane Gray
   B. Jane Austen
   C. James Clavel
   D. Jane Seymour

2. Laissez-Faire is a concept associated mostly with the work of_____.
   A. Adam Smith
   B. David Ricardo
   C. Robert Malthus
   D. Karl Marx

3. John Stuart Mill, a foe of intolerance, contributed to the literature of liberalism and intolerance with his famous work(s)_____.
   A. *Essay on the Subjugation of Women*
   B. *On Liberty*
   C. *On Slavery*
   D. Both A and B

4. Among the early socialists are a number of utopianists such as_____.
   A. Robert Owen
   B. Charles Fourier
   C. San Simon
   D. All of the above

5. In 1819, Britain forbade the employment of children in cotton mills who were under the age of_____.
   A. Fifteen years
   B. Nine years
   C. Twelve years
   D. Thirteen years

6. One of the most celebrated French writers in the second half of the 19th century whose works included the famous *Hunchback of Notre Dame* was_____.
   A. Victor Hugo
   B. Charles Fourier
   C. Jean Jacques Rousseau
   D. Charles Dickens

7. Alexander Pushkin, one of the leading Russian novelists, authored all of the following except_____.
   A. *Eugene Onegin*
   B. *War and Peace*
   C. *Queen of Spades*
   D. *Letters of Alexander Pushkin*

8. The *Symphonie fantastique* was composed by_____.
   A. Chopin
   B. Schubert
   C. Berlioz
   D. Rossini

## Answers and Explanations

1. B. Women of the well-to-do classes attended to their households, supported by maids; they occupied themselves with gardening, reading, writing (as did Jane Austen, d. 1817; *Pride and Prejudice),* and social gatherings. The political role of women in the United States was similar. But, as in other pioneering societies, the influence of women, especially in frontier regions, was considerable. Living conditions were largely determined by their activities and decisions.

2. A. In line with liberal trends, and inspired by Adam Smith's laissez-faire views, economists defended modern capitalism and private property. They extolled the division of labor and investigated the economics of money, rent, labor, and value. Most of them held to the liberal proposition that the free play of economic activities would bring the most favorable general conditions. They also believed that individuals are the best judges of their own interests, and that individuals serve society best when they promote their own interests.

3. D. John Stuart Mill, a foe of intolerance *(On Liberty, Essay on the Subjection of Women),* somewhat later insisted, like List, that a measure of regulation and social reform directed by the state was necessary to guarantee the freedom of the individual. Most of them recognized that the availability of industrial goods created "needs" that had not been felt before, and that consumption would rapidly increase.

4. D. Of special importance were the "utopians" who, believing in the goodness of people if wisely led, expected a better future from the full development of their rational and moral qualities. Robert Owen, an English textile worker who had become owner of a mill, best represented their views and aims. A more scientific approach than Owen's can be ascribed to Saint-Simon. This noted Frenchman, a wealthy count and devoted Christian who sacrificed all his possessions for his ideals, taught that society must be scientifically planned, that true freedom consists in serving the community, and that spiritual values depend upon economic conditions. He held that property corrupts people. In this, his compatriots, Fourier and Proudhon, agreed with him. The latter two did not expect salvation from society, church, or state, who were considered agents of law, protectors of property, and, therefore, vicious.

5. B. In 1819, Britain forbade the employment of children less than nine years of age in the cotton mills. Factory codes (1833) and other laws for the protection of women and children followed, even though enforcement was slack. By 1847, a maximum working day of ten hours had been established for women and minors in certain trades. All European governments, however, held out against recognition of the workers' right to form associations or to resort to strikes.

6. A. Perhaps the most important of the writers of the late 19th century was Victor Hugo *(The Hunchback of Notre Dame),* who lived until 1885, and whose historical novels have continued to enjoy wide popularity.

7. B. Like the United States, Russia entered the world's literary stage as a newcomer. Its writers displayed unique artistic gifts. Pushkin (d. 1837; *Eugene Onegin, Queen of Spades*) with his exquisite lyrics, powerful dramas, and enchanting stories stands at the beginning of a long list of Russian artists of outstanding genius.

8. C. Outside of Germany, Berlioz composed the *Symphonie fantastique.*

**CHAPTER 14**

# The Bourgeois Era and Revolution (1830-1848)

**1831** Faraday's experiments with electromagnetism
**1832** First Reform Bill in England
Goethe, *Faust* (second part)
Beginnings of "Young Italy" movement (Mazzini)
**1833** *Zollverein* founded in Germany
**1834** Ranke, *History of the Popes*
**1835** David Friedrich Strauss, *Life of Jesus*
**1837** Invention of telegraph by Morse
**1838** Dickens, *Oliver Twist*
**1839** British-Chinese Opium War
Belgium established as independent neutral state
**1841** Straits Convention
Carlyle, *Heroes and Hero-Worship*
**1842** Chartist risings in England
Comte, *Cours de philosophie positive*
**1845** Texas annexed by U.S.A.
Poe, *Tales*
Dumas, *Count of Monte Cristo*
**1846** Repeal of Corn Laws of England
**1847** Helmholtz, *On the Conservation of Energy*
**1848** February Revolution in France
Revolutions in Italy and Germany
California, New Mexico, etc., incorporated by U.S.A.
First Pan-Slav Congress
Marx, *Communist Manifesto*
Balzac, *Comedie humaine* completed
Mill, *Principles of Political Economy*

*In international affairs, the period from 1830 to 1848 was one of the quietest in European history. This proved the wisdom of Europe's most prominent statesman of the age, Prince Metternich. Despite his conservatism, he had succeeded in establishing a balance of power that created a lasting peace for Europe. Internal affairs in the various European nations did not bear the same peaceful stamp. The conservatism of their statesmen acted as a brake on normal progress and as a stimulus for radicalism.*

## ■ NEW CONSERVATISM VERSUS NEW LIBERALISM

As soon as the upper-middle classes had attained positions of leadership in most of Western Europe via the revolutions of 1830, they became more conservative. In the meantime, liberals continued to push for greater individual liberty and were motivated by idealism and conviction.

### Britain

Changes resulting from the growth of industries placed Britain in a precarious situation. Shifting social stratification, transformation of the British countryside, and new objectives in both economic and international affairs created a variety of problems to which satisfactory answers could be found only slowly.

### *General Problems*

During the early 1830s, the British were plagued by tensions between industrial workers, new entrepreneurial groups, and the landowning nobility. In addition to the political Reform Bill of 1832, some social reform legislation was passed. Parliament published factory codes, improved health and sanitation systems, imposed church and municipal reforms, and made long-overdue arrangements to abolish slavery throughout the empire. All this was insufficient, however. Numerous problems remained, including those associated with urbanization, poor relief, and the questions of free trade or protective legislation, centralized or decentralized government, and numerous humanitarian issues. Riots occurred, and the threat of general revolution persisted.

### *Political Parties*

Under these circumstances, political leaders could no longer defer taking further steps toward modernization. In 1837, the accession to the throne of the young queen, Victoria, marked the turning point. Dissolute and extravagant court life was reformed, and the governing parties were reorganized. The old Tories split, and a "Conservative party" emerged. This party—opposed as it was to the increasingly important bourgeoisie, the rich industrialists in the Midlands, and the ambitious merchants—promoted mainly the interests of the large landowners. Occasionally, under the influence of Shaftesbury, the Conservatives sought to make an alliance with the working class. The Whigs also reformed. They came to be known as the "Liberal party." True to the nature of liberalism, they found themselves divided into numerous factions. Some of the best-known members, like Grey, Palmerston, and Melbourne, were close in their thinking to the more progressive Conservatives. Others were radicals and insisted on speedy reforms, and still others, like the Irish leader, O'Connell, espoused special interests. Essentially, the Liberals stood for *laissez-faire*, trusting that the greatest progress would result if substantial freedom of action were allowed to the individual. Backed by a majority of the voting public, they formed several successive cabinets.

Neither they nor the Conservatives represented industrial workers, however. Consequently, other groups and movements arose, generally opposed to extreme liberalism and to conservatism. Some of them were anti-capitalistic. Among these groups was the Anti-Corn Law League, which wanted to abolish the tariffs on grain that protected the landed gentry but adversely affected the industrial workers and industrial entrepreneurs alike. Another was the Chartist group, which included factory workers, miners, and intellectuals who devoted themselves to the causes of humanitarianism and democracy. The Chartists demanded economic improvement for the workers, social equality for all, and radical changes in the electoral system, including universal male suffrage. They did not agree as to the means—peaceful or revolutionary—by which to achieve their aims, however. They lacked sufficient funds to build an organization that would enable them to gain control of the government. Yet, they succeeded in keeping alive the issue of social reform. Millions of petitions were sent to the House of Commons to advocate their cause. Well-known public figures, including the reformer, Edwin Chadwick, and leaders of the Anti-Corn Law League supported their program. Almost a century was to pass before their major proposals were to be carried out.

### *Internal Reforms*

The internal realignments, the formation of new leagues and parties, and the vigorous political propaganda accompanying the changes could not help but increase general unrest, and by the middle of the 1840s, this convinced the ruling forces to make further concessions. Factory codes were improved, and laws were enacted to provide more adequately for the protection of workers. Most important, in 1846, when Peel was prime minister, the Conservative Party, though split, had the Corn Laws repealed. A chief grievance of business and industrial workers was thus eliminated.

However, the repeal had many untoward consequences. It caused distress among the farmers, especially in nonindustrialized Ireland where potato blight and subsequent famine were already in strong evidence. The repeal also eventually led Britain to adopt a more aggressive colonial policy to safeguard its imports of foodstuffs and its markets for industrial goods. It tempted the government to engage in wars that were both costly and damaging to its reputation. Once the repeal of the Corn Laws had been achieved, Chartists continued to demand further reforms. When another revolution broke out in France (the February Revolution of 1848), and danger of violence threatened England as well, the reform movement was interrupted. The government preferred to use repressive measures, a policy which caused widespread resentment. Many left the country to seek a better life in the New World or in Australia.

### *Foreign Affairs*

British problems created by the rapid growth of industry, finance, and trade led the government to formulate a specific type of foreign policy. For example, Britain isolated itself even more from Continental affairs, satisfied that the existing balance of power was a guarantee of safety. It concentrated on overseas policies and the protection of the sea routes to its various colonies. It expanded its Asiatic possessions by penetrating into Burma. In the 1840s, it launched an attack on China. The attack was prompted by a Chinese law, which prohibited opium imports from India, and also by the destruction of English-owned opium stores in China. This attack, which was widely condemned because it implicitly coerced the Chinese to allow the sale of the dangerous drug that was banned elsewhere, came to be known as the "Opium War." China, defeated, was forced to pay damages, to revoke its prohibition of opium, to open a number of ports to British traders, and to grant them numerous privileges on Chinese soil.

## France

In France, a conservative course was taken during the reign of Louis Philippe. This king wisely turned his back on doubtful battlefield glory. His government, led in the 1830s by the historian Thiers, worked for internal prosperity. During Louis Philippe's reign, the French population continued to grow. Public works were sponsored, schools were founded, and relations with the Catholic Church were normalized. The arts flourished, and France once more took its place as an outstanding cultural center of the Western world.

However, dissatisfaction grew among certain groups. Reactionary royalists who supported the claims of the deposed Bourbons, nationalists who dreamed of Napoleonic glory, liberals who demanded wider constitutional rights than the Charter provided, and socialists who wanted political power for the workers never reconciled themselves to Louis Philippe's rule. Within a few years, newspapers began to ridicule the king for his "bourgeois" ways and views, and Louis Philippe found no better means of dealing with the situation than to reenact repressive legislation.

This only increased resistance. Thiers resigned, and another historian, Guizot, became prime minister. Through unpopular measures, including his opposition to the Church, his refusal to enlarge the franchise, and his dishonesty in dealing with the parliament, Guizot contributed to a further decline of Louis Philippe's prestige. By the end of 1847, the opposition organized large public banquets that provided the opportunity for revolutionary speeches. When, on February 22, 1848, one such banquet was to be held, the government forbade it. This was the signal for open revolt. A third French revolution, the "February Revolution" of 1848, began.

## Germany

As in France, so in Germany, The period from 1830 to 1848 was one of external calm and internal seething. The influence of Metternich prevailed throughout, however, and notwithstanding minor modifications, his system remained basically as he had planned it.

### *Internal Conditions*

Most of the German states were governed efficiently, albeit in the tradition of enlightened despotism rather than according to liberal standards. Industrialization, with its initial social effects, had not occurred in Germany to the same degree as in England and France. Economic conditions were comparatively favorable. German philosophers, poets, and musicians were admired everywhere; German universities, with their eminent men of science and great scholars in the humanities, drew students from all parts of the world. Underneath the surface, however, much dissatisfaction smoldered. There was little acknowledgment of national aspirations or liberal social demands. The cause of representative government made little progress. For example, newspapers and books remained subject to censorship. In most places, the nobility, with its agrarian interests, retained the highest administrative, military, and diplomatic positions, while the bourgeoisie played a subordinate role.

### *Nationality Problems*

Economic and social questions were complicated by problems of nationality. In the Hapsburg areas of the German federation, the numerous non-German nationality groups—Italians, Czechs, Hungarians, and others—began to clamor for self-government. However, the Germans in most areas agitated for a closer union and for one great Germany. Fearful that the latter demand would endanger their multinational empire, the Hapsburgs opposed all unification attempts. Vying for leadership within a German federation, Prussia, however, identified itself to a certain extent with the aspirations for one united nation.

The conflict dividing the Hapsburgs and Prussians into hostile camps was sharpened by their divergent attitudes in social and political matters. Austria appealed to the conservative forces and to the vanity of the small princes. Prussia aligned itself with the forces demanding change, established the *Zollverein* (customs union), and introduced trial by jury and freedom of the press. When general unrest mounted in 1847, the King of Prussia even called for a parliament composed of representatives of the people. His measure was halfhearted, however, and no legislative powers were vested in the parliament, nor was a constitution adopted. Thus, nowhere was real progress made toward the solution of critical problems. When the February Revolution broke out in France, unrest in Prussia was as great as it was in Austria. The call to revolution found a wide and enthusiastic echo everywhere in German lands.

## Italy

Like Germany, Italy was disunited as a nation. In addition, most of its territory was subject to foreign rule: Sicily and Naples to the Spanish Bourbons; the Central Provinces (Parma, Modena, Tuscany) to various Austrian princes; and Lombardy and Venetia to the Hapsburg Empire. Only Piedmont and the Papal States had Italian rulers—the one, the House of Savoy, the other the pope. All parts of the nation were badly administered. Progressive forces were suppressed economically as well as politically. The population was divided over political and religious questions. Neither industry and agriculture nor political institutions prospered, and poverty was widespread. Intellectual activities were important only among the small, higher class groups of the population. The anti-Catholicism feelings among many people in this upper class prevented much contact between them and the masses.

Further, unity did not exist among the leaders. Some were republicans, some royalists, and some supported a unified Italy ruled by the pope. Still others were without any plan. A movement called "Young Italy" envisioned a *Risorgimento,* a rebirth of the nation, but it remained weak. Rebellions, which occurred at regular intervals, achieved little. Thus, a revolt, which was undertaken by a young enthusiast, Garibaldi, in Genoa in 1834, resulted in failure and the exile of its leader.

In 1846, new hopes for change were aroused by the election of a rather young pope, Pius IX, who was credited with liberal leanings and administrative ability. Metternich was not disturbed. He remarked cynically that "a liberal pope is inconceivable." The expectations of the patriots were not realized. They could look for leadership only from Piedmont, the one other independent Italian state. The House of Savoy, which ruled Piedmont, saw its opportunity and began, like the Prussian royal house in Germany, to move ahead on the road of liberal reform. It even granted a constitution. Although its sincerity about reforms remained as doubtful as that of Prussia, it could, because of the national issue, assume the desired role of leadership in Italy when the February Revolution began in France.

## Russia

During the period from 1830 to 1848, economic conditions and political trends were working slow changes in other parts of Europe, accumulating enough pressure to cause revolutionary outbreaks. Conditions in Russia, however, remained stagnant.

### *Internal Policies*

After suppressing the Dekabrist revolt, Russia restored tsarist power, keeping intact the rule of the landlord class and the institution of serfdom. Adopting the slogan "autocracy, orthodoxy, nationality," the government made few progressive moves. It did adopt a new code of laws along the lines proposed by the old statesman, Speransky. It also improved public finance, modernized the administrative organization, extended some civil rights to the wealthier classes, and accepted more of the principles of private capitalism. However, it suppressed all demands for constitutional government, social change, and religious freedom. It did little to check corruption. Serfdom, which was the most critical problem and which was a hindrance to Russia's modernization and economic growth, was left untouched. Constant local peasant uprisings occurred. Equally ignored was the question of nationalities within the empire.

In vain did some of the greatest Russian writers raise their voices in criticism. They were silenced and exiled, and their works were suppressed. Groups expressing concern about political problems were banned. The movement of the Slavophils, which sought progress through reviving a mythical Russian spirit believed to manifest cooperation and true Christianity, was viewed with disfavor. Another group that received a similar reaction was the Westernizers, who also advocated social changes paralleling western European scientific and liberal trends. Universities were kept small, and their students were closely supervised. Courses, particularly science courses, were considered dangerous to traditional views and were sharply restricted.

### External Policies

Nationalistic external policies were vigorously, though not successfully, promoted. An expansionist drive was launched southeastward into the Transcaspian regions and central Asia, but the expeditionary force perished in the steppes. Another advance was attempted in the direction of the Turkish Straits, stimulated by the fundamental aim of Russian policy to rule the coasts of the Black Sea and eventually gain domination of the straits of the Bosporus and the Dardanelles.

Under Nicholas I, the Russians came close to fulfilling their aim. In 1829, the Peace of Adrianople and, subsequently, the Treaty of Unkiar Skelessy (1833) gave them not only territorial concessions, but also special rights in the straits and a voice in internal Ottoman Turkish affairs. In 1841, however, this southward penetration came to an end. When new troubles in Turkey occurred, England, Prussia, and Austria insisted on joint international action rather than unilateral action by Russia alone. This represented a turning point in the development of Russia's foreign policies.

## United States

Unencumbered by existing and long-established aristocratic traditions, the United States, a republic in a world dominated by monarchs and vested landed interests, continued to escape most of the complex social problems confronting other Western nations during the period from 1830 to 1848.

### Internal Conditions

The United States's population enjoyed civil rights. Hereditary, privileged classes did not exist. The franchise, accorded in England or France to no more than a tenth or a twentieth of the population, only benefited the male population, but the government and law courts were democratically organized. A new bank system was introduced. It provided for an independent treasury department. Canals were built. The settlement of western lands continued to act as a powerful force for democratization. Although life was comparatively hard and competition was sharp in most areas—a notable exception was found in the upper-middle class of the eastern states and the plantation owners of the South—America held out promise for all. A growing number of immigrants continued to arrive, even though a long depression hit the country in the late 1830s and many of them, particularly to Catholics, were victims of discrimination.

Serious issues persisted, but they were of a different sort than those raised in other parts of the Western world. Among them were race problems and slavery, which also involved the question of unity between the agricultural South and the increasingly industrial North. The issue was sharpened through the introduction of the cotton gin, which altered labor conditions in the South. Those who wanted to retain slavery were opposed by numerous antislavery groups in the North. Likewise, women's rights groups started to organize. The issue of protective tariffs remained unsettled, as did matters involving centralized government and the lagging enforcement of the law.

### Foreign Policy

Despite its safe geographic location, the United States showed strong nationalistic tendencies. Fearful of European colonialism, it proclaimed the Monroe Doctrine in 1823. This was aimed at preventing foreign powers from gaining additional footholds in the New World. The successful development of the nation stimulated nationalistic feelings and a measure of imperialism. The expansion westward was accompanied by the eviction or extermination of Native Americans. Economic imperialism was reflected in the tremendous growth of the lumber industry and in the swift development of mining for copper, silver, and gold. War was used to annex territory: Texas in 1845 and other large Mexican areas in 1848. Treaties, such as the compact with England regarding the Canadian border, likewise served the purpose of expansion. Thus, while domestic unrest and international calm marked the European scene, in North

America the situation was somewhat reversed. Internally, the country progressed without revolutionary outbreaks, but externally, expansion and wars marked the period from 1830 to 1848.

## ■ REVOLUTIONS OF 1848

The revolutions of 1848 were not as dramatic as the great Revolution of 1789 in France. Their effect, however, was hardly less incisive. The French Revolution of 1789 came at the end of a period, the *ancien regime* with its feudal heritage. The revolutions of 1848 occurred at the beginning of a new age and introduced the socialistic element into the political arena of the bourgeois world.

It was the year Karl Marx published his *Communist Manifesto*. The same industries that gave the middle class its strength also imposed deplorable conditions on workers. Thus, there quickly arose a challenge to middle-class predominance. The benefits of the bourgeoisie's liberal creed proved to be illusory in many ways. Instead of furthering "the greatest happiness of the greatest number," the unregulated functioning of the economy created unexpected misery and necessitated an early modification.

### Revolution in France

When, in February 1848, the forbidden banquet was held in defiance of the regime, cries of "*Vive la république*" were heard in the night, and street fighting began. Anxious to avoid any shedding of blood on his account, the king abdicated and fled to England, just as Charles X had done eighteen years earlier. A republic was declared. Lamartine, a historian, and Louis Blanc, a socialist, along with several other liberals, formed a provisional government.

#### *Provisional Government*

The new government was handicapped from the beginning. It had inherited an almost bankrupt treasury and could do nothing about the crop failures and business stagnation that had preceded its assumption of power. Dissension quickly became evident. Socialists like Blanc and Ledru Rollin demanded immediate changes in the economic structure of the country. They insisted on the establishment of national workshops that would provide employment—no matter how unproductive—for those without work. They demanded high taxes from the wealthy, the nationalization of the means of production, and equal civil rights for all. They raised the red flag of revolution and formed radical clubs along patterns established in 1789.

Moderates agreed to the establishment of the national workshops, and concentrated on political reform, civil rights, universal suffrage, and democratization of the National Guards. In April, elections were held in which moderates scored an overwhelming victory over the still small industrial working class. Now in control, they excluded the socialist representatives and rejected antiliberal and anticapitalistic proposals. Their policies led to another rebellion. In May, a mob invaded the new assembly.

#### *June Days*

The uprising was followed by further disturbances and a wave of arrests. The workshops were now closed, and the jobless were sent to the provinces or drafted into the army. Agitation mounted, hunger riots broke out, and the leftist opposition joined forces with the reactionary right, both bent upon the overthrow of the provisional government. Toward the end of June, the government was unable to subdue an organized rebellion and it ultimately granted dictatorial powers to an army general, Cavaignac.

Under his regime, the revolutionaries were defeated, civil liberties were suppressed anew, and a constitution acceptable to the right and the center parties was drafted. Then, new elections were held to choose a president for the republic. The people in the provinces, eager to restore national unity and prestige, and the bourgeoisie in the cities, who wanted a government strong enough to deal with labor revolts, voted against the provisional government. On December 10, 1848, Louis Napoleon was elected head of the Second Republic.

## Revolution in Germany

As soon as news of the February Revolution reached Germany, rebellions began there. The long-suppressed opponents of the government believed the time for introducing liberal institutions had come at last.

### End of Metternichism

In Vienna, liberals petitioned for a constitutional government and civil rights. They were joined by members of the numerous nationalities that formed the Hapsburg domains, who also demanded autonomy. Barricades went up in the streets. In March, there was violence in Berlin and in the Rhineland. Outbreaks in Dresden, Munich, and other capitals followed. In Budapest, liberals and Magyar nationalists, under the leadership of Louis Kossuth, rebelled. The whole Metternich structure toppled, and the aged minister was forced to resign and flee. Everywhere, German princes granted constitutions to their peoples. Even the emperor of Austria signed a constitution and acknowledged the autonomous status of Hungary and Bohemia. These actions failed to satisfy the liberals, however, and they demanded, as a right of free citizens, constitutions of their own design. New revolts occurred in Vienna, Budapest, Prague, and Milan. The Slavs in Bohemia organized the first Pan-Slav Congress, and the Italians, under Piedmontese leadership, declared war on Austria.

The emperor fled, and in December 1848, he was forced to abdicate. His Prussian colleague, Frederick William IV, proved more pliable, however. Unencumbered by nationality problems—except in some eastern areas where many Poles lived—he survived two days of violence and humiliation in March. He promptly permitted a diet to meet and then watched it waste time on a number of radical but unimportant acts, such as the abolition of titles and orders. By autumn, he had recovered control. He granted a constitution which, with its liberal stipulations, surpassed the expectations of even the most radical groups. Having taken the wind out of the sails of the liberal movement, he began to rebuild his own power. In a similar way, other German princes retained their thrones and regained authority.

### Frankfurt Parliament

The revolutions in Germany were influenced not only by the liberal forces, but also by the problem of nationalism. In May 1848, the diet of the federation was replaced by a new, nationally elected parliament. Liberals, who dominated the assembly, promptly attacked the problem of the unification of the country. They prepared a constitution that was to extend civil rights, suffrage, and personal liberties to all German peoples, and they discussed various plans for a united Germany. They discussed whether it should be a firm union or a loose federation, a monarchy or a republic, and whether Hapsburg-Austrian territories and their numerous foreign dominions should be included to form a "Greater Germany" or excluded, leaving a "Little Germany" under Prussian leadership.

However, since parliament lacked executive power, the dualism of Austria and Prussia proved to be an insurmountable obstacle. Too late did the advocates of the *klein-deutsche* (the "Little Germany") solution prevail. In April 1849, they offered the imperial crown to the King of Prussia, but he refused to take it from the hands of the representatives of the people instead of the princes. Participation in a war against Denmark, which supported the North German province of Schleswig, did nothing to further the cause of unification. Thus, the energies of the parliament were wasted, and soon it was again reduced to insignificance.

### Revolution in Italy

Revolution in Vienna prompted uprisings of nationalists and liberals in Italy. In January 1848, revolts occurred in Sicily, and the ruling Bourbons granted a constitution. In the beginning of March, many of the larger towns were ablaze: Naples, Rome, Florence, Venice, and Milan. Hard-pressed, Piedmont declared war on Austria. Simultaneously, patriots under the leadership of Mazzini and Garibaldi attacked the Papal States.

However, the poorly organized forces gained only temporary successes. In the north, the rebels were routed by Austrian Field Marshal Radetzky in the battles of Custozza and Novara, and Piedmont had to sue for peace. Resistance collapsed in Venice, too. In the central region, Mazzini and Garibaldi took Rome, the pope fled, and a Roman republic was established. However, the two leaders proved incapable of organizing an effective government, and their republic came to an early end when French and Austrian troops came to the aid of the pope. In 1850, Pius IX returned. In the south and in Sicily, the revolt was suppressed by the former rulers. Everywhere, the old institutions were revived, and nationalistic and liberal aspirations had to be deferred.

### Revolution in the Smaller Countries

Revolutionary fever spread to many of the smaller nations of Europe. In Switzerland, a new constitution was drafted to firmly establish as European the unique multinational and multilingual republic. The country was based on democratic principles and committed to permanent neutrality, to which Switzerland still adheres. In the Scandinavian countries, and in Holland and Belgium, too, institutions were brought into conformity with the demands of the age. A constitutional government was introduced in Hungary under Kossuth, but it did not last. The Austrians invaded Hungary. When they were unable to deal with the Hungarian forces, they appealed to the Russians, whose tsar, Nicholas I, assumed the role of "*gendarme*" of Europe. With the help of his troops, the rebellious forces were subdued, and Kossuth was forced to flee.

Repercussions of the February Revolution were felt in the Slavic nations that were subject to Turkish rule and in Spain and Portugal. Thus, with the exception of Russia, where autocracy and the police force cut the roots of every liberal movement, and the United States, where citizens already possessed what European liberals were fighting for, the age of revolution encompassed most of Western civilization.

### Effects of the February Revolution

Historians have considered the revolutions of 1848 largely a failure, pointing out that the order in existence from 1830 or earlier was not shattered. The upper bourgeoisie remained in control in Western Europe, and the middle class failed to win control of central Europe. Liberalism and nationalism continued to be the dominant trends of the age, and the political map of Europe was not altered.

Yet, a significant change had occurred. The working class had emerged as a claimant to power. Egalitarian trends increased. Liberal constitutions were adopted in most European countries. Serfdom disappeared in all areas except Russia and Ottoman Turkey. A more pragmatic climate of opinion now prevailed, checking the overly optimistic beliefs of the liberals. Nationalism, though still unsuccessful in both Germany and Italy, had shown its strength and intensified among the peoples of these countries and many additional national groups. Finally, the failure of the revolutions drove thousands of individuals to the United States, where their enthusiasm, skills, and labor helped to build the firm foundations for a society that conformed to their principles.

### Perspective

*With the end of the revolution of 1830, a new period of comparative quiet began. Conservative governments held political changes in check, but technological advances forced social change upon them.*

*England, in particular, was exposed to such pressures. A rapidly growing proletariat made reform necessary, and the Whig party, replacing the Conservatives, carried out some reforms. Other European countries were under less pressure, but there, too, unrest increased.*

*In 1848, outbreaks resulted, and they were far more violent than those in 1830. Once again, they erupted in France, but this time, with the exception of Russia, they engulfed all of Europe. The Metternich system collapsed. Karl Marx published his* Communist Manifesto, *and Socialist doctrines were added to the demands of leading liberal thinkers. Although the revolutions were ultimately suppressed, it was not before compromises were made. Many countries adopted constitutions and broadened welfare legislation. Social movements, largely purged of utopian aims, focused on practical reforms instead, and they gained in strength and influence.*

## Selected Readings

Albrecht-Carrie, Rene. A *Diplomatic History of Europe* (New York: Harper and Row, 1973).

Breunig, Charles. *The Age of Revolution and Reaction* (New York: Norton, 1970).

Cipolla, Carlo M., ed. *The Fontana Economic History of Europe.* 6 vols. (New York: Barnes & Noble, 1977).

Craig, Gordon. *Europe Since 1815* (Hinsdale, IL: The Dryden Press, 1972).

Cobban, Alfred: *History of Modern France*, 2 vols. (Baltimore: Penguin Books, 1961).

Hobsbawn, E. J. *The Age of Revolution: Europe, 1789–1848* (Cleveland: World Pub., 1970).

Stearns, Peter N. *1848: The Revolutionary Tide in Europe* (New York: Norton, 1974).

Tipton, Frank. *A History of Modern Germany Since 1815* (Berkeley: University of California Press, 2003).

Macartney, C. A. *The Hapsburg Empire, 1790-1918* (New York: Macmillan, 1969).

Tombs, Robert. *France, 1814–1914* (New York: Longman, 1996).

Sarti, Ronald. *Mazzini: A Life for the Religion of Politics* (Westport, Conn.: Praeger, 1997).

## Test Yourself

1. The Anti-Corn Law League aimed at_____.
   A. The abolition of slavery
   B. The abolition of tariffs on grain
   C. The abolition of voting rights
   D. None of the above

2. After China's defeat in the Opium War (1839), China_____.
   A. Was forced to pay damages
   B. Revoked the prohibition on opium
   C. Closed ports to British traders
   D. A and B

3. In 1846, new hopes for change in Italy occurred with the election of_____.
   A. Pope Pius IX
   B. Pope Pius XII
   C. Pope Julius I
   D. Pope Benedict XVI

4. The Treaty of Unkiar-Skelessy of 1833 between the Russians and the Ottoman Empire granted Russia_____.
   A. Special rights to the Bosporus and the Dardanelles
   B. Access to the Siberian peninsula
   C. Part of Istanbul
   D. None of the above

5. The Revolutions of 1848 originated in _____.
   A. France
   B. Austria
   C. Prussia
   D. Russia

6. The 1848 revolutions were preceded by the publication of Karl Marx's_____.
   A. *On Liberty*
   B. *Das Kapital*
   C. *Communist Manifesto*
   D. *On the Origin of Species*

7. Louis Napoleon (Napoleon III) was elected head of the Second French Republic on December 10_____.

    A. 1840
    B. 1848
    C. 1865
    D. 1880

8. The movement called "Young Italy" was led by a young enthusiast named _____.

    A. Mussolini
    B. Cavour
    C. Garibaldi
    D. Mazzini

## Answers and Explanations

1. **B.** The Anti-Corn Law League aimed at the abolition of the tariffs on grain that protected the landed gentry but adversely affected the industrial workers and the industrial entrepreneurs alike. Another was the Chartist group, which included factory workers, miners, and many intellectuals who devoted themselves to the cause of humanitarianism and democracy.

2. **D.** In the 1840s, Britain launched an attack on China, prompted by a Chinese law prohibiting opium imports from India and by the destruction of English-owned opium stores in China. This attack, which was widely condemned because it implicitly coerced the Chinese to allow the sale of the dangerous drug, came to be known as the "Opium War." China, defeated, was forced to pay damages, to revoke the prohibition of opium, to open a number of ports to British traders, and to grant them numerous privileges on Chinese soil.

3. **A.** In 1846, new hopes for change were aroused by the election of a rather young pope, Pius IX, who was credited with liberal leanings and administrative ability.

4. **A.** In 1827, the Peace of Adrianople and, subsequently, the Treaty of Unkiar Skelessy (1833) gave them not only territorial concessions, but also special rights in the straits and a voice in internal Ottoman Turkish affairs. In 1841, however, an end was put to this southward penetration. When new troubles in Turkey occurred, England, Prussia, and Austria insisted on joint international, instead of unilateral Russian, action. Thus, a turning point was reached in the development of Russia's foreign policies.

5. **A.** The revolutions of 1848 were not as dramatic as the great Revolution of 1789. Their effect, however, was hardly less incisive. The French Revolution of 1789 came at the end of a period, the *ancien regime* with its feudal heritage; the revolutions of 1848 occurred at the beginning of a new age. They introduced the socialistic element into the political arena of the bourgeois world.

6. **C.** In 1848, Karl Marx published his *Communist Manifesto*. The same industries that gave the middle class its strength also created deplorable working conditions. Thus, there quickly arose a challenge to middle-class predominance. The benefits promised to all by the liberal creed proved to be in many ways illusory. Instead of furthering "the greatest happiness of the greatest number," its unregulated functioning created unexpected misery and necessitated an early modification.

7. **B.** New elections were held to choose a president for the republic. The people in the provinces, eager to restore national unity and prestige, and the bourgeoisie in the cities, who wanted a government strong enough to deal with labor revolts, voted against the provisional government. On December 10, 1848, Louis Napoleon was elected head of the Second Republic.

8. **C.** A movement called "Young Italy" envisioned a *Risorgimento,* a rebirth of the nation, but it remained weak. Rebellions, which occurred at regular intervals, achieved little. Thus, in 1834, a revolt undertaken in Genoa by a young enthusiast, Garibaldi, resulted in failure and the exile of its leader.

**CHAPTER 15**

# Political Reorganization (1848-1870)

1849 Frankfurt Assembly dissolved
1848 Macaulay, *History of England*
1850 Cavour becomes prime minister of Piedmont
1852 Napoleon III becomes emperor
   Harriet Beecher Stowe, *Uncle Tom's Cabin*
1854 Start of Crimean War
   Opening of Japan to the West
1857 Peace of Paris
   Bessemer process for steel manufacturing invented
1857 Indian Mutiny
   Dred Scott decision
1858 Treaty of Tientsin: opening of China to the West
1859 War between Austria and Piedmont
   Mill, *Essay on Liberty*
1860 Chevalier-Cobden Treaty between France and England
1861 Kingdom of Italy founded
   Death of Cavour
   Outbreak of Civil War in U.S.A.
   Emancipation of serfs in Russia
1862 Bismarck becomes Prussian prime minister
1863 Emancipation Proclamation by Lincoln
   Revolt in Poland
1864 Danish-German War for Schleswig-Holstein
   French expedition in Mexico (Emperor Maximilian)
   "First International" (workers' association)
   Pius IX, "Syllabus of Errors"

*The dynamic changes of the quarter-century following 1848 contrast sharply with the relative lack of change prevailing during the preceding quarter-century. In 1850, Cavour became prime minister of Piedmont, and in 1852, Louis Napoleon made himself emperor of France. The "tsar-liberator," Alexander II, came to the throne of Russia in 1855. Abraham Lincoln was elected president of the United States in 1860, and, in 1862, Bismarck became prime minister of Prussia. Most of these leaders worked to transform the existing institutions rather than preserve them. In the pursuit of their aims, all except the Russian emperor resorted to force. While not of continental or global scope, wars mark the period between 1848 and 1870.*

*By 1870, the balance of power as established by Metternich had changed. The previously existing societal structures in East and West, in Russia and the United States, were altered in the wake of emancipation movements. A new and aggressive spirit expressed itself in the renewed expansionist drive of Western societies to other continents.*

## ■ EUROPE FROM 1848 TO 1870

The first few years after 1848 seemed to bring a renewal of reactionary political policies. However, this mood soon vanished. Progressive trends were increasingly felt in most European countries. The strength of both liberals and socialists increased, and concessions had to be made to the very forces that had been defeated in the revolutions of 1848. Constitutions were liberalized. The right to vote was extended to larger segments of the populations everywhere. Social legislation was broadened, and nationalistic ambitions were furthered.

*Figure 15–1 The German Confederation, 1848–1858*

## France

The republican dream of the French enthusiasts of 1848 was short-lived. Within three years, the president of the Second Republic, Louis Napoleon, making free use of bribery and violating the constitution through arbitrary changes in the electoral law, had himself elected to another ten-year term as president. A year later, in December 1852, he proclaimed himself the emperor, "Napoleon III."

### Napoleon III (1852-1870)

Napoleon set to work shaping public opinion to suit his ambitions. He won over the well-to-do middle class by pledging to restore order. He gained support from the working class by publicizing the socialistic leanings of his youth. He obtained the good will of monarchists, Napoleonists, and army officers by promising them glory. To the bureaucracy, he granted higher salaries, and he pacified the clergy by supporting the papacy against Italian nationalists and republicans. To all, he promised peace.

Once in power, he muzzled the press, harassed the universities, exiled opponents, and permitted the schools to revert to Church supervision. He tried to control judicial decisions. He reintroduced universal suffrage, but the representative assembly was given no more than a shadowy existence. Yet, statesmen gave him the support they withheld from his amiable predecessor and thus enhanced his prestige. In some respects, he is considered the model for later totalitarian rulers.

### Height of Napoleonic System

During Louis Napoleon's first ten years of rule, France prospered. Banks and credit institutes were organized, and industries were encouraged. The fashion industry was promoted by his wife, Eugenie. Railways and telegraph facilities were built, and new methods in agriculture were sponsored. An economic boom promised to mitigate some of the hard conditions experienced by laborers. Mutually advantageous low tariffs were negotiated with neighbors. For example, the Chevalier-Cobden Treaty of 1860 provided for free trade with Britain. Broad new boulevards were constructed to beautify Paris and simultaneously served as a precaution against possible insurgents. A great international exposition and festivals, which were organized to encourage trade, made France the focus of world attention.

Ominous signs appeared with Napoleon's ambitious foreign policies, however, which brought war after war. Within two years of his accession to the throne, France, in alliance with Britain, invaded Russia. After victory was won, a peace congress was held in Paris, but the French gained little but vain prestige. Senegal in Africa was annexed. An extremely bloody war waged in Italy against Austria in 1859 brought the acquisition of the Italian territories of Savoy and Nice.

### Decline of Napoleonic System

The experience of the Italian war, Napoleon III's ill health, and the fear of mounting discontent created some relaxation in the Napoleonic system after 1860. Attempts were made to liberalize the government. Press and parliament were given greater freedom and influence. Greater attention was paid to the grievances of the working class, whose right to strike was formally recognized in 1864. New foreign adventures wrecked the empire, however, and wars broke out in Morocco and Syria. Amman was invaded in 1862, and large funds were invested in the construction of the Suez Canal. When the United States became involved in civil war, a French expedition was sent to conquer Mexico.

The disastrous expedition to Mexico began with the conquest of Mexico City and ended with defeat and the execution of Napoleon's puppet emperor, Maximilian. Another blow came in 1866, when Prussia defeated Austria, and by means of generous peace terms, put an end to the internal German rivalry that had always been of benefit to France. Napoleon tried in vain to strengthen his position by offering further concessions within France and by attempting to obtain compensation from Prussia for French neutrality during the Prusso-Austrian war. In 1870, a new issue, the succession to the Spanish throne, led him to risk another war, this time against Germany. Within little more than a month, Napoleon was captured. While a prisoner in Germany, he was deposed, and for the third time, France became a republic.

## Germany

The Revolution of 1848 created a setback for German national aspirations, as well as for liberal hopes. It had demonstrated the weakness of both the middle class and proletariat, a weakness that came from the initially slow development of industry and business and the lack of great social leaders who might have inspired the middle class. The year 1849 had brought new uprisings in Vienna, new conflicts in Italy, and a resumption of the revolution in Hungary. All were in vain.

### Reaction

In Austria, the new minister, Schwarzenberg, understood how to carry on the traditions of Metternich. He made minimal concessions to the new spirit. Rather, he helped reestablish the authority of the emperor and the prestige of the Hapsburgs within the German federation. He revived the conservative spirit of pre-revolutionary days. Prussia likewise failed to promote either liberal or national institutions. Although the Prussian king perceived that the unification of the German states might make his state the leader of a new Germany, he was forced, after a conference with Austria at Olmtitz in 1850, to give up such aspirations. Hopes disappeared both for a liberal Germany and for a united Germany under a constitutional monarchy. The southern German states followed the political example of Austria. Nothing survived other than the existing loose federation with its ineffectual Frankfurt parliament.

The next decade was conservative in political affairs despite the fact that in 1850, the King of Prussia granted a constitution providing for universal suffrage, although by classes. Progress was made in the economic sphere. Particularly in western Germany, industrialization grew apace; coal mining and steel production greatly increased. As in France, banks were founded, railways built, and the postal service, which was once in private hands, improved and expanded. Foreign trade also grew. The sciences flourished. The high standards of the German universities continued to make the country an important center of scholarship in the West. Only when a crisis occurred in Prussia over an army budget did grave political issues again stir the country. A succession of rapid changes took place, however.

### Bismarck

In 1861, Prussia's parliament refused to appropriate funds demanded by the king for a new army program. The liberals tried to use this occasion to gain political concessions in exchange for support. The army, however, was of decisive importance to Prussia, and as a last resort, the king appointed Otto von Bismarck as prime minister in 1862. He had been a representative at Frankfurt, ambassador to Russia, and then ambassador to France.

Bismarck's father was a small landowner, a nobleman, and a conservative. Bismarck solved the budget problem by unconstitutional means through the collection of the necessary taxes without parliamentary authorization. He strengthened Prussia's position by helping Russia subdue a Polish rebellion in 1863. Then, he induced Austria to join Prussia in settling another problem. The German provinces of Schleswig and Holstein had long been united dynastically with Denmark, even after the German states had supported a Schleswig revolt in 1848. However, when the Danish ruling family died out in 1863, the Danes decided to annex Schleswig completely. Bismarck took advantage of this situation to whip up national enthusiasm against annexation. War was declared, and, despite a valiant defense by the Danes, the provinces were conquered. The administration of the territory was then divided between Austria and Prussia. Dissensions arose and gave Bismarck an opportunity to settle the issue of Prussian versus Austrian leadership in Germany.

Figure 15-2 Otto Von Bismarck, 1815–1898

### Solution of Austro-Prussian Dualism

War broke out in 1866. To the surprise of all Europe, Prussia defeated the Austrians and their South German allies within seven weeks. The excellence of the Prussian army, its use of the newly invented needle gun, and the brilliant strategy of General Moltke were responsible for the victory in the one decisive battle at Sadowa. Peace followed promptly. Acting with prudence, Bismarck made no demands on Austria except that it would not oppose the rearrangement of German affairs contemplated by Prussia The only territorial loss incurred by Austria was the surrender of Venice to Italy, which had been induced to attack Austria from the south.

As a result, the Hapsburgs withdrew from involvements in internal German affairs and devoted their attention to reconstituting their empire. A dual monarchy was established—Austria-Hungary. The two areas were governed by the same ruler and pursued a common policy in public finance and foreign relations, but each managed its internal affairs independently. The Hapsburgs failed, however, to extend similar local autonomy to the Slavs, and thus implemented their reorganization only halfway.

In the meantime, Bismarck set to work on the reconstruction of Germany. North German states that had supported Austria were incorporated into Prussia. South German states were left independent, but made secret military alliances with Prussia and, in 1867, joined the Prussian Customs Union. The North German *Bund,* a new federation under Prussia's presidency, was formed, and a common parliament was established.

### Founding of the German Empire

It was then that, alarmed by the emergence of a greatly strengthened Prussia, Napoleon III asked for territorial compensations in Germany. He made several suggestions, but were all rejected. The position of France was further weakened when the possibility arose of a new dynastic combination, Prussia and Spain, which could menace France from two sides. Having had their own revolution, the Spaniards offered their vacant throne to a Hohenzollern prince who was distantly related to the Prussian king. The French protested. In July 1870, they ordered their envoy to ask the Prussian king, who was vacationing at Bad Ems, to withhold his consent. The king telegraphed his prime minister, and the telegram—the famous *Ems depeche*— was edited and published by Bismarck in such a way as to inflame national feelings in both Berlin and Paris. Mass hysteria seized Paris.

In the confusion, the French declared war, and the Franco-Prussian War began. World opinion was mainly on Prussia's side. Prussian troops were joined by those of all other German states and overwhelmed the French forces. Two entire French army corps were taken prisoner—one in which Napoleon III was captured at Sedan, and the other at Metz. When the German armies were at the gates of Paris, Bismarck arranged for the crowning achievement of his policies: a united "German Empire" was proclaimed in the French palace of Versailles, and the Prussian king was designated as its emperor.

The nation was established as a constitutional monarchy—a union of some twenty states that included all German peoples except those living in the Hapsburg Empire. Shortly thereafter, Paris was taken. France agreed to German demands to pay an indemnity of $1 billion within three years. This indemnity was fully paid before the term expired. Alsace was ceded to Germany except for the Territory of Belfort and a large part of Lorraine. The latter provision was included more for strategic than nationalistic reasons, as well as for the sake of the rich iron mines of the region.

## Italy

Italy's path to unification was much more circuitous than that of Germany. Among the most serious obstacles were subjection to foreign rule, slow economic development, a lack of capable leaders, and the existence of the Papal States. The success of unification efforts hinged upon the role of Piedmont. Yet, in 1849, Piedmont itself was defeated in war and torn by inner struggles.

### *Cavour*

Count Cavour changed the situation and prepared Piedmont for Italian leadership. Beginning his career as prime minister in 1850, he proved to be one of the most astute statesmen of his time. He realized that only liberal policies and economic strength could give Piedmont the necessary prestige and influence. Hence, he reduced tariffs, entered into favorable commercial treaties with neighboring countries, encouraged railway building, improved Franco-Italian relations by tunneling the Alps at Mont Cenis, and modernized the army. He made concessions to the liberals, such as legalizing civil marriage and suppressing mendicant religious orders, such as the Franciscans and Dominicans. He protected Church life where it did not interfere with politics, however.

### *Steps to Unification*

Cavour also applied his energies to external policies. His first objective was to "put Italy on the map." For this purpose, he joined England and France in the Crimean War, which demanded many sacrifices. However, it served Italian interests by enabling the king of Piedmont, after the victory, to show himself triumphantly in Paris and London and to have Piedmont participate in the Peace Congress of Paris in 1857. There, Cavour brought up the Italian problem, extolled Piedmont's future role, and laid the groundwork for an alliance with France, which was consummated two years later.

Once this was achieved, he provoked war with Austria. Supported by Napoleon III, the Italians defeated the Austrians in two extremely bloody battles at Magenta and Solferino. It was at Solferino that a young Swiss banker, Dunant, conceived the idea of organizing a relief institution for prisoners and the wounded. Subsequently, Dunant founded the Red Cross.

The French emperor deserted the Italian cause shortly after Solferino. Fearing that Italy might become too powerful or that Prussia might intervene, he concluded a peace treaty with Austria at Villafranca. This treaty secured the province of Lombardy for Piedmont, but did not bring unity to the whole of Italy. Disheartened, Cavour resigned.

Yet, the process of unification had been set in motion. Within a year, Cavour returned to his premiership. The Central Provinces revolted against their various Austrian rulers and, by plebiscite, also joined Piedmont. In order to secure Napoleon's recognition of this second step in Italian unification, Italy had to cede Savoy and Nice to France.

Almost simultaneously, a third step was taken. With the support of Cavour, Garibaldi led a band of a "thousand" volunteers into Sicily and quickly succeeded in driving out the Spanish Bourbon rulers. Crossing back to the mainland, Garibaldi occupied Naples; simultaneously, Piedmontese troops coming from the north seized part of the Papal States. In 1861, the king of Piedmont was proclaimed king of Italy, Florence became the capital, and a constitution was drafted. Only Venetia and Rome were still lacking to complete Italian unity. In the same year, Cavour died.

### Fulfillment

In 1866, after Prussia's victory, Italy seized Venice. The capture of Napoleon III in 1870 enabled Italy to take Rome. As soon as the French emperor could no longer protect the papacy, the Italians invaded

*Figure 15–3 The Unification of Italy, 1870*

the city and put an end to the temporal (or civil) power of the popes. A history of more than a thousand years was thus concluded. Denouncing the "evil" spirit of the time, Pius IX retreated into the Vatican. He refused ever to set foot again on the soil outside, thus making the popes voluntary prisoners for more than half a century. Rome became the capital of Italy. Many problems remained. Italy had achieved unity only with foreign help, its national strength remaining at a low level. It had not made peace with the papacy. Its economy, though improving, offered no firm foundation for a prosperous commonwealth. Jurisdiction did not include Italian populations in the southern part of South Tirol, in Dalmatia, Savoy, Nice, Corsica, or Malta. Yet, Italy had become an independent, united country with a constitutional monarchy. It had attained a certain amount of stability and could take its place among the modern nations of Europe.

### Britain

While the period from 1848 to 1870 witnessed great innovations in France, Germany, and Italy, it brought few changes in Britain. Enjoying its "splendid isolation," its industrial wealth, and its "Victorian" way of life, Britain continued on the path of gradual democratization and colonial expansion. With the backing of industrialists in the manufacturing cities of the Midlands, in Manchester, Birmingham, and Sheffield, the Liberal party stayed in power. Prime ministers of considerable ability—Russell, Derby, Palmerston, and, later, Gladstone—directed the government. Consistent support was given to business, and various regulations helped to improve conditions for the working class. In 1867, when the Conservatives under Prime Minister Disraeli were in power for a short time, a second Reform Bill was passed. It extended the franchise to large additional segments of the middle class. Emigration to all parts of the empire was encouraged so that ties with Britain would be strengthened and markets for British goods would be developed.

In foreign affairs, a vigorous colonial policy was pursued. British nationalistic sentiments were aroused, and the various governments, especially in Palmerston's time, appealed to them. In Africa, British holdings were extended through the work of missionaries and merchants, who were followed by occupation troops: "the flag following trade." New concessions were demanded from China. In India, an uprising of the natives in the British army in 1857, known as the "Mutiny," was fiercely suppressed, whereupon the administration of India was put entirely under the direction of the British government.

In Canada, reforms were undertaken. In order to retain Canada's loyalty, Britain gave the country control of its internal affairs in the 1850s. The British North American Act of 1867 recognized the change, and Canada became a "Dominion." Special attention was paid to safeguard the communication lines between Britain and its colonies. Russia was prevented from gaining free access to the Mediterranean by the Crimean War. Subsequent wars and treaties with Persia and Afghanistan also prevented Russia from reaching the land route to India.

## ■ RUSSIA AND AMERICA

The years from 1848 to 1870 were also of importance to Russia and the United States. Decisive events included the abolition of serfdom in Russia and the abolition of slavery in the United States.

### Russia

For Russia, the decisive moment came with the Crimean War. It revealed the backwardness, inefficiency, and corruption of Russian institutions and forced the government to undertake long-overdue reforms.

#### *Crimean War and Russian Expansion in Asia*

The Crimean War (1854–1856), which was provoked by Napoleon III's meddling in Turkish affairs, but essentially reflected British-Russian rivalry, brought little glory to any participant. Russian soldiers fought valiantly; their defense of the fortress of Sebastopol has become famous. However, their leaders and their equipment were lamentable. Motley French, British, Italian, and Turkish troops, though just as badly led, were able to defeat Russia and impose stifling peace conditions. Russia was deprived of all the special rights it had enjoyed on Turkish soil. It was forbidden to maintain fortifications along its Black Sea border or to keep warships there. Earlier conquests were restored to Turkey. With its drive southward stalled, Russia renounced further advances in Europe and turned its attention eastward. There, it met with better success. Penetrating the central Asiatic regions, it occupied Tashkent, Bokhara, Samarkand, and Khiva. It also sent troops and settlers under Count Muraviev into the Amur region, forcing China to relinquish the territory. In 1860, Russia built the harbor of Vladivostok on the Sea of Japan. It penetrated Manchuria and occupied Sakhalin.

These successes in the East, compensating somewhat for the failures in the West, did not allow the government to overlook the need to correct the country's internal weaknesses, however. Nicholas I had died during the Crimean War. His son, Alexander II, faced the difficult task of converting Russian institutions to meet the demands of modern times.

### *Emancipation*

The defects of the Russian system were rooted in the institution of serfdom, which made it impossible to modernize and industrialize the country. Serfdom was universally condemned by economists, sociologists, and idealists. It was the chief target of the "intelligentsia," an important group of the educated population. Composed largely of members of the free professions, students, and merchants, the intelligentsia had been driven more and more into opposition to all aspects of the existing political system. Many of them came from the ranks of the high nobility, but they, too, preferred exile and disgrace to living under the existing conditions, no matter how much, personally, they could have profited by them. The literary critic Belinsky, the politician Herzen, the social philosopher Samarin, the anarchist Bakunin—these intellectuals and innumerable others unceasingly protested against the evils of autocracy and its counterpart, serfdom.

Alexander may not have listened, but the lesson of the Crimean War could not be ignored. In 1856, he appointed a commission to prepare the necessary reform work. He insisted that any plan include provisions to give the peasants (1) freedom, (2) an economic basis for their lives (namely, land), and (3) due compensation to the former owners whose land was to be transferred to peasants. Owing to the steadfast cooperation of progressive landowners, the gigantic task of liberation was accomplished within five years. Neither fear of its possible revolutionary consequences nor opposition from reactionary quarters could stop the work. Additionally, it could not be stopped by lack of financial means, bureaucratic impediments, or difficulties resulting from the diversity of conditions in the various parts of the empire.

On February 19, 1861, 23 million serfs and their families were declared free and received land allotments. A transitional period, however, was provided. During this period, the peasant did not gain actual ownership of the land, but remained a member of a village community *(mir)* in which ownership was vested and which provided for communal cultivation of the fields. The *mir* received certain rights of jurisdiction over its members. It was responsible for the special "redemption tax," which, in the course of some 40 years, was to reimburse the state for compensation paid to the landowners.

### *Financial and Judicial Reforms*

Once the government abolished serfdom, it proceeded rapidly with additional reforms. It reorganized state finances and the tax system, created a state bank, and set up a regular budget. It abolished state monopolies and made numerous personnel changes. Educational reforms followed. Universities were given more freedom, women were admitted to schools of secondary education, and public education was extended. Censorship regulations were modified.

In the political and judicial sphere, district assemblies *(zemstvos)* were established to decide local issues. Equality before the law was formally acknowledged, and secret interrogation and flogging were prohibited. A jury system was introduced, and judges were freed of governmental control. Municipalities received charters for self-government. Finally, through universal conscription, the arbitrary levying of troops was ended. Reform measures were slowed by a revolt of the Poles in 1863 and an attempt on the life of the tsar in 1866, but by 1870, Russia had, without civil war or revolution, achieved a reorganization that enabled it to enter the Modern Age.

## United States

In the United States, foremost in the practice of liberal democracy, the same issue of involuntary human servitude and its economic consequences was the most inhibiting factor and burning problem during the period between 1848 and 1870. The issue concerned a smaller sector of the population than it did in Russia, but the practice of full "slavery" in the U.S., as opposed to "serfdom," was more revolting to the conscience of modern people. It was also more complicated. It had an effect on the entire political scene, aroused regional jealousies, and involved racial antagonisms.

### *Emancipation*

During the 1850s, the United States experienced a rapid development of its productive forces. Output in industry and mining increased, and railway construction proceeded rapidly, which stimulated the giving of land grants as gifts to the railway builders. Additional areas of public land were sold at minimal prices, opening the way to even more speculation and corruption, while providing pioneers with farmland. The discovery of gold in California released a stream of prospectors to the West, rapidly populating it with Americans and many newly arrived immigrants. National wealth grew, and liberal political institutions continued to foster an enterprising, inventive spirit.

Grave problems remained unresolved, however. Ideology divided the northern and the southern states. Divergent economic interests between an industrialized North and an agricultural South could not be reconciled. The routing of railways across the continent, important for future development as well as the personal gain of entrepreneurs, caused bitter disputes. Slavery and the status of fugitive slaves who sought shelter in the North also created divisions. In 1854, the Missouri Compromise was repealed. Thus, at the very time when European nations were maintaining relatively stable governments, the United States experienced widespread controversy and dissension that threatened the peace of the land.

Into this atmosphere, Abraham Lincoln was elected to the presidency in 1860. Within a few months, the southern states seceded from the Union. At that point, the issue of preserving the union came to overshadow the issue of slavery. The Civil War began. Both sides were poorly organized, but the North was better equipped and richer. Owing to the ruthless use of modern weapons, the war caused extremely heavy casualties on both sides and especially terrible devastation in the South, where unarmed civilian inhabitants suffered incredible brutality. Victory for the industrially stronger North did not come until 1865. However, in 1863, about two years after Russia's freeing of the serfs, Lincoln issued his Emancipation Proclamation. It freed the slaves. In contrast to the laws passed in Russia, this measure failed to provide the freedmen with land as a basis for their economic future. It did not, in fact, even gain for them the equal rights set forth in subsequent amendments to the Constitution. More Americans were killed in the course of the Civil War than in the two later world wars combined. When Lincoln was assassinated soon after the end of the war, the South was treated as a conquered country. Confiscations, discrimination, and military occupation were imposed upon the vanquished. As to the slaves, their segregation was not ended, but personal slavery was abolished. The country was reunited politically, and the balance of power shifted decisively in favor of the North. In the long run, the way was now open to further modernization and national prosperity.

## Expansion

The vigorous United States pushed on to new tasks. In 1867, the government purchased Alaska from Russia, and in 1869, the first transcontinental railway was completed. The government made available new territories for farming and encouraged business enterprise by passing more effective protective tariffs. The subsequent economic boom helped even the defeated South to regain economic health and contributed immensely to the political strength of the nation.

## ■ THE WEST, ASIA, AND AFRICA

Events during the period from 1848 to 1870 changed the political and social structure of both the European continent and North America. They also transformed the relationship between Western civilization and the rest of the globe. A new era of expansion in Western countries began, and their scientific methods and techniques spread to other lands. This process took place not only in regions completely or partially under Western domination, but even in independent nations that adopted Western ways on their own initiative.

### Asia

The course of Westernization in Asia is most manifest in Japan. The Japanese succeeded in introducing many Western ways without becoming colonized. During the regime of Emperor Meiji, Japan, having been forced to open its ports to Western traders in 1854, averted the dangers of domestic revolution and foreign subjugation by adopting reforms in the European model.

Other peoples of Asia had to accept Western ways involuntarily through a combination of economic and military penetration. The Dutch occupied Sumatra and other parts of Indonesia, which were rich in sugar and coffee. They arbitrarily imposed Dutch customs and institutions. Weak, impoverished China, torn by internal disorders and rivalry between conservative and reform factions, had to establish diplomatic relations with the West. Forced to grant extraterritorial rights, China was also made to cede ports to Western governments. It even had to renounce many old ties with other Eastern nations. Only constant bickering among the Europeans themselves saved China from losing its independence. As it was, Britain, which had instigated the Opium War, attacked the country once more. Together with French contingents, British troops looted Peking in 1860.

In India, after the Mutiny of 1857, the British imposed their jurisdiction and customs. Their policy of "salutary neglect," which meant indifference to the domestic needs of the country, was combined with a gradual enforcement of Western political and legal concepts. A portion of the upper class was slowly Anglicized. Many Indian students received an education in England. Indian markets and resources were integrated into the British economy. In Persia and Afghanistan, both England and Russia exerted a dominant economic and political influence.

### Africa and the Americas

In Africa, the northern coast became the chief objective of European colonization. Construction of the Suez Canal began in 1859, and it was opened for international navigation in 1869. French, English, and Spanish interests were established among the Muslims of North Africa—then largely under Ottoman Turkish rule.

The Western nations also expanded their activities and influence in North and South America. Immigration, the settlement of vast areas, the building of railways, and the integration of the entire region into the Western economy acted as powerful forces, spreading to all parts of the Western Hemisphere the concepts, social customs, and industrial techniques of the West.

## Imperialism

In the late19th century, imperialism meant the building of European empires by embracing weaker, mainly underdeveloped, colonial nations. It constituted a violent form of nationalism. Like all colonizers, the imperialist nations often brought a modicum of order, law, and certain ethical and religious precepts. They also brought a measure of education to their colonial areas. However, in their search for raw materials, industrial markets, fiscal revenues, and national prestige, the imperialists often ruthlessly exploited the inhabitants of these areas. For the sake of maintaining control over them, many wars were fought, and many injustices were committed. Independence movements were suppressed.

## Perspective

*After the revolutions of 1848, important changes occurred in the European political arena. Governments in most European countries took further steps, through action "from above," toward the introduction of constitutions which, though still limited in scope, included important moves toward representative government. France experienced a brief period of social and economic progress followed by a decline, mainly owing to the ambitious foreign policies of Napoleon III. Germany, resolving the leadership dispute between Prussia and Austria in favor of Prussia, progressed toward unification. Italy likewise made great strides in the same direction.*

*The greatest changes occurred in Russia and the United States. Both countries, Russia peacefully, the United States in a devastating war, put an end to serfdom in Russia and slavery in America. Both enlarged their territories through wars, penetration, and settlement on their respective continents. Imperialism triumphed in England and France as it did in Russia and the United States. Western economic, diplomatic, military, political, and missionary institutions spread around the globe. Imperialism wove "a close net of common behavior and thought patterns" of Western origin around all parts of the five continents.*

## Selected Readings

Blum, Jerome. *Lord and Peasant in Russia* (New York: Atheneum, 1964).

Dehio, Ludwig. *The Precarious Balance: Four Centuries of European Power Struggle* (New York: Knopf, 1962).

Hearder, H. *Italy: A Short History* (Cambridge: Cambridge University Press, 2001).

Hofstadter, Richard. *The American Political Tradition and the Man Who Made It* (New York: Knopf, 1979).

Kann, Robert A. *History of the Habsburg Empire 1526–1918* (Berkeley: The University of California Press, 1974).

Raisanovsky, Nicholas V. *A History of Russia* (New York: Oxford University Press, 1984).

Kolchin, Peter. *Unfree Labor: American Slavery and Russian Serfdom* (Cambridge: Harvard University Press, 1987).

Mack Smith, Denis. *Cavour* (New York: Knopf, 1985).

Morison, Samuel E. *The Oxford History of the American People* (New York: Oxford University Press, 1965).

Pipes, Richard. *Russia under the Old Regime* (New York: Scribner, 1974).

Plessis, A. *The Rise and Fall of the Second Empire, 1852–1871* (Cambridge: Cambridge University Press, 1985).

Lerman, Katherine. *Bismarck* (New York: Pearson Longman, 2004).

Webb, R. K. *Modern England, from the Eighteenth Century to the Present* (New York, Harper & Row, 1980).

## Test Yourself

1. In 1862, Prussia was led by Prime Minister_____.
   A. Adolph Hitler
   B. William I
   C. Otto von Bismarck
   D. William II

2. In the Franco-Prussian War of 1870, the French were_____.
   A. Victorious
   B. Defeated
   C. Forced to pay indemnities
   D. Both B and C

3. Italian unification hinged upon the role of_____.
   A. The Pope
   B. Sicily
   C. Piedmont
   D. Rome

4. The Crimean War (1854-1856) was fought mainly between_____.
   A. Russia and France
   B. Russia and England
   C. Russia and Austria
   D. Russia and the Ottoman Empire

5. Abraham Lincoln was elected to the presidency of the United States in_____.
   A. 1860
   B. 1865
   C. 1862
   D. 1880

6. The American Civil War was fought during the period_____.
   A. 1862-1868
   B. 1861-1865
   C. 1860-1865
   D. 1850-1877

7. In 1867, Great Britain was led by a conservative prime minister named_____.
   A. Gladstone
   B. Lord Palmerston
   C. Benjamin Disraeli
   D. None of the above

8. During the period leading to the American Civil War, the issue of preserving the union came to overshadow the issue of_____.
   A. Liberty
   B. States Rights
   C. Slavery
   D. Tariffs

## Answers and Explanations

1. **C.** In 1861, Prussia's parliament refused to appropriate funds demanded by the king for a new army program. The liberals tried to use this occasion to gain political concessions in exchange for support. The army, however, was of decisive importance to Prussia and, as a last resort, the king appointed Otto von Bismarck as prime minister in 1862. He had been a representative at Frankfurt, ambassador to Russia, and ambassador to France.

2. **D.** The French declared war, and the Franco-Prussian War began. World opinion was mainly on Prussia's side. Prussian troops, joined by those of all other German states, overwhelmed the French forces. Two entire French army corps were taken prisoner—one in which Napoleon III was captured at Sedan, the other at Metz. When the German armies were at the gates of Paris, Bismarck arranged for the crowning achievement of his policies: A united "German Empire" was proclaimed in the French palace of Versailles, and the Prussian king was designated as its emperor.

3. **C.** Italy's path to unification was much more circuitous than that of Germany. Among the most serious obstacles were subjection to foreign rule, slow economic development, a lack of capable leaders, and the existence of the Papal States. The success of unification efforts hinged upon the role of Piedmont. Yet, in 1849, Piedmont itself was defeated in war and torn by inner struggles.

4. **D.** Provoked by Napoleon III's meddling in Turkish affairs, but essentially reflecting British-Russian rivalry, the Crimean War (1854–1856) brought little glory to any participant. Russian soldiers fought valiantly; their defense of the fortress of Sebastopol has become famous. Their leaders and their equipment were lamentable, however. Motley French, British, Italian, and Turkish troops, though just as badly led, were able to defeat Russia and impose stifling peace conditions.

5. **A.** Abraham Lincoln was elected to the presidency in 1860. Within a few months, the southern states seceded from the Union.

6. **B.** The Civil War began in 1861. Both sides were poorly organized, but the North was better equipped and richer. Owing to the ruthless use of modern weapons, the war caused extremely heavy casualties on both sides and fearful devastation in the South, where even unarmed civilian inhabitants suffered incredible brutalities. Victory for the industrially stronger North did not come until 1865.

7. **C.** In 1867, when the Conservatives under Prime Minister Disraeli were in power for a short time, a second Reform Bill was passed to extend the franchise to large additional segments of the middle class. Emigration to all parts of the empire was encouraged so that ties with Britain would be strengthened and markets for British goods would be developed.

8. **C.** Abraham Lincoln was elected to the presidency in 1860. Within a few months, the southern states seceded from the Union. At that point, the issue of preserving the union came to overshadow the issue of slavery.

# CHAPTER 16
# Revaluation of Values (1848-1870)

**1865** End of American Civil War
Lincoln assassinated
Maxwell, *Treatise on Electricity*
**1864** Tolstoy, *War and Peace*
**1866** Austro-Prussian ("Seven Weeks")
War Italy annexes Venetia
Dostoevsky, *Crime and Punishment*
**1867** Dual monarchy of Austria-Hungary established
Invention of dynamite (Nobel)
Second Reform Bill in England
Marx, *Das Kapital*
Ibsen, *Peer Gynt*
Purchase of Alaska by U.S.A.
**1869** Opening of Suez Canal
**1870** Jules Verne, *Twenty Thousand Leagues under the Sea*
Outbreak of Franco Prussian War
Napoleon III made prisoner by Germans, deposed by French
End of Papal States: Rome becomes Italian capital
Dogma of papal infallibility
**1871** Founding of German Empire
Revolt of the *Commune* in Paris
Impressionist exhibition in Paris
Verdi, *Aida*

*The rapid transformation of the political stage of the West by the thought, fervor, and endeavors of statesmen like Cavour, Bismarck, Napoleon III, and others, and by events like the emancipation of serfs and slaves in Russia and America, was duplicated in the contemporary cultural scene by equally rapid changes. In the sciences, Darwin's theory of evolution changed previously held concepts far beyond the field of biology for which it was conceived. In the arts, the traditionalism of a century was overturned by the impressionists. In literature, the novels of Dostoevsky and Tolstoy opened up new vistas into human nature, human passions, and the human subconscious. In the religious field, scholarly research and historical criticism of the Scriptures attacked inherited views, and a conflict took shape between a society trusting in science and progress and individuals vigorously reaffirming Christian tenets and creeds.*

*Finally, the whole social pattern of Western civilization was called into question and repudiated by the work of Karl Marx.*

## ■ DEVELOPING PATTERNS

The period from 1848-1870 witnessed several developing patterns in the fields of social and natural sciences. As a result, many European societies experienced rapid socio-economic and political transformations.

### History

The study of history took on a particularly important new role, in line with scientific views, in the middle of the 19th century. A growing consciousness developed about the significance of the past to conditions in the present. Avoiding the often utopian, idealistic, and imaginative approach marking the Age of Enlightenment, historians now used scientific methods. They engaged in conscientious study of sources on which they based their writings. In general, they followed the principle stated by Ranke—to describe "what actually happened." Their method came to be applied in various fields outside the study of history as well, but they combined their aim of pure scholarship with that of the *philosophes* of the 18th century, who had been ready to interpret, to educate, and to indoctrinate. Historical writings, therefore, became a force of national significance in preserving national traditions and promoting national consciousness. Especially influential were Carlyle and Macaulay in England and Bancroft and Parkman in the United States. On the Continent, Mommsen's masterful work on Roman history, written with detachment, was supplemented by historians like Sybel and Droysen, who acclaimed the Prussian state, and by Thiers and Michelet in France, who presented to their compatriots the glories of the French Revolution and Napoleon.

### Literature

European literature generally followed paths established earlier in the century. Germany continued to add to its past accomplishments. France continued to maintain a high level of prose fiction through the works of Zola, Maupassant, and others. Britain had a number of skilled essayists and critics, as well as several excellent novelists and poets—the latter including Tennyson and Browning. The United States contributed the poems of Whitman and Longfellow, the novels of Melville and Hawthorne, and the essays of Thoreau and Emerson.

A considerable number of significant works were created by women. In Britain, it was George Eliot and Elizabeth Browning, in Germany Droste-Hülshoff, and in America, Emily Dickinson and others put their imprint on the literature of the age. A special place belongs to Harriet Beecher Stowe, who, with her moving *Uncle Tom's Cabin,* appealed to the conscience of the American people with regard to the abolition of slavery. Her work evoked worldwide sympathy.

In terms of the achievements of individual nations, however, it was Russia that produced the outstanding masterpieces of the time. In Russia, dissatisfaction with prevailing conditions led to a grave spiritual crisis. Out of the crisis emerged the searching, penetrating social and psychological novels of Turgenev *(Fathers and Sons),* Dostoevsky *(Crime and Punishment, the Brothers Karamazov),* and Tolstoy *(War and Peace, Anna Karenina).* On the whole, it was the novel that appealed to a large and literate public, a major part of which belonged to the upper-middle class.

### Music

In the field of music, post-1848 Europe maintained remarkably high standards with brilliant performers such as Liszt. Through his new harmonic conceptions, he also contributed much to the art of composition. Still more significant were the achievements in opera. The 19th century found operatic creation at its apex. Towering over the excellent French composers, such as Gounod *(Faust)* and Bizet *(Carmen),* were the two mighty figures of Wagner and Verdi *(Rigoletto, La Traviata, Aida).* Verdi devoted himself to Italian opera, with its emphasis on voice and melody, and brought it to new heights through the greatness of his art. Wagner *(Tristan and Isolde, Nibelungen Ring, Parsifal, Meistersinger)* traveled an independent path based on his view of opera as a musical drama that demanded serious texts of poetic worth. Wagner wrote his own librettos and allocated to the orchestra a more essential role than previous composers had done. His work, based on sagas and folklore, shows many romantic traits, yet it constitutes one of the most beautiful and enduring expressions of the age. The symphonic and concert music of the mid-19th century likewise attained excellence with works by Brahms, the foremost symphonic composer of his time, and significant contributions by Berlioz and other composers, such as Bruckner and Johann Strauss.

## Arts

Painting, too, received new inspiration, which led to lasting achievements. Neoclassic, neo-Gothic, pre-Raphaelite, and other contemporaneous and often imitative art movements, as their names imply, were denounced by a younger generation. Some of the great painters of the middle 19th century staged a revolt against the traditional approach. Artists in Paris took the lead. Paris had grown steadily important as an art center where masters such as Corot, Millet, and the caricaturist and critic Daumier produced and exhibited their works. Now, a new school of art, "impressionism," was developed by Manet, Monet, Degas, and other brilliant artists. They sought an artistic expression that departed sharply from the fashions, habits, and techniques of the past. Developing new concepts in the use of color and reproducing the luminous quality of the air, they depicted human life and nature in so fresh and inspiring a manner that they stimulated many disciples to carry forward the task of artistic reinterpretation.

By the mid-19th century, the arts began to reach a still wider public through new channels than in the preceding two centuries. In the Middle Ages and early Modern Age, it had been the churches, foremost the Catholic and Orthodox Churches, which had, in the West, communicated philosophical thought and the great works in music, art, and architecture to the populations. They appealed to rich and poor alike. The same was true in Reformation times, but, later, it was principally only select audiences that could follow the philosophical developments and enjoy the arts in salons, academies, and social gatherings in the homes of the elite. Now a wider public was reached once more. New outlets became available: concert halls, operas and theaters, and museums. Free lectures were given for the general public in special auditoriums, and newspapers reported and evaluated current political and cultural events.

## Philosophy

In the field of philosophy, rationalist tendencies, which had steadily grown since the late Middle Ages, attained a final triumph. Despite the acceptance of numerous traditional concepts in metaphysics, rational analysis had, in the 17th century, characterized the works of Descartes, Spinoza, and Leibnitz. Eighteenth-century philosophers of the Enlightenment had similarly put their trust in reason rather than faith; following them—despite idealistic and ethical differences—Kant, Hegel, and Fichte had also emphasized the function of reason.

This trend came to a climax in the mid-19th century with the philosophy of Comte, who rejected all views based upon metaphysical speculation. In his "positivist" system, he described metaphysics and religion as evidence of primitive stages of human development. To him, the future was to be shaped by science and based on logic and observable facts. Only through science would the human race reach its highest achievements. A scientific approach also underlay the empiricism of John Stuart Mill, who directed his attention to social organization. Mill became an advocate of democratic and liberal concepts—even though he distrusted their effect on the human spirit.

The same confidence in reason as the best guide to truth inspired David Friedrich Strauss. He applied the scientific method to the Scriptures, which he subjected to a searching criticism. This investigation led him to challenge the historical accuracy of many parts of the Bible. In the record of Christ's life, Ernest Renan saw the story of an extraordinary human being and the exposition of the highest ethical code. Together, Strauss and Renan added strength to a movement which rejected traditional, and especially transcendental, beliefs and which looked to science, logic, and reason for guidance.

## Science

Western civilization, having developed a steadfast confidence in reason and science, pressed forward in its investigations of nature. It searched for laws governing natural phenomena and sought to apply scientific knowledge to practical problems.

### *Physical Sciences*

In chemistry, Mendeleev, one of the first great Russian scientists, drafted the periodic table of the elements at the same time as the German, Meyer. There were many basic discoveries in both inorganic and organic chemistry. Liebig laid the foundations for a broad application of chemical knowledge to agriculture. A petroleum industry was founded. In physics, fundamental principles were discovered (especially thermodynamics and electricity). Large industries applying the new knowledge evolved, including those developing new inventions (e.g., telegraphy and photography).

### *Medical Sciences*

Of the most immediate benefit for people were the scientific advances in medical sciences. Researchers studied physiology, especially the human cellular structure and nervous system. They also investigated problems of nutrition. Pasteur and Koch made fundamental contributions in bacteriology, and the germ theory of diseases was widely disseminated. Long-established theories of spontaneous generation were conclusively discarded.

As the causes of dread diseases were traced to bacteria, antitoxins and other means of preventive and curative treatment were developed. Epidemics such as cholera still occurred in many countries, but sanitation improved and, with it, public health. Antisepsis came into general use, and anesthesia prevented untold suffering. Similarly, in embryology, insights of lasting benefit were achieved.

### *Biological Sciences*

The most notable advance leading to new insights of basic significance was made in biology. Many scientists, studying the life histories of plants, lower animals, and human beings, had concluded that an evolutionary process was taking place. Scientists like Erasmus Darwin and Lamarck, poets like Goethe, philosophers like Hegel, and social thinkers like Malthus had foreshadowed such views. The decisive step, however, was taken when Erasmus Darwin's grandson, Charles, explained life in terms of a struggle for existence in which the weak members among plants, lower animals, and humans are constantly being eliminated, while only the "fittest" survive. Thus, it was shown that a natural selection takes place and, through heredity, the natural qualities of the survivors are passed on from generation to generation until new, better-adapted species have evolved. This theory of evolution was promoted with almost religious fervor by a number of Darwin's disciples. Darwin's work brought a deeper understanding of nature's evolutionary processes. Additionally, it led to a rethinking of traditional beliefs outside the field of natural sciences.

## Religion

No area of human endeavor was more deeply affected by evolutionary views than that of the Christian churches. The whole of science, scientific methodology, historical criticism, and the climate of opinion of the Age of Liberalism and Nationalism posed a challenge. The Catholic and Protestant followers were now forced to face a world where scientific explanations were accepted for the evolution of the universe, the creation of the human race, and the relationship of humans and nature. They also had to consider the various modern theories about the connections between the individual and human society and between the psychology of people and their natural heritage.

### *Catholic Attitude*

In the presence of such issues, the Roman Catholic Church, under the firm hand of Pope Pius IX, who had disappointed the expectations of liberal and progressive thinkers, took a resolute stand. Since the Age of Enlightenment, the Church had fought a new wave of irreligion and atheism. In the first half of the 19th century, it had succeeded, despite the progress of science, in making new conversions, including the Anglican churchman John Henry Newman in England, who had converted to Catholicism. It had the satisfaction of seeing the emancipation of the Catholics in England in 1829 and the reestablishment of the Catholic hierarchy in 1850. The Church had normalized its relations with France, and it had survived the onslaughts of the Italian nationalists and their occupation of Rome in 1848. It met with a friendlier spirit even among some of the foremost religious thinkers of Orthodox Russia.

The Church, therefore, felt equal to dealing with evolutionary and other scientific views. Unconcerned with conflicting scientific interpretations, the pope put forth in 1854 the dogma of the "Immaculate Conception" of Mary. In 1864, he issued his "Syllabus of Errors." In 80 short statements, he stated that science and reason are unable to explain all natural forces, that salvation cannot be gained outside the Roman Catholic Church, that the Church cannot dispense with temporal or worldly power, that marriage cannot be a Christian marriage without Church rites, and, in the last, most important paragraph, that progress, liberalism, and modern civilization are altogether at variance with the teachings of the Church. This strong statement, rejecting any thought of compromise, was followed in 1870 by the declaration of the "infallibility" of the pope in *ex-cathedra* pronouncements—pronouncements made from the altar of St. Peter's in Rome—on matters of faith and morals.

### *Protestant Attitude*

Papal indictments of and warnings against the unrestricted belief in science, in human progress, and in contemporary civilization shocked many Catholics. They found even less approval among many Protestants. Divided as Protestants were into a multitude of groups—liberals with vague pantheistic ideas, fundamentalists with belief in the literal truth of the Scriptures, and a majority holding to the middle ground—they could take no united stand. As a whole, they found themselves less at odds than the Catholics with the climate of the time, which was colored by capitalism, industrialism, liberalism, and nationalism. However, science raised problems for Protestants, too. In particular, Strauss's historical criticism and Charles Darwin's evolutionary theories were difficult to reconcile with their traditional teachings. Indeed, scholarly investigation, unconcerned with Christian ethics, and Darwin's implication that organisms evolve in response to natural conditions, led to a stronger reaction among many Protestants than among Catholics.

## Social Theory

Science and evolution necessarily had an impact also upon social theory and were used by some radical thinkers to support their condemnation of existing social conditions. Socialists, in particular—who often found themselves in conflict with nationalism and liberalism, with religion, and with all traditions—gladly spread the scientific creed.

## Anarchism

The most extreme socialist wing, the anarchists, rejected everything that was held in esteem, in Western civilization except modern science. Following Proudhon, the anarchists saw the "root of all evil" in the state. By coercion, the state corrupted people; its laws served only a small, propertied ruling group. Utopians at heart, including men like the Russian aristocrats Bakunin and Kropotkin, the anarchists expected progress and morality to arise in a scientific age when all peoples would enjoy complete political and economic freedom. By persuasion, or preferably by a cleansing revolution, they wished to create a new society in which law would be replaced by voluntary contracts. Only a completely free society, one in which only state, family, marriage bonds, property and law would exist, and where science and rationality would reign; only such a society, they thought, could be expected to bring perfection to humanity.

## Marxism

In contrast to the utopianism of the anarchists, another socialist trend was based on the scientifically conceived ideas of Karl Marx. A German by birth, Marx collaborated with his friend, Friedrich Engels, in writing the *Communist Manifesto,* which was published in 1848. In 1867, while he was living in England, the first volume of his famous work, *Das Kapital,* appeared.

Marx's teachings are complex and open to various interpretations. With their emphasis on economic forces, they reflect the climate of his age and have become of fundamental importance in later times. Marx insisted that "history is the history of class conflicts," that the means of production and changing economic processes determine the law, politics, and morals of each succeeding society. He believed that,

*Figure 16–1  Karl Marx, 1818–1883, and Friedrich Engels, 1820–1895*

with capitalism, the world had entered a stage that would bring forth the last and greatest class conflict. He asserted that capitalism is interested in profits and not in the satisfaction of human needs. It deprives workers of an adequate share of the profits from their production by reserving for the capitalist all "surplus value" resulting from the laborer's toil.

Capitalism would lead increasingly to the concentration of wealth in a few hands and to greater misery for the masses. Labor had become a mere commodity available for the benefit of the capitalist. Dangerous business cycles would continue to haunt the world until the proletariat, the workers of all countries, had united, revolted, and brought about the collapse of the capitalistic system. Thus, through a dialectical process, according to which everything produces the seeds of its own destruction, capitalism would destroy itself. The state would wither away, and all workers would be compensated for their labor according to their effort and their needs.

## Socialism in Action

If other socialist or communist theories had inspired many revolutionary outbreaks through the ages, Marxism, with its more scientific investigation of the relationship of economics and history, laid the foundations for a far more relentless and thoroughgoing movement. Its practical effects were correspondingly far-reaching.

### *Formation of Socialist Parties*

By the time the full impact of Marxism was felt, the situation of the working class had greatly changed from what it was during the early stages of industrial development. Socialists had gained strength through union. Toward the middle of the century, they had forced state authorities to recognize the right of collective bargaining. Then, realizing that political control was necessary for the emancipation of the workers, socialists began to form their first political parties. They sought representation in parliaments, where they opposed liberal as well as conservative aims. They rejected military appropriations and denounced the churches and nationalism. While thus repudiating the major creeds and loyalties of the age, they undertook to build a new loyalty to the international working class. For this purpose they founded, in 1864, the "First International" of labor unions.

### *La Commune*

A new opportunity to strengthen the socialist cause, which had been profoundly influenced by Marx's teachings, came in 1870. Promptly upon the defeat of the French at Sedan and Metz and the collapse of the French Empire, revolutionary outbreaks occurred in Paris. Clubs on the order of the Jacobins were formed, and subsequent elections brought a great increase of socialist strength in the National Assembly. In March 1871, when many social and political ties were broken, and a victorious foreign army stood at the gates of Paris, organized revolution began. The government was forced to flee to Versailles. A city council (the *Commune*), composed of radical and international socialists, was established as the executive agency. This revolution was of unique importance. Whereas the revolutions of 1789 and 1830 had been sponsored by the bourgeoisie against the "old regime," and that of 1848 was sponsored by an alliance of the bourgeoisie and the proletariat, the Revolution of 1871 was undertaken by the proletariat against the newly dominant bourgeoisie. Bakunin and many other socialists and anarchists took an active part in it, while Karl Marx, though considering it premature, applauded the aims of the revolutionaries.

The course of the uprising was tragic, however. Both sides committed incredible atrocities. When the bourgeois government of France under the aged Thiers finally put down the *Commune*, a legacy of hatred remained that was to poison class relationships not only in France, but throughout the Western world.

## Perspective

*Russia gave the world some of the most outstanding works of fiction, presenting social, political, and religious topics with insights into the predicaments of the human condition in stories of unique artistry and depth. High literary standards were also maintained in other Western countries, particularly in an ever-increasing number of published novels and dramas. Yet, in many ways, it was music, art, and science that marked the cultural world in the middle and late 19th century. Wagner and Verdi, Darwin and Marx, the Impressionists, and many scientists in physics, chemistry, and medicine all made a most significant impact.*

*Religion attracted new attention via its critics and defenders. On one hand, there were Strauss and Renan or, in sharper form, Karl Marx, who challenged religious beliefs; on the other hand, there were those who held firmly to traditional values. Foremost among the latter was Pope Pius IX, who rejected the tendencies of modern times and tried to reassert the role of the Catholic Church as arbiter of faith, morals, and the values that the modern world should maintain.*

## Selected Readings

Wood, Allen W. *Karl Marx* (Boston: Rutledge, 1981).

Marx, Karl. *The Communist Manifesto/Karl Marx and Friedrich Engels*; edited and translated by L. M. Findlay. (Peterborough, Ontario: Broadview Press, 2004).

Craig, Gordon A. *German History, 1866–1945* (Oxford: Oxford University Press, 1978).

Hobsbawn, E. J. *The Age of Capital, 1848–1875* (New York: Scribner, 1975).

Gay, Peter. *The Enlightenment: An Interpretation* (New York: Knopf, 1969).

Lindemann, Albert S. *A History of European Socialism* (New Haven: Yale University Press, 1984).

Mason, Stephen F. *History of the Sciences* (New York: Collier Books, 1962).

Porter, Andrew N. *European Imperialism, 1860-1914* (Houndmills, Basingstoke, Hampshire: Macmillan, 1994).

Jenkins, Philip. *A History of the United States* (New York: Palgrave Macmillan, 2003).

## Test Yourself

1. According to the philosophy of Comte, all views based on metaphysical speculations are_____.
   A. Rejected
   B. Accepted
   C. Modified
   D. None of the above

2. The abdication of the scientific method to the Scriptures was advanced by_____.
   A. Auguste Comte
   B. David Frederick Strauss
   C. John Stuart Mill
   D. None of the above

3. Protestant traditional teachings conflicted with scholarly investigations such as_____.
   A. Christian ethics
   B. Comte's Positivism
   C. Darwin's evolutionary theory
   D. The Theory of Relativity

4. Karl Marx argues in his writings that labor had become_____.
   A. A mere commodity available for the benefit of the capitalist
   B. Enriched peasantry's wealth
   C. A means of uniting workers and capitalists
   D. None of the above

5. In 1870, the Catholic Pope made several pronouncements on matters of faith and morals also known as_____.
   A. The Declaration of Independence
   B. The Declaration of Infallibility
   C. The Declaration of Rights
   D. The Vatican Declaration

## Answers and Explanations

1. **A.** This trend came to a climax in the mid-19th century, with the philosophy of Comte, who rejected all views based upon metaphysical speculation. In his "positivist" system, he described metaphysics and religion as evidence of primitive stages of human development. To him, the future was to be shaped by science and based on logic and observable facts. Only by science would the human race reach its highest achievements.

2. **B.** The same confidence in reason as the best guide to truth inspired David Friedrich Strauss. He applied the scientific method to the Scriptures, which he subjected to a searching criticism. This investigation led him to challenge the historical accuracy of many parts of the Bible.

3. **C.** Science raised problems for Protestants. In particular, Strauss's historical criticism and Charles Darwin's evolutionary theories were difficult to reconcile with traditional teachings. Indeed, scholarly investigation, unconcerned with Christian ethics, and Darwin's implication that organisms evolve in response to natural conditions, led to a stronger reaction among many Protestants than among Catholics.

4. **A.** Capitalism would lead increasingly to the concentration of wealth in a few hands and to greater misery for the masses. Labor had become a mere commodity available for the benefit of the capitalist. Dangerous business cycles would continue to haunt the world until the proletariat, the workers of all countries, had united, revolted, and brought about the collapse of the capitalistic system. Thus, through a dialectical process, according to which everything produces the seeds of its own destruction, capitalism would destroy itself. The state would wither away, and all workers would be compensated for their labor according to their effort and their needs.

5. **B.** This strong statement, rejecting any thought of compromise, was followed in 1870 by the declaration of the "infallibility" of the pope in *ex-cathedra* pronouncements—pronouncements made from the altar of St. Peter's in Rome—on matters of faith and morals.

# CHAPTER 17
# The Era of Bismarck (1870-1890)

**1872** Three Emperors' League (Germany, Austria, Russia)
*Kulturkampf* in Germany
**1875** British purchase of Suez Canal shares
**1876** Bell, telephone
**1877** Outbreak of Russo-Turkish War
Edison, phonograph
**1878** Congress of Berlin
**1879** Ibsen, *The Doll's House*
**1880** Edison invents electric light bulb
**1881** Assassination of Alexander II of Russia
Tunisia under French protectorate
**1882** Triple Alliance established (Germany, Austria, and Italy)
British occupy Egypt
Beginning of Bismarck's social
**1883** Germany acquires colonies legislation in Germany
**1884** Nietzsche, *Thus Spake Zarathustra* completed
**1887** German-Russian Reinsurance Treaty
U.S.A. passes Interstate Commerce Act
**1888** Van Gogh, *Sunflowers*
**1890** Dismissal of Bismarck

*A definite configuration in Western civilization is traceable during the period between 1870 and 1890. Politically, nationalism was strong everywhere. Democracy was stronger the farther west one looked; autocracy, the farther east. Economically, industrialism, based on scientific attitudes and technical inventions, was the chief manifestation of the age. It advanced quickly in the northern and Protestant countries, more slowly in the south and where Catholicism dominated. Culturally, the trend was toward wider participation of all groups of the population in national affairs. There was also a trend toward the expansion of literacy, toward science, and away from traditional metaphysical beliefs. The arts flourished, but strong utilitarian tendencies were felt in many areas.*

*As a result, there developed numerous new tensions—internally between workers and entrepreneurs, externally between nations. No major revolution occurred, and there was no all-embracing war. With the help of uncommonly able and responsible statesmen in the key countries, progressive legislation brought improvements for the less privileged classes. Capable diplomats aided in the settlement of international disputes.*

## ■ THE EUROPEAN STATES AND THEIR ALLIANCES

The era after 1870 is frequently named for Bismarck, who became Germany's first chancellor in 1871 and remained the dominant figure on the international political stage until 1890. Having achieved the unification of Germany by means of three wars, he devoted himself for almost two decades to the preservation of a European peace that was to permit the consolidation of the newly founded German Empire. "Seldom," the liberal *Manchester Guardian* once wrote, "has power so vast been employed so well." The "Era of Bismarck" is marked by the growth and rooting of constitutional government in many countries, by worldwide industrialization and social progress, and by struggles between states and the Catholic Church as well as between capitalistic governments and socialist parties. Diplomatically, it witnessed a broad international system of alliances that replaced the old balance of power that had been Metternich's aim.

### Germany

The German Empire created in 1871 consisted of some 20 states, most of them ruled by local princes. Owing to the enterprising spirit of its merchant class, the strength of its military establishment, and the efficiency of its administrative apparatus, it quickly attained a position as one of the great world powers.

#### *Internal Affairs*

In Germany, the period from 1870 to 1890 was marked by economic growth and by the flourishing of intellectual, and especially scientific, studies in the universities. On the other hand, events of these two decades reflected exaggerated nationalistic trends. They demonstrated the weakness of the constitutional order as conceived by Bismarck. They brought to the fore the specific problems of Catholicism and socialism.

#### Constitutional Arrangements

The German emperor, who was simultaneously King of Prussia, acted within the limits of a constitution that gave him authority to direct military and foreign affairs and to appoint ministers. Legislative power, however, was vested in the *Bundesrat* and the *Reichstag*. The former, having limited functions, was meant to constitute a conservative force. The great political struggles were fought out in the *Reichstag,* the popular representation of the German people. The *Reichstag* was made up of conservative, liberal, Catholic, and socialist parties. Its members were elected by the entire male population.

#### Problem of National Unity

Bismarck's task of welding Germany into a powerful unit was not unlike that facing the United States and its sectional interests. The problems confronting the chancellor were rooted in differences of economic conditions between an agricultural East and an industrial West; in dissimilarities of religion, customs, and political traditions between southern and northern German states; and in nationality issues involving Poles and Danes living in eastern and northern border regions and French inhabitants in Alsace-Lorraine. Alsace-Lorraine did not become a separate state of the union. It was ruled from Berlin and, for some time, was administered poorly. Yet, the population in all the states took pride in Germany's prestige,

*Figure 17-1 The Unification of Germany, 1871*

its economic progress, its army, and its educational system. A shared interest in German culture facilitated the task of unification.

## Economic Conditions

Unification allowed the rapid expansion of Germany's industrial capacity. In steel production, Germany soon challenged and then surpassed Britain. Owing to its growing population and excellent scientific research, Germany's chemical, electrical, and machine industries flourished. The organization of cartels and the modernization of techniques made production more economical and efficient. The merchant marine grew, and a nationalized railway system proved successful. Trade connections with all parts of the world were established and, during the 1880s, colonies were acquired. Despite a number of financial crises—including one crisis generated by the sudden influx of gold from payments of France's war indemnity—German banks and holding companies proved sound and gained worldwide importance.

Yet, agriculture suffered reversals as occurred in many other newly industrialized countries. Much concerned, Bismarck vacillated between a policy of protective tariff legislation to further agriculture and a policy of low tariffs to further the new industries.

**Confessional and Socialistic Issues**

During Bismarck's administration, two great issues disturbed Germany's internal peace. One was the issue of the proper relationship between the state and the Catholic Church, and the other was socialism. The "infallibility doctrine" of the Church had raised grave misgivings throughout the Western world because it seemed to demand a double allegiance from Catholic citizens. Bismarck, in particular, was disturbed, inasmuch as separate Catholic interests in predominantly Protestant Germany could endanger the unity of the country. His misgivings increased when a Catholic political party, the "Center," was founded, and a struggle between Bismarck's government and the Catholics, *a Kulturkampf,* ensued.

The struggle centered on educational facilities. Bismarck wanted to see Catholic institutions under state supervision. He had stringent laws enacted against sectarian schools, and he sought to bar or control Catholic religious orders. Everywhere, the liberties of the Catholics were infringed upon. Since Bismarck's repressive policy, which was supported by liberals, did not succeed, he took advantage of the first opportunity—the death of Pius IX—to make a compromise. He revoked the restraining laws and sought the support of the Center party in order to fight a potentially more dangerous enemy: socialism.

After 1875, the various socialist groups had gained in power by merging into a "Social Democratic Party." This party had won a number of seats in the *Reichstag,* where it opposed much of imperial legislation and all military bills. The chancellor met this threat by means of two seemingly contradictory policies. On one hand, he used force to impede freedom of speech and the press and to exile or imprison socialist leaders. On the other hand, he tried to deflate the program of the socialist party by satisfying as many of its demands as seemed justified. This latter policy led him to institute a bold program of social legislation that was to become a model for all nations. In 1883, he introduced compulsory health insurance for workers; in 1884, accident insurance; and in 1889, old-age insurance. Employers and employees had to share with the government the costs of such insurance. Similar social insurance systems were subsequently adopted by most Western nations and by Russia.

### Foreign Affairs

In foreign affairs, Bismarck hoped to achieve European peace and German security by isolating France and building German alliances with other nations. He sought friendly relations with England. He cooperated with the British in numerous practical issues and exercised restraint in regard to German demands for colonies. In 1873, he drew Austria-Hungary into a close alliance for which he had prepared the ground by using moderation in the war settlement of 1866. He induced Russia to join this alliance, and thus formed a "Three Emperors' League," despite Russo-Austrian rivalry and the agitation of Pan-Slaves, who advocated a commonwealth of all Slavic peoples and constituted the extreme nationalist wing among Russia's political forces. In 1882, he negotiated a second alliance system, which included Germany, Austria, and Italy, later known as the "Triple Alliance." He made treaties with Romania and other small nations. All in all, friendly ties connected Berlin with London, Vienna, St. Petersburg, Rome, Bucharest, and other capitals.

Yet, Bismarck did not succeed in maintaining all such ties intact. Relations with England cooled during the 1880s. Those with Russia likewise weakened. The Three Emperors' League was threatened in 1875 because of personal jealousies. It was suspended in 1878 when, following a victorious Russian war against Ottoman Turkey, Bismarck failed to support Russia's demands for spoils. Furthermore, because of the incompatibility of Russian and Austrian aims, the league was allowed to expire in 1887. Although Bismarck considered Russia the "pivot" of German security, he succeeded in replacing the league only by a shaky and secret German-Russian "Reinsurance Treaty," which survived no more than three years. In 1890, the 75-year-old chancellor was dismissed from office by the young emperor William II, who had succeeded to the throne in 1888, and who refused to renew the Reinsurance Treaty. This brought to an end Bismarck's international system.

## France

Germany's vigorous economic and political growth from 1870 to 1890 was not paralleled in France. The required initiative was lacking. The population hardly increased. France continued to devote itself primarily to agricultural pursuits, whereas industries developed slowly. The war of 1870–1871 had left France without a legitimate government. The National Assembly was obliged to conclude the Peace of Frankfurt with Germany.

Not until 1875 was a regular government organized, and not until 1879, after many attempts by royalists to reintroduce a monarchy, was the "Third Republic" established. A parliamentary regime, with two legislative chambers, was established, with the members being elected by general male suffrage on an equalitarian basis. The legislature included many divergent forces—monarchists, liberals, republicans, and socialists. The president of the republic became a mere figurehead.

### *Internal Affairs*

A number of years elapsed before the new government earned respect and confidence at home and abroad. Corruption marked its first two decades. Scandals occurred over the sale of Legion of Merit awards and over the building of the Panama Canal. In 1887, General Boulanger, aided by nationalists, threatened to set himself up as a dictator. Moreover, disunity was created by widespread materialism and religious skepticism among liberal bourgeoisie and the workers. Both clashed with the Catholic traditions of the conservatives and the peasantry and led to much anticlerical agitation. Disunity was further increased by repressive acts against socialists.

Yet, beneath the surface, France did make progress in numerous respects. Its army was reorganized. Its economy recovered from the disasters of war and revolution. Living conditions for workers improved. Civil rights were no longer violated as they had been in Napoleonic times. Artistic life continued to flourish and to attract foreign visitors. Advances in education were substantial.

### *External Affairs*

In external affairs, France was held down in Europe both by its own dreams of a *revanche* (revenge) for 1870 and by the strength of Germany on the Continent and of England on the seas. France failed to adjust to the new international situation. Moreover, by seizing Tunisia, which Italy coveted, and by establishing a French protectorate there, France incurred the hostility of the Italians. For two decades, France remained isolated. Yet, its Tunisian conquest compensated to a degree for the failure of some of its nationalistic plans. The Tunisian conquest was followed by an act incorporating Algiers into the empire. There, as in Tunisia, French law was introduced. Many settlers from France spread French customs, language, and culture.

## England and the British Empire

The British Isles had remained untouched by the wars of France, Italy, Germany, Austria, and Denmark. In "splendid isolation," though carefully watching events on the Continent, Britain continued to devote itself to the affairs of its own empire.

### *Internal Affairs*

After 1870, conservative and liberal governments alternated more rapidly than in preceding years. Both parties had outstanding leaders: the Conservatives had Disraeli, and the Liberals had Gladstone. Though wholly opposed in their attitude toward life, both leaders worked diligently and with success for the aggrandizement of their country. They introduced urgently needed improvements in the educational system, which lagged behind those of the Continental powers. The economy made rapid progress. Measures for the protection of business interests and *laissez-faire* policies were now increasingly accepted by Conservatives; the unfair taxation system was revised. The workers gained by the legalization of labor unions, and relief finally came for the textile workers.

Additionally, progress was made toward broader democracy through the introduction of the secret ballot. In 1884, a Third Reform Bill was passed. While it still did not make the right to vote universal, it did confer this right on those who paid taxes. This meant that about three-quarters of the male population received that right. Anti-Jewish legislation, as it still existed in England, was eliminated, but nothing was done for women. Thereafter, radicalism became less extreme in its demands. Instead, a mild socialism was promoted by the "Fabian Society," which was founded in 1883. It was to usher in a socialist society by peaceful evolution rather than by violent revolution.

The problem of Irish self-government, which had long poisoned the relations between Irish and English, remained unsolved. Against much opposition, Gladstone sought to settle the conflict by concessions. Land laws were passed in favor of Irish peasants. Religious peace was sought on the basis of an act, passed in 1869, that provided for the disestablishment of the Church of Ireland. However, as an essentially agricultural land with an almost medieval system of British landlords and Irish peasants, Ireland was bound to suffer from English policies, which were keyed to the trading and exporting of manufactured goods. Conditions of starvation had existed since the potato famine of 1845. Irish hostility, derived from alien rule and kept alive by economic difficulties, smoldered.

### *External Affairs*

In external affairs, Britain pursued a vigorous imperialistic policy. It also became increasingly dependent upon its empire. The British consolidated their holdings in the Far East and built up their trade with China and Japan. They maintained their position in India by strengthening their lines of communication and by acquiring, in 1875, controlling shares of stock in the Suez Canal Company. They purchased the shares from the Egyptian king, who had received them in exchange for his permission to allow the construction of the canal through his territory. However, his love of luxury depleted his finances and forced him to sell the securities. Next, the British named Queen Victoria the "Empress of India." They extended their sphere of influence into Afghanistan and Persia, thereby preventing a Russian route to India, and they vigorously increased their colonizing activities in Africa. Britain also made an agreement with the Portuguese that made it possible for them to expand their acquisitions on Africa's western coast. Finally, when the ruthless exploitation and outrages of the Belgian king in the Congo became known, the British attended a congress convened by Bismarck in Berlin (1885), where an international agreement regarding more humane treatment of the natives of Africa was concluded. Principles for the colonization of Africa were laid down. Soon, the map of Africa showed no unclaimed space.

Moreover, in 1882, at a time of discontent in Egypt, the British navy took advantage of the situation and suddenly shelled Alexandria. This caused a substantial loss of life in the population and inflicted great damage to property. Britain then followed up on this action by seizing the entire country. British rule in

Egypt continued until 1952 when an Egyptian revolutionary movement seized power and negotiated an end to British occupation of the country.

## Italy

Between 1870 and 1890, Italy experienced unique difficulties that adversely affected its political, economic, and cultural life.

### *Internal Affairs*

Inexperienced in self-government, Italy struggled to create an efficient administration. Capable leaders and a sound bureaucracy were lacking. Funds were wasted, and corruption prevailed. Illiteracy was so widespread that it took a long time to build a working parliamentary system. National pride demanded that a powerful army and navy be maintained, and this involved huge costs and excessive taxation for an effort that was hardly warranted.

More fundamental were other handicaps. The population increased rapidly. Because scarcity of raw materials prevented industrial development, poverty, too, increased. Many enterprising citizens chose to immigrate to America. Others joined radical parties that encouraged riots and peasant revolts, and the anarchist movement grew. Finally, through a unilateral "Law of Guarantees," the Italian government accorded sovereignty of the Vatican to the papacy, paid an indemnity, and allowed religious institutions to function.

### *External Affairs*

An Italian foreign policy could only evolve slowly; none had existed before Italy became a nation. Friendship with England and an alliance with Germany eventually formed the basis of Italian policy. The British had been supportive of Italian national ambitions. British good will continued to be important for Italy, and since the British dominated the Mediterranean Sea and Malta, they could have become a threat along the extended Italian coastline. Germany had proved equally sympathetic. Despite Italian-Austrian rivalry over territories claimed by "irredentist" Italian nationalists, who sought the annexation of all territories where Italian people lived, the Triple Alliance was concluded between Italy, Austria, and Germany in 1882. A treaty of friendship was also negotiated between Italy and Russia.

Only with neighboring France did relations remain precarious. The attitude of the French had vacillated during Italy's reunification struggle. France had seized Italian territories and had competed with Italy in colonial areas. In 1881, France took Tunisia.

## Russia

The evolution of Russia from 1870 to 1890 continued to follow a path that differed from that of Western Europe. Intellectual movements asserted themselves, claiming for Russia a unique role in world history. Revolutionary and conservative groups shared these pretensions, though for divergent reasons. They expected their country to defeat the materialism of the West. Russia, they claimed, was animated either by the spirit of true Christianity or by that of communistic, neighborly love and cooperation that could spread antimaterialistic, humane ideas. Significantly, such beliefs were held in the face of the deep national and social rifts that existed within the country, strong economic pressures toward greater Westernization, and Pan-Slav expansionist ambitions.

### *Internal Affairs*

Few institutions existing in Russia in 1870 qualified the nation to take the leadership role either among the Slavic countries or among the world powers. Although, after emancipation and reform, the way was open for economic readjustment, autocracy was preserved, and political modernization was slow.

### Economic Conditions

Foreign capital, foreign entrepreneurs, and foreign technicians helped to develop Russia's natural resources. Numerous industries were founded. Coal, steel, and oil production rose, and copper and gold mining increased. Soon after 1870, a vast railroad-building program was undertaken, serving, as elsewhere, both economic and military aims. The network was expanded southward in order to facilitate the export of grain and oil via the Black Sea, as well as to prevent a repetition of the military disasters experienced in the Crimean War.

### Social Conditions

As a result, new social problems developed. Increasingly affected by Western trends, the growing and ambitious bourgeoisie found itself more and more in ideological conflict with the autocratic government. A similar conflict existed between the government and the factory workers. The workers suffered as elsewhere from the hardships of early industrialization, and they aspired to obtain political rights and economic improvement.

Still more dangerous to existing institutions was the dissatisfaction of the peasants. Legal restrictions and burdens weighed heavily upon them. Their individual holdings were generally too small for adequate subsistence. The redemption tax was high. Most peasants or village communes found it difficult to acquire sufficient additional land and to introduce modern techniques. The institution of the *mir*, with its collectivism, hindered initiative, reduced profits, led to much strife. Moreover, certain enterprising peasants (the *kulaks*) understood how to exploit the situation to accumulate large acreages purchased from others who were unable to make an independent living. This *kulak* class became important as a psychological factor in arousing resentment among the masses.

The government tried to meet the emergency by applying both progressive and repressive measures. It continued the reform work, passed social legislation, reduced the redemption tax, gave more independence to the *mir*, and improved the *zemstvo* system. On the other hand, it maintained the autocracy of the tsar. It refused an extension of civil rights and did nothing to eradicate the corruption permeating the entire bureaucracy. It intensified police methods, built up its espionage network in town and country, and continued the fearful system of exiling opponents to Siberia while leaving their families destitute at home.

### Political Conditions

Under such circumstances, a threatening mood of resistance grew among all social classes. Idealists among the nobility, middle-class people desiring political rights, workers in need of further social legislation, peasants burdened by taxes and poverty, religious groups dissenting from the official orthodoxy, Jews agitating for equality, Poles and Finns and other aliens resenting both Russian domination and intensified "Russification" policies, all were united in assailing the existing institutions.

The intelligentsia became leaders of the discontented masses. Artists and writers, who played a more prominent role than ever before, often devoted their works to social criticism. To most of the reformers, a constitutional system in line with Western customs hardly seemed sufficient. Many felt that social rejuvenation would be possible only through revolution. In the 1870s, anarchists, whose primary desire was to destroy the state completely, gained an importance equaled nowhere else in Europe. Nihilists rejected all traditional values, and terrorists insisted that the times called for practical revolutionary deeds instead of mere theories. Together, nihilists, anarchists, and terrorists arranged for the assassinations of leading officials, which culminated in 1881 with the murder of Tsar Alexander II. Marxists carried the teachings of Marx and Engels to the industrial workers.

Populists *(narodniki)* sought to gain salvation for Russia by winning over the peasants. The radicals instituted the *v narod*("to the people") movement, which had two purposes: (1) young intellectuals were to live with peasants and become familiar with their ideas and needs; and (2) they were to propagate revolutionary ideas among the peasants. After the assassination of Alexander II, nihilism, terrorism, and populism abated somewhat in spite of the stern measures of his successor, Alexander III, who fostered his grandfather Nicholas's aim of "autocracy, orthodoxy, nationality"; Marxist socialism continued to grow. In 1883, an all-Russian socialist organization, forbidden at home, was founded abroad by Georgi Plekhanov. It devoted its efforts to spreading Marxist ideas among the Russian workers. Socialists agitated for shorter working hours and higher wages and sponsored strikes.

## *External Affairs*

In foreign affairs, Russia sought to cooperate with Germany. It used the Franco-German War as a pretext to abrogate the Black Sea Clause imposed at the Peace of Paris. After Germany's victory, Russia formed the Three Emperors' League with Germany and Austria. By concluding this alliance and, subsequently, by making separate arrangements with Austria, Russia prepared to pursue its major aim: the resumption of its drive southward toward Constantinople.

The old aim of gaining control of Constantinople and the straits had become a major objective for the newly influential nationalistic forces in Russia, especially the Pan-Slavs. Ever since the first Pan-Slav Congress in Prague in 1848, they had looked forward to a mighty Slavic commonwealth under Russian leadership. When, during the 1870s, southern Slavic nations rebelled against Turkey, and a "Young Turk" movement endeavored to modernize the country, an activity which would have interfered with Russian intentions regarding Constantinople, the Pan-Slavs seized the opportunity and began to agitate for war. It soon materialized (Russo-Turkish War of 1877-1878). Technologically backward and weakened by the administration of corrupt and inefficient sultans, Ottoman Turkey was quickly defeated. It was forced to sign a peace treaty at San Stefano whereby it had to surrender most of its European possessions, to grant independence or autonomy to its Slavic groups, and to agree to the formation of a Greater Bulgaria as a substantial power. It also had to give the Russians special rights in the straits and relinquish part of the Southern Caucasus.

This treaty aroused fears in England and Austria, which wanted to preserve Ottoman Turkey as a buffer, and the British insisted on the treaty's cancellation. They forced the Turks to cede Cyprus to them and then undertook to defend the freedom of the straits. Thus threatened, Russia agreed to an international congress, which Bismarck was persuaded to convene in Berlin. The Peace of San Stefano was set aside, and the formation of Greater Bulgaria, which would have had an outlet to the Mediterranean Sea via the Aegean, was prevented. International control of the straits rather than Russian was arranged. Russia only gained some territory in the Caucasus and in Bessarabia, as well as the recognition of the independence of Serbia and Romania. The outcome of the congress, which seemed to have rendered most of the sacrifices of war futile, embittered Russia not only against England and Austria, but also against Germany because, in order to prevent a general European conflict, Germany had supported England. Not until 1881 was the Three Emperors' League renewed—and then only because of Russia's dependence upon German markets for its grain exports and on German supplies for its industrialization.

Frustrated in Europe, Russia resumed its Asiatic ventures. By 1884, Russian troops stood at Mew, not far from the Indian border. This advance led to further conflict with England and, in turn, brought another renewal of the Three Emperors' League. The league lasted until 1887 and was then replaced by the Reinsurance Treaty, which lasted until 1890.

## ■THE UNITED STATES

In the period 1870 to 1890, developments in the United States became more and more like those in Europe. With the worldwide progress of democratization, including measures in behalf of civil rights, political differences diminished. In the economic sphere, the two decades witnessed, in America as in Europe, a rapid expansion of business and industry. Population growth was, however, more rapid in the United States, whose low death rate and high birth rate, combined with steadily rising immigration, resulted in an annual increase far above the rate in other Western countries. These demographic and economic factors enabled the United States to play an increasingly important role in world politics.

## Internal Affairs

In addition to corruption and graft, material progress during the two decades after 1870 was enormous. Manufacturing and mining flourished. Large private fortunes were accumulated, while "equality of opportunity" became a watchword. Notwithstanding continued disagreements in the 1880s concerning the relative advantages of free trade and high tariffs, trade generally expanded. Farming expanded, as well, and it remained the chief occupational pursuit. Introduction of technical innovations—the telephone, phonograph, typewriter, gas lighting, sewing machines, among others—helped to establish the United States as a leading industrial nation. Urbanization accelerated.

This situation led to the emergence of numerous problems, some of which the United States shared with European countries. The United States, too, was beset by labor problems involving wages, working conditions, and spread of slum areas and strikes. Numerous riots, some bloody, occurred. In the 1880s, an immigrant, Samuel Gompers, founded the American Federation of Labor.

Under such circumstances, the challenge of extreme liberalism had to be met, and a beginning was made with restrictive government legislation. A large bureaucracy was created to enforce the legislation. In 1883, the government enacted laws governing civil service. In 1887, the Interstate Commerce Act was passed to regulate the railroads, and in 1890, the Sherman Anti-Trust Act passed for the purpose of preventing business monopolies.

Moreover, a number of developments and problems peculiar to America emerged, primarily concerning (1) the aftermath of the Civil War, (2) the expansion of agriculture and the settlement of western areas, (3) the challenge of immigration, and (4) the promotion of financial stability. In contrast to European limitations, the agricultural area could be increased. Between the Mississippi River and the Rocky Mountains were vast regions where Native Americans lived among the buffalo herds, and these lands could be seized. Gradually, these Native Americans were assaulted and largely exterminated. Their lands were fenced in with barbed wire. The buffalo herds were likewise nearly exterminated, and the land was converted to cattle grazing and agriculture. As these regions became increasingly populated by American settlers, new states were formed and admitted to the Union.

The new problem of immigration now had to be addressed. The bulk of the newcomers no longer came from northern Europe, but from the southern and eastern European countries. They possessed a racial, social, and language background different from that of earlier immigrants. More of them settled in urban centers than rural districts, and they were often exploited by irresponsible politicians who bought their votes and thereby vitiated the democratic process. Their integration into the mainstream life of the country was thus delayed.

Last, economic and financial developments gave rise to other serious problems. During the later part of the 19th century, the United States remained a debtor nation. This resulted in agitation to promote the use of silver as the basis for the currency, instead of strict adherence to the gold standard that prevailed in most European countries.

## External Affairs

In general, European problems in international relations held little interest for Americans. The United States entered into no alliances. It remained disinterested in the distribution of power overseas. For the most part, it stayed out of the race for territory. Nevertheless, it became involved in a number of foreign issues.

Population shifts to the West Coast and the acquisition of Alaska, as well as the occupation of the Midway Islands west of Hawaii, which had taken place in 1867, forced upon the nation a more active role in the Pacific area where American interests impinged upon those of Japan, England, Russia, and Germany, and necessitated both commitments and international conventions. A fear of "the Yellow Peril" resulted. Economic strength brought greater interest in Latin American countries and led to the First Pan-American Congress in 1889. The westward expansion within the United States and controversies with England dating back to the Civil War period made new agreements with England necessary. These were eventually achieved through arbitration by the German emperor and through the so-called "Halifax award," which settled the questions of the Oregon boundary and of the Newfoundland fisheries, respectively.

## THE SMALLER NATIONS

The trends and problems of the great powers were duplicated among the smaller nations. However, few of these countries played any influential role on the international stage. Only in the Balkan nations did problems arise that led to wars. Only Portugal, Holland, and Belgium were active in colonial affairs. In all cases, a regulating influence was exercised by the great powers. Thus, in the Balkans, peace arrangements were dictated by the large nations. As a rule, the smaller countries devoted their attention to internal improvements. Switzerland and Denmark set an example with their advanced educational systems. They and other small countries succeeded in creating living conditions for their peoples that were often more satisfactory than those of larger countries. Democracy was strong in the small western and northern countries, while patriarchal and absolutist forms of government continued to prevail among Russia's and Turkey's neighbors in Eastern Europe.

Unique roles were played by Switzerland, which had the most nearly perfect democracy in Western civilization; by Spain, which failed to rid itself of obsolete feudal institutions and which missed modernization in economic affairs as well; and by Latin American countries, where geographical disadvantages, underdeveloped economic resources, and political inexperience created favorable conditions for the rise of dictatorships. Even in Mexico, where a vigorous reform movement was led by Juarez, and after him by Diaz, progress in the direction of modern liberal institutions was slow.

### Perspective

*Under the influence of Bismarck, peace was maintained in Europe. Only on the fringes did warfare erupt, as it did between Russia and Turkey. Outside of Europe, force was employed by the various colonial imperialistic nations. Internally, considerable social advances were made. Most countries followed Bismarck's example and introduced old-age, health, and accident insurance, as in Germany. Rapid changes in industrial life brought new problems, which neither conservative nor liberal governments could satisfactorily solve. Socialism, seeking to address the problems by introducing greatly altered social organization, was opposed in Germany, France, Russia, Italy, and elsewhere, but it gained in strength. Social democratic parties were founded and began to win seats and representation in constitutional assemblies.*

*In the meantime, the United States, where socialism did not become an issue, concentrated on perfecting its own internal organization and dealing with the numerous problems that came in the wake of the Civil War and the rapid industrialization of the country. A stream of immigrants came to the country.*

### Selected Readings

Cobban, Alfred. *A History of Modern France* (New York: Braziller, 1965).
Craig, Gordon A. *German History, 1866-1945* (New York: Oxford University Press, 1981).
Killinger, Charles. *The History of Italy* (London: Greenwood Press, 2002).

Eyck, Erich. *Bismarck and the German Empire* (London: Allen & Unwin, 1960).

Hargreaves, David. *Bismarck and German Unification* (Basingstoke: Macmillan, 1991).

Lukacs, John A. *The Great Powers and Eastern Europe* (New York: American Books Company, 1953).

Robert, J. M. *The New History of the World* (New York: Oxford University Press, 2003).

Roessler, Shirley Elson & Miklos, Reny. *Europe, 1715-1919: From Enlightenment to World War* (Oxford: Rowman & Littlefield Publishers, Inc., 2003).

Sheehan, J. J. *German Liberalism in the Nineteenth Century* (Chicago, The University of Chicago Press, 1978).

Taylor, A. J. P. *The Struggle for Mastery in Europe, 1848–1918* (Oxford: Clarendon Press, 1954).

Zeldin, T. *France, 1848–1945. 2 vols.* (Oxford: Oxford University Press, 1984).

## Test Yourself

1. The German unified states established in 1871 consisted of _____.
   A. Fifty states
   B. Twenty states
   C. Thirty states
   D. Fifteen states

2. During Bismarck's administration, two great issues disturbed Germany's internal peace. One was the issue of proper relationship between the state and the Catholic Church, and the other issue was_____.
   A. Communism
   B. Anarchism
   C. Socialism
   D. Liberalism

3. The Fabian society in England, founded in 1883, promoted a mild form of _____.
   A. Communism
   B. Democracy
   C. Anarchism
   D. Socialism

4. In 1882, the British Navy invaded_____.
   A. The United States
   B. Egypt
   C. Russia
   D. France

5. The Russian word *kulaks* also means_____.
   A. Enterprising peasants
   B. Bankers
   C. Capitalists
   D. Kings

6. The Russo-Turkish War of 1877-1878 ended with the signing of a peace treaty at_____.
   A. San Simon
   B. St. Petersburg
   C. San Stefano
   D. San Martin

7. The American Interstate Commerce Act of 1887 was passed to_____.
   A. Regulate highways
   B. Regulate ocean commerce
   C. Regulate mule trains
   D. Regulate railroads

8. The Sherman Anti-Trust Act of 1880 was passed for the purpose of_____.
   A. Preventing capitalism
   B. Preventing communism
   C. Preventing business monopolies
   D. Preventing labor strikes

## Answers and Explanations

1. **B.** The German Empire created in 1871 consisted of some 20 states, most of them ruled by local princes. Owing to the enterprising spirit of its merchant class, the strength of its military establishment, and the efficiency of its administrative apparatus, it quickly attained a position as one of the great world powers.

2. **C.** During Bismarck's administration, two great issues disturbed Germany's internal peace. One was the issue of the proper relationship between the state and the Catholic Church, and the other issue was socialism. The "infallibility doctrine" of the Church had raised grave misgivings throughout the Western world because it seemed to demand a double allegiance from Catholic citizens. Bismarck, in particular, was disturbed, inasmuch as separate Catholic interests in predominantly protestant Germany could endanger the unity of the country; and his misgivings increased when a Catholic political party, the "Center," was founded, and a struggle between Bismarck's government and the Catholics, *a Kulturkampf*, ensued.

3. **D.** Instead, a mild socialism was promoted by the "Fabian Society," which was founded in 1883. It was to usher in a socialist society by peaceful evolution rather than by violent revolution.

4. **B.** In 1882, at a time of discontent in Egypt, the British navy took advantage of the situation and suddenly shelled Alexandria. This caused much loss of life among the population and inflicted great damage to property. Britain followed up this action by seizing the entire country. British rule in Egypt continued until 1952 when an Egyptian revolutionary movement seized power and negotiated an end to British occupation of the country.

5. **A.** Certain enterprising peasants (called the *kulaks*) understood how to exploit the situation and to accumulate large acreages purchased from others who were unable to make an independent living. This *kulak* class became important as a psychological factor in arousing resentment among the masses.

6. **C.** When, during the 1870s, southern Slavic nations rebelled against Turkey and a "Young Turk" movement endeavored to modernize the country, an activity which would have interfered with Russian intentions regarding Constantinople, the Pan-Slavs seized the opportunity and began to agitate for war. It soon materialized (Russo-Turkish War of 1877-1878). Technologically backward and weakened by the administration of corrupt and inefficient sultans, Ottoman Turkey was quickly defeated. It was forced to sign a peace treaty at San Stefano whereby it had to surrender most of its European possessions, to grant independence or autonomy to its Slavic groups, and to agree to the formation of a Greater Bulgaria as a substantial power.

7. **D.** In 1887, the Interstate Commerce Act was passed to regulate the railroads.

8. **C.** In 1890, the Sherman Anti-Trust Act was passed to prevent business monopolies.

# CHAPTER 18

# Economic and Cultural Trends (1870-1914)

**1891** Franco-Russian Alliance
**1894** Dreyfus affair in France
**1895** Jameson Raid
Discovery of X-rays by Roentgen
**1898** European powers occupy Chinese ports
U.S.A. annexes Hawaii
Spanish-American War
Discovery of radium by the Curies

*The period from 1870 to 1914 has been frequently criticized as an era of "bourgeois complacency." Actually, a measure of complacency did prevail among the middle class—and perhaps justifiably. Having gained dominance and influence in the state, its well-to-do members were proud of their material wealth and comfort, the economic growth and prestige of their various nations, and their personal standards of "solidity and propriety." From education and literacy, they expected general progress in political and moral behavior. They celebrated important scientific discoveries, insights gained into the workings of nature, and the achievements of contemporary writers and painters.*

*Far too often, however, they ignored many disturbing underlying conditions and avoided the currents that indicated growing dissatisfaction. These currents were felt not only by the less favored classes, but also by the privileged. Many leading thinkers questioned the possibility of continuous progress, whether it came, as many liberals believed, from the innate morality and good sense of people, through science and education, or as socialists believed, through revolution and emancipation, which they considered an inevitable result of an evolutionary process. Philosophers of the late 19th century reflected a deep pessimism. Many social thinkers were attracted by nihilistic views.*

## ■ ECONOMIC CHANGES

In the five decades before 1914, sharp competition among private enterprises and among nations led to enormous industrial expansion in most Western countries. This "second industrial revolution" is marked by the growth of chemical and electrical industries. Agriculture absorbed an ever-decreasing share of the available labor force and capital. Industrialization was materially beneficial, although the benefits did not reach the less favored classes until mass production became possible. Socially and politically, the effects seemed less promising. Class antagonisms increased. Socialist propaganda accused industrialists of exploiting the worker, gaining undue influence in political affairs, promoting colonialism, and instigating wars. Business affairs absorbed the energies of many outstanding figures: Carnegie, who built a steel empire; Nobel, who invented dynamite and built large munitions plants; Krupp, who presided over huge steel, armament, and machine industries; Rockefeller, who founded the Standard Oil Company; Alfred Mond, who organized vast chemical enterprises; and Werner von Siemens and Emil Rathenau in the electrical industry. Competition eliminated some individuals while bringing others to the forefront; unlike the former nobility, these captains of industry depended upon individual inventiveness and personal ability to maintain their positions, rather than class, birth, or even inherited wealth.

## Population

The rapid increase of productivity was made possible by population growth. Despite emigration, the population in such countries as Germany, England, and Russia gained about sixty-five percent from 1870 to 1914. By then, about 425 million people lived in Europe, with another 135 million Europeans residing in overseas territory, making up a record one-third of the global population.

Many capitals with millions of inhabitants had arisen in the West: London, Paris, St. Petersburg, Berlin, Vienna, and Rome. City life offered excitement, opportunities, educational facilities, and independence, but also hurried competitive, unhealthy, and insecure conditions. Still, migration from country to town continued unabated.

## Industry

Urbanization not only facilitated industrialism and economic growth, but also made them inevitable. Innumerable technical inventions were devised. Heavy industries increased manifold. Chemical industries began the large-scale production of both medical preparations and synthetic materials used in manufacturing. Aspirin was discovered in Germany. The rubber and oil industries gained special importance, benefiting mainly the United States and England, as well as enterprising small countries, such as Holland. To some extent, steam power was replaced by electric power. In 1914, Germany produced one-third of the world output in electricity, with the United States a close second. Even small countries like Sweden and Switzerland, owing to natural resources, gained worldwide importance as producers of electricity and electrical machinery. Old industries found new markets—such as the textile industry after the invention of the sewing machine. New industries developed in the field of communications: the wireless and motion-picture industries. The transportation industry expanded. Trains and ships were improved in speed and comfort. The first electrical streetcars appeared in Berlin in 1879. Bicycles became a popular means of transportation, and after the German Nikolaus Otto had developed the first internal combustion motor, the first modern automobiles were built in the 1890s. Eventually, airplanes were constructed. In the United States, the Wright brothers undertook the first flight in 1903; within six years, the Frenchman Bleriot crossed the Channel to England.

Progress in transportation supported numerous auxiliary industries, the construction of highways, the extension of railways, and the building of canals—such as the Panama Canal and the various inland waterways. The pace of life accelerated.

## *Finance*

Industries grew rapidly, but business cycles increasingly caused uncertainties. Inventors and producers often did not have the funds to finance their business ventures. Through borrowing, they became dependent upon banks, trusts, and holding companies; power came to be concentrated in the hands of financiers and promoters. Financial institutions began to determine business policies. They put their representatives on boards of directors. They exerted pressure on their clients to conclude mergers and market-sharing agreements, or to form cartels. Small independent businesses diminished in number and influence. Large corporations, with limited liability, predominated. A comparatively small minority of stockholders exercised control, despite a wide distribution of shares. Fluctuations of the market and business cycles speeded the process of consolidation into large units. London became the main financial market, but individual banks, such as the Credit Lyonnais in France, gained power as well.

## Agriculture

While industry was the most dynamic part of Western economy, agriculture still comprised the largest sector. Only in England, where urbanization had progressed furthest and where half of the country's arable land was owned by less than one percent of the population, was the small landowner almost entirely eliminated. In Germany, a large percentage of the population still owned landed property or worked on the land. In France and the United States, more than half of the population derived their livelihood from agriculture; in Russia, almost three-quarters were peasants.

But, so far as increase in productivity is concerned, agriculture lagged behind industry. Age-old farming methods were widely retained in many regions. The system of agricultural holdings—whether those of large, almost feudal estates in eastern Europe or those of small individual peasant estates in western Europe—was not adequately modified to meet the new conditions. Although machines, particularly harvesting machines, came into widespread use, technical knowledge was not widely disseminated. Agricultural banks, credit institutes, and cooperatives, which sought to provide capital and efficient marketing organizations, achieved only limited success.

## Economic Effects on the International Situation

The shifts in the national economies affected the international scene, destroying the existing power balance of the nations. Industrialization allowed "younger" nations to come to the forefront, while some older ones declined. Britain's position was particularly affected. It still had certain advantages: its colonial empire, London's financial prestige, and substantial profits from its carrying trade, foreign investments, and worldwide insurance. But as its share in world exports was reduced, its political influence diminished. The distribution of British manufactures (steel products, cutlery, machinery, and even textiles) encountered difficulties. Because of its dependence upon foreign markets and imports, England could not easily protect itself by means of protective tariffs. Britain's most successful competitors, Germany and the United States, had begun to industrialize late; they had benefited from British experience. They proved less conservative. They acquired more modern machinery; they more readily adopted new inventions and new techniques of production and distribution. They protected domestic manufactures with tariff walls. The United States, like Russia, had never accepted free trade; Germany, though vacillating, imposed higher duties than those in effect before 1870. Both countries used their newly gained economic dominance to further their political aims.

As for France, its wealthier classes proved overcautious. Instead of investing in speculative industries, they preferred safe investments that yielded high returns. They thereby prevented the country from gaining the position that brisk economic activity could have given it, even after the political debacle. France, too, steadily increased its tariffs during the 1870-1892 period.

Russia also increased its productive capacities. However, it gained little prestige in the world economy. The size and needs of its domestic market made it impossible for Russia to become a leading exporter of any products except grain and textiles. Its infrastructure remained weak.

## Economic Effects on Social Conditions

Economic changes affected the social power and prestige of nations; they also affected the life of the individual. More money was made available, and money could buy goods and services undreamed of in previous centuries. However, the social distance between the upper and lower classes steadily widened. People in the lower classes could scarcely earn their subsistence. During depressions, such as those of the middle 1870s and the early 1890s, many of them lost their only capital—the opportunity to work gainfully. During the boom periods that prevailed in the years before the First World War, the same people suffered from swift inflation. Moreover, early in the 20th century the use of assembly-line methods of production reduced the need for skilled labor, speeded up manufacturing operations, made work monotonous and exhausting, and created additional unemployment. The workers, who were often led by idealistic members of the well-to-do classes, intensified their struggle for improvement by utilizing unions, strikes, political parties, and propaganda.

### *Effects on Social Legislation*

The most important social consequence of the economic situation was the introduction of social-security legislation. The German government had been first to realize both the value of satisfactory labor conditions to the state itself and the responsibility of the state toward its less fortunate members. In a series of persuasive speeches, Bismarck convinced the members of the *Reichstag* that fear of a "socialistic element" should not check laws promoting the welfare of all citizens. He therefore advocated income taxes that put the main tax burden on those who possessed capital; in the years from 1881 to 1889, the government passed laws for state-guaranteed accident, old-age, and health insurance, covering low-income industrial workers. This insurance plan was broadened and improved in subsequent years, and was imitated in most Western countries. In France, which had recognized labor unions since 1884, a series of factory codes was promulgated in 1892. Laws providing for workmen's compensation appeared in 1898. Old-age pensions were introduced between 1893 and 1910. In Russia, during the same time period, government decrees brought the improvement of labor conditions and the adoption of various types of social insurance. Britain moved ahead more slowly. Yet by 1911, it had not only passed social-welfare laws dealing with old-age pensions, workmen's compensation, and national insurance, but had also introduced staggered income taxes, land and inheritance taxes, and unemployment benefits.

Among the great powers, only the United States failed to follow the trend toward social legislation. The imposition of a federal income tax required a constitutional amendment that was not ratified until 1913. Federal inheritance taxes were not levied until after the First World War. Social insurance legislation was not enacted until the Great Depression of the 1930s.

### *Effects on Attitude of the Churches*

The spirit behind social legislation was consistent with many demands of the principal religious denominations. Among Russian Orthodox and Protestant groups, it was mainly a few individuals and reform groups who associated themselves with political forces demanding social improvement and social security. As to the Catholic Church, Pope Pius IX had (in his *Syllabus of Errors*) denounced the uninhibited liberal view, and his successor, Leo XIII, had published an encyclical *(Rerum novarum)* in 1891 in which he repeated Pius's condemnation of socialism, communism, and unchecked liberalism. Yet, simultaneously, Leo XIII pointed out the moral obligations of the wealthier classes. He also approved governments' determined efforts to improve the living conditions of the masses and to restrict business practices harmful to the working class.

### *Effects on Socialist Parties*

Significantly, the endeavors of governments and churches to improve social conditions did not stop the growth of socialism. On the contrary, the socialist movement accelerated. Workers used prosperous times to withhold their labor, a weapon that, however, misfired in times of depression. Still, socialism gained from the growing consciousness that industrialism had created problems that needed society's attention. Everywhere, socialist parties secured wide influence.

In Germany, the Social-Democratic party, founded by Lasalle in 1863, sent two representatives to the first imperial diet in 1871. When Bismarck's repressive laws were abolished in the 1890s, the party sent more than forty representatives to the diet, and in 1914, their numbers grew to more than a hundred representatives, almost thirty percent of the total. In France, despite equally vigorous suppression in the 1870s, the development was similar. Around 1900, a socialist was chosen as a cabinet minister. The same trends were witnessed in the smaller countries of northern and western Europe. In Russia, moderate and radical socialists were elected to the Russian parliament, the *Duma,* where they had considerable influence.

In Britain and the United States, however, the socialists failed to secure representation. Socialist Labor parties were founded in both countries before the turn of the century. However, Marxist ideology lacked appeal to the factory worker, especially in America. In both countries, the tradition of a two-party system hindered the representation of smaller groups and prevented socialists from making much headway in elections. Yet, in Britain as well as in the United States, the socialists achieved some of their aims. The British Socialists contributed indirectly to the victory of the Liberal party in 1906, bringing Asquith and Lloyd George into power. The American Socialists supported Populists and other third parties in their efforts to accelerate reform legislation.

### *Effects on Socialist Programs*

All socialist parties steadfastly advocated the abolition of private property. They continued to oppose colonialism and militarism. They also worked for international cooperation of the laboring classes. In 1889, they organized a "Second International" of Labor, which identified itself with Karl Marx's teachings.

As time went on, however, it became increasingly difficult for them to preserve a united front. To many, Marx's theory that the class struggle is unavoidable and revolution inevitable seemed more and more doubtful. The skeptics organized a "revisionist" movement in Germany (with Karl Kautsky and Eduard Bernstein proposing modifications of Marxism), a Fabian Society in England, and a moderate "Menshevik" wing of the Socialist party in Russia. The anarchists lost whatever strength they had gained. In fact, not the radicals, but those socialist groups that advocated a transformation of society by legal and democratic means, gained the leadership of the labor movement.

## ■ CULTURAL CHANGES

In the period from 1870 to 1914, much fundamental theoretical work in science was accomplished. The investigation of radiation and atomic structure achieved important results. Einstein formulated his relativity theory. Attention was being given to applying the newly acquired theoretical knowledge to the solution of practical problems. Many technological inventions were made that affected every aspect of Western life.

Insight into the social and spiritual condition of the individual did not advance correspondingly, however. Nihilistic tendencies appeared in various humanistic fields. The generation maturing around 1900 (the generation of the *fin de siecle*) has often been described as wanting in spirit and enthusiasm, as well as showing decadence. This notion was not confirmed in the art world. Shortly before World War I, when the social world that had been created in the 18th and 19th centuries was crumbling, impressionist and expressionist artists were creating meaningful original work.

### Science

The last quarter of the 19th century and the years before World War I brought a revolution in science comparable to that caused by Newton's discoveries in the 17th century. Scientific methods had been perfected. With the help of new instruments (themselves the result of scientific advances), observations were made that traditional Newtonian concepts could not explain, especially in atomic physics. The work of Planck and Einstein offered solutions and new understanding. Similarly, in the biological sciences, the conflicts with Darwinism regarding the struggle between science and the supernatural were recognized; new hypotheses were formulated to explain facts obtained by means of new observations.

## Biology and Medicine

In biology, Huxley and other disciples spread the theories of Darwin. They influenced the various subdivisions of biology, as well as anthropology, physiology, and sociology. The scientific data concerning plants or whole species of animals could not with certainty be applied to humans. Darwin's views needed to be supplemented. The mid-century discoveries of the Austrian monk Mendel, who formulated laws of heredity, contributed to a better understanding of evolutionary issues. The German Weismann disproved the inheritance of acquired characteristics. The Dutch botanist De Vries demonstrated that sudden variations (mutations) occur rather frequently in the evolutionary process. Biological investigations helped to redirect medical research. Diseases affecting human tissues were studied in the light of newly developed cell theory. Lister, Pasteur, Koch, and their numerous disciples made great strides in the field of bacteriology. There was notable progress in surgery; Virchow and other pioneers undertook daring operations. Public health conditions were improved in response to a growing realization of the need for sanitation. The average life span increased further. Problems of nutrition were scientifically investigated, and the importance of certain vitamins became recognized.

Most significant was the study of the nervous system, which in turn led to radical changes in the field of psychology. The Russian Pavlov described conditioned reflexes. The Austrian Sigmund Freud investigated the subconscious mind and began to develop the techniques of psychoanalysis.

Considerable thought was given to ethics in medicine. Views that disease was a divine punishment for sin had to make room for those emphasizing the obligation of doctors to cure disease, whether or not the patient was responsible for his or her own disease, whether it was inherited, contracted during an epidemic, or "psychological." These considerations also involved modern government, which gradually came to shoulder responsibility for public health and for maintaining it in the interest of the entire population.

## Chemistry and Physics

Research in the field of chemistry brought extensive knowledge, which was found useful in practical applications. Of no less importance was the fundamental work accomplished in physics. Photography was developed in France around 1840. In rapid succession, Roentgen discovered X-rays, and Hertz identified and analyzed electric waves. The atomic structure of matter was investigated; Roentgen, Thomson, Millikan, and others explored the functions of electrons. Becquerel discovered radioactivity.

In 1898, the Curies found radium; they showed that matter disintegrates spontaneously, releasing enormous amounts of energy. The work of the Curies stimulated further studies of matter (more specifically, the structure of the atom), of radiation, and of wave systems. In 1899, Planck published his fundamental work on quantum theory, which proposed that energy is emitted by atoms not in a constant flow, but in an irregular pulsating movement. Planck called the amount of energy emitted a "quantum."

His theory was in turn followed in 1905 by Einstein's relativity theory. Einstein demonstrated that time and space are not absolutes, but that they are relative to the observer. He worked out a fundamental equation ($E = mc^2$), which stated the relationship between matter and energy. His findings, comparable in importance to Newton's discoveries more than two centuries earlier, were of fundamental significance not merely for pure physics, but also for astronomy and new insights into the structure of the universe.

## Philosophy

Scientific attitudes and methods impressed themselves so deeply on the thinking habits of Western society that the whole discipline of traditional philosophy had to be rethought. Metaphysical speculations were increasingly rejected. Empiricism—the attempt to use experience alone as a basis for an explanation of "reality"—spread. The Austrian Mach taught that even our understanding of nature and its laws is limited by our imperfect sense of perceptions. Only observation and logical thought can act as trustworthy guides to knowledge. Embracing this premise, utilitarian concepts seemed to constitute the most reliable teacher of the philosopher, and a form of pragmatism, as taught by William James—the major American contribution to philosophy—was widely accepted. There were also many adherents of a rigid determinism who believed that laws such as evolution governed events in history and nature; such laws allowed little scope for free will. This view led many to accept a relativistic philosophy in which objects of philosophical investigation throughout the ages, such as ethics and morals, wisdom, truth, freedom, and goodness, were no longer significant. Such an attitude negated religious doctrines and encouraged men such as Spencer and Haeckel to develop the new field of sociology.

Few voices rejected the mechanistic concepts underlying all these interpretations. For example, the Frenchman Henri Bergson reemphasized metaphysical ideas, postulating that an *élan vital*, or creative impulse, was passed on from generation to generation and constituted the main force in human evolution. More representative of the age was the German philosopher Friedrich Nietzsche. He attacked the Christian creed and both traditional and contemporary concepts of ethics. He called instead for a repudiation of conventional values, a "transvaluation" of values. He described the individual's will to power, especially the exceptional individual's will to power, as the source of great deeds and as the standard by which a person and his work should be judged ethically.

## Education

The extension of knowledge and the acceptance of pragmatic and democratic attitudes created a need for changes in education. Elementary education became a necessity; compulsory schooling was introduced widely on the Continent. In 1911, England followed suit with the necessary legislation. Simultaneously, the United States, Russia, Brazil, and other countries of great size and multinational composition sought solutions befitting their special situations. Elementary education alone did not suffice, however; to disseminate new ideas and discoveries, revisions had to be made in the material taught in higher schools and universities. Knowledge was no longer, as in the Middle Ages, one body of data based on one set of premises. With the secularization of learning, a great variety of subjects and concepts had appeared; specialization increasingly marked the intellectual world. Disciplines such as chemistry, literature, and history had to be subdivided into numerous branches.

As a result, the universities began to organize specialized "institutes," while the secondary schools were divided into two groups: one stressing natural sciences, the other emphasizing humanistic studies. Instruction in religion was left largely to church schools. Art and music, once an integral part of higher education, were slighted or even eliminated. Attempts of outstanding scholars to achieve a new unity were futile in the face of the necessities that the development of economic, scientific, and political endeavors had created.

## Literature, Art, and Music

The *Zeitgeist* (or intellectual climate of the era) influencing science, philosophy, and education left its imprint on the world of literature and the arts. By 1870, the "Victorian style" (named after the English queen, Victoria) had become dominant. It was exemplified in architecture. Architecture symbolized the way of life and the aspirations of the most successful members of the well-to-do bourgeoisie. Only slowly did a reaction develop against the ideology underlying the Victorian style, and only at the turn of the century did this critical attitude begin to show itself in works of an experimental nature—leading to "modernism," as it emerged in literature, painting, and music, as well as architecture.

## Literature

The literary developments between 1870 and 1914 clearly indicated this changing intellectual climate. During the first period, a poet such as Tennyson represented the Victorian style. Romantic novelists, such as the younger Dumas, continued the traditions of the great French romantics in the age of Balzac and Stendhal. However, gifted younger writers turned increasingly to penetrating analysis of human nature, to naturalism and criticism of society. Most prominent were the French novelist Zola, the outstanding Norwegian playwright Ibsen, and Ibsen's disciples: the Swede Strindberg, the Irishman Shaw, and the German Hauptmann. Their influential social descriptions and their interpretations are in contrast with the pessimism and frequent cynicism that characterize the works of others representative of the *fin de siécle*. To a certain extent, Strindberg and Ibsen, but perhaps more so the French novelist Maupassant and also Anatole France, had represented this later trend. The Russian Chekhov belonged also to the group that marked the "end of the century," and perhaps even Mark Twain, despite his earlier inclinations toward affirmation of life and humor. Other authors, such as Lagerlof (Swedish), Kipling (English), and Conrad (Polish-English), who continued the great tradition of writing imaginative fiction, gave—sometimes within the Romantic mode—a sharp and sober picture of human character, longings, and weaknesses.

More experimental was a third group of authors, who began to win fame shortly before World War I. Partly under the influence of Dostoevsky and Tolstoy (who remained the towering figures on the literary stage after 1870), they sought for entirely new forms to express their deep, psychological investigations of the human predicament, of human inner contradictions and the tragedy of life. Probing into the last recesses of the soul, into feelings of anxiety, fear, and guilt, writers such as Kafka *(Metamorphosis)* and Proust *(Remembrance of Things Past)* attempted a new approach in what came to be known as the "surrealist" manner. But it was hardly appreciated for at least a generation. Newspapers and journals came to exercise, through their art and literary criticism, a growing influence on public taste, in addition to that on political and social attitudes.

## Painting, Sculpture, and Architecture

Comparable changes took place in the fine arts. After 1870, the work of the impressionist school with its emphasis on light and color continued. Then, toward the end of the century, there emerged the neo-impressionists and the "Fauvists" (van Gogh, Gauguin, Seurat, Cezanne, and Matisse) and, following them, the "expressionists," such as Kandinsky and Klee. It has been said that during the period 1870 to 1914, contrary to the democratic trend of the age, "a split occurred between artists and public" and that only an "elite" could grasp the meaning of many of the new paintings and their symbolism. But such splits and such limitations are, perhaps, in the nature of all works of art. In all times, many facets of artistic endeavor have been grasped first, if at all, by only a few people. No new situation was created when some of the greatest painters at the turn of the century found little appreciation among the public.

In fact, by turning away from classical as well as 19th-century traditions and by seeking to give expression to emotion and to reveal intrinsic meanings and to demonstrate their social consciousness, rather than merely depicting the visible environment, the expressionists seem to have anticipated a world of which subsequent generations would become more fully aware. They left a more lasting impression and exerted a deeper influence than other fine artists, such as the Americans Whistler and Homer, who proceeded along more conventional paths.

In sculpture, France produced the extraordinary artist Rodin. In architecture, numerous innovators who paved the way for modernism and to whom proportions and lines meant more than detail and ornamentation challenged the Victorian style. The newly appearing skyscraper gave a special character to the environment.

## Music

Similarly, in symphonic and chamber music, the reaction against the Romantic spirit and against sentimentalism brought a sequence of masters, consisting of impressionist, then neo-impressionist, and eventually—in the last few years before the war—expressionist composers. Romanticism was still evident in the works of the Austrian Bruckner and later in those of the Bohemian Mahler and the Norwegian Grieg. Impressionism was represented by the Frenchmen Debussy and Cesar Franck. Expressionism, with its new concept of atonality, came to the fore with the German Schonberg. At that time, there was also a long line of extraordinary Slavic (most of them Russian) composers, including Dvorak, Mussorgsky, Rimsky-Korsakov, and also Tchaikovsky, who tended to be, more than the others, in the Western tradition. The opera continued in the meantime along traditional lines, perhaps with the exception of Mussorgsky's *Boris Godunov*. In Italy, the best-known operas were composed by Puccini *(La Boheme, Tosca)*, and in Germany the outstanding works were contributed by Richard Strauss *(Salome, Rosenkavalier)*.

## Religion

In the face of the secularization of Western culture, the churches found their hold on their members (especially the youth) increasingly difficult to maintain. The "conflict between science and religion" began to manifest itself in many directions. Some of the foremost contributors to the natural and social sciences sharpened the conflict by characterizing religion as a mere survival of old superstitions. Actually, the process of secularization did not require a denial of the ethical demands of Christianity or of the need for inspirational and charitable functions exercised by the churches. On the contrary, so deeply were the basic humanitarian sentiments and moral principles of Christianity embedded in the Western world, after almost two thousand years of its history, that they automatically became a function of the now all-powerful states. It became the task of secular authorities to provide social legislation (in lieu of Christian charity), to spread education, and to support the arts.

## State and Church

During the transition from religious to secular sponsorship, many conflicts arose. Catholics, especially, proved less willing than protestants or the adherents of the Greek Orthodox Church to subordinate themselves to national political institutions. Examples included the *Kulturkampf* in Germany, the struggle between Catholics and atheists in France, the controversies between the papacy and the new regime in Italy, and other conflicts between materialists and the Roman Catholic Church, such as those in Spain and Latin America. In some instances, the secular authorities consented to compromises favorable to a church, but even then the governments achieved their objectives on many points of disagreement. The materialistic trend generally assured them of victory in the battles against a church hierarchy.

In Germany, the *Kulturkampf* brought church property under laymen control; all marriages performed by civil authorities became legal, and the training of the clergy was placed under governmental control. In France, a comparable struggle led to the expulsion of the Jesuits in 1880, the elimination of religion from primary schools a few years later, taxation of all ecclesiastical wealth, and finally, in 1905, separation of state and church. In Italy, despite the prevalence of strong nationalistic and atheistic tendencies, attempts to separate church and state failed. The government retained possession of the city of Rome, however. It insisted on the legality of civil marriages and asserted its right to determine the relationship between state and church. Unilaterally, it decreed the neutrality of the Vatican and guaranteed the possessions of the Roman Catholic Church.

*Spiritual Renewal*

These new relationships between state and church enabled religious institutions, particularly the Catholic Church, to rid themselves of political responsibilities and devote all their attention to spiritual matters. Consequently, a religious revival got under way. The Catholic hierarchy, while reaffirming traditional doctrines, concentrated on improving the education of the clergy and extending their missionary activities. In line with Leo XIII's *Rerum novarum,* the Church continued to oppose merely utilitarian principles. The Protestant churches experienced a similar spiritual revival, which was reflected in the formation of numerous fundamentalist groups or organizations, such as the Christian Science Church and the Salvation Army. There was also intensified religious activity within the Orthodox Church.

In Russia, the state-dominated church was opposed not only by the numerous atheist Marxists, but also by the "Old Believers." Some ten to twenty million strong, their fervor for a dedicated Christian life only increased with discrimination and persecution. The works of outstanding Russian philosophers bore a strong religious imprint. Tolstoy, Vladimir Soloviev, and Berdyaev infused Russian thought with the spirit of Christian love and Christian wisdom.

## ■ EXPANSION OF WESTERN CULTURE

Despite ideological conflicts and its many problems, Western culture was diffused so widely during the half-century from 1870 to 1914 that adoption of Western scientific thought, Western technology, and Western institutions became necessary for the survival and freedom of every civilization. Nowhere else did Westernization occur voluntarily except in Japan. Western ways were imposed upon the native populations everywhere else, including China, Persia, Africa, the Arab countries, and the Latin American hinterland. They became either completely or partially subservient to European nations.

*Figure 18–1 Europe's Colonial Possessions, 1900*

Emigration to many parts of the globe contributed to Westernization. The U.S.A absorbed half of the emigrants. Most of the newcomers came from Great Britain, Germany, Russia, Italy, and Spain. Sometimes adverse conditions at home, sometimes the attraction of the New World, and often individual, private reasons, such as lust for adventure, animated the people. Yet, up to a fourth of those who left eventually returned to their homeland.

## Western Influences on Outside Culture

Wherever it penetrated, Western civilization brought new patterns of culture through the preaching of Christianity, the introduction of humanitarian laws and European educational views, the teaching of European languages, and the dissemination of Western political ideologies. The contributions of Western civilization were numerous and varied—ranging from new inventions, techniques, and products (in transportation, manufacturing, agriculture, and mining) to improvements in health and medicine, and even to new modes of dress. Modern concepts of sanitation were widely introduced; the supply of trained doctors proved a blessing to millions.

On the other hand, Westernization had its negative side for the native populations; many of their useful customs were disrupted. Although the Westerners helped to wipe out old diseases, they brought new ailments with them. Hasty changes in long-established habits of life and work wiped out some native populations. Neither were new methods in political affairs an unmixed blessing. The old forms of human exploitation by native rulers were often merely replaced by equally cruel alien ones.

## Western Exposure to Outside Influences

While spreading to all parts of the world, Western civilization was, itself, subject to the influence of foreign cultures; it was compelled to solve new challenging problems. Expansion had its disadvantages. Expenses for investments and for defense were often higher than the rewards. Most colonies failed to drain off the surplus populations of Europe. Instead, they attracted limited numbers of often the most independently minded, venturesome people. The colonizing nations also continued to engage among themselves in costly struggles for economic and military power. Often, they failed to achieve the economic independence they had expected to derive from colonization. In fact, they became more dependent than ever before upon distant sources of raw materials and income.

Of course, colonization also had advantages for the West. The home countries were able to obtain needed commodities that contributed to their economic growth and profits, as well as a higher standard of living. Financiers and other leaders in the community made fortunes from the exploitation of colonial resources. The possession of rich colonies made it possible for small European powers, such as Holland, to attain world prestige and influence.

Moreover, the expansionist drive aroused the imagination of many people who were dedicated to a cause, such as "the white man's burden," of bringing the assumed virtues of Western civilization to the "natives" and of converting the heathen to Christianity. A missionary spirit went hand in hand with the mercantile spirit. Native religions, customs, art, and even food habits had an invigorating influence on Western people. They fired curiosity. Without consideration of economic gain, adventurous people set out to explore the unknown.

## New Western Horizons

Thus, after exploring various regions for material profits, Westerners turned to those that offered intellectual or emotional rewards. Scholars and adventurers sought satisfaction of their urge to know and learn. Expeditions to unknown regions flattered their vanity, or catered to their national ambitions and desire to plant their nation's flag on untouched soil. For such reasons, Livingstone searched for the source of the Nile, while Stanley sailed to face terrible hardships in the Congo. Sven Hedin explored the arid inner regions of Asia and Tibet and visited Lhasa. English, German, and Austrian mountain climbers scaled the icy peaks of the Alps and Himalayas.

Extraordinary exploits were undertaken in the Arctic and Antarctic regions. Peary is said to have reached the North Pole in 1909. A whole group of intrepid Scandinavians achieved what for centuries had seemed impossible; the *Fram,* a ship equipped by Nansen, drifted from Norway to Labrador, almost by way of the North Pole; Nordenskjold accomplished the first Northeast Passage, Amundsen the first Northwest Passage. In 1911 Amundsen, in a brilliant achievement, reached the South Pole.

## Perspective

*In the 45-year period preceding the First World War, peace reigned in Europe. New industries developed and new industrial products supplemented old ones. Further fundamental advances in science and in analyzing nature's forces were made, as well as in important inventions that could find practical applications. Financial institutions serving industries prospered. Agricultural production increased with the introduction of machinery and chemical fertilizers, reducing the need for hard labor. Transportation was modernized and speeded up. Migration from the land to the cities and emigration overseas accelerated. Living conditions for the masses improved.*

*The modern way of life was, however, criticized by the Catholic Church and, more effectually, by the strong socialist movement. Labor unions and political parties gained votes. The turn of the century brought a feeling of widespread "malaise," as expressed in philosophical and sociological treatments. The uneasiness filtered down to the masses that, by then, were more literate; they were influenced by the ever-widening stream of books, newspapers, and journals. Art, music, and literature reflected these feelings. The trend in art was toward nontraditional ways of representation, as shown by expressionists, painters, and architects, as well as in opera, polytonality and twelve-tone music, drama, and literature. Both normal and abnormal psychology were studied in new ways.*

*Government establishments seldom took an active part in furthering new intellectual trends. They concentrated their attention on their customary administrative tasks and their worldwide ambitions. They helped to spread the traditional principles of Western civilization and sought old ways of exploitation. Whether in America or Europe, governments paid little attention to Eastern or African lifestyles. But a desire for exploits in foreign lands continued to animate scientists and explorers. They made discoveries in the tropics, arctic climes, the deserts, and they penetrated to the most remote corners of the globe.*

## Selected Readings

Blue, Gregory, et al., eds. *Colonialism and the Modern World: Selected Studies* (New York: M. E. Sharpe, 2002).

Geary, D. *A Social History of Western Europe, 1848–1945* (1985).

Kaelble, Hartmut. *A Social History of Western Europe, 1880-1980* (Savage, MD.: Barnes and Noble, 1990).

Hayes, Carlton J. H. *A Generation of Materialism* (New York: Harper & Brothers 1963).

Milward, Alan S. and Saul, S. B. *The Development of the Economies of Continental Europe, 1850–1914* (Cambridge: Harvard University Press, 1977).

Pollard, Sidney. *Peaceful Conquest: The Industrialization of Europe, 1760–1970* (Oxford: Oxford University Press, 1981).

Russell, Bertrand. A *History of Western Philosophy* (New York: Simon and Schuster, 1972).

Shryock, Richard H. *Development of Modern Medicine* (Philadelphia: University of Pennsylvania Press, 1936).

## Test Yourself

1. In 1898, the United States went to war against which European Power_____?
   A. France
   B. England
   C. Spain
   D. Italy

2. Pope Leo XIII published in 1891 an Encyclical in which he repeated his predecessor's condemnation of_____.
   A. Socialism, Communism, and unchecked Liberalism
   B. Socialism, Communism, and Capitalism
   C. Democracy, Socialism, and Communism
   D. None of the above

3. In 1906, the British Parliament was led by _____.
   A. The Whig Party
   B. The Liberal Party
   C. The Tory Party
   D. The Republican Party

4. In Germany, the Social Democratic party was founded in 1863 by_____.
   A. Lasalle
   B. Bismarck
   C. Hitler
   D. None of the above

5. The study of the central nervous system was advanced by the work of_____.
   A. The German Weisman
   B. The Russian Pavlov
   C. The Russian Mendelev
   D. The Englishman Darwin

6. The techniques of psychoanalysis were developed by_____.
   A. Isaac Newton
   B. Albert Einstein
   C. Karl Marx
   D. Sigmund Freud

7. The Theory of Relativity was developed in 1905 by_____.
    A. Karl Marx
    B. Albert Einstein
    C. Sigmund Freud
    D. Frederich Nietzsche

8. Writers such as Franz Kafka and Proust attempted a new approach in what came to be known as_____.
    A. The New Age
    B. The Surrealist manner
    C. The Socialist manner
    D. The Anarchist manner

## Answers and Explanations

1. **C.** In 1898, the United States went to war against Spain, and its victory and acquisition of Spanish territories helped make the U.S. an imperialist power.

2. **A.** Leo XIII published an encyclical *(Rerum novarum)* in 1891 in which he repeated Pius's condemnation of socialism, communism, and unchecked liberalism. Yet, simultaneously, Leo XIII pointed out the moral obligations of the wealthier classes. He also approved the government's determined efforts to improve the living conditions of the masses and to restrict business practices harmful to the working class.

3. **B.** The British Socialists contributed indirectly to the victory of the Liberal party in 1906, bringing Asquith and Lloyd George into power. The American Socialists supported Populists and other third parties in their efforts to accelerate reform legislation.

4. **A.** In Germany, the Social-Democratic party, founded by Lasalle in 1863, sent two representatives to the first imperial diet in 1871. When Bismarck's repressive laws were abolished in the 1890s, it sent more than forty representatives to the diet, and in 1914 their numbers grew to more than a hundred representatives, almost thirty percent of the total.

5. **B.** Most significant of scientific advances during this period was the study of the nervous system, which in turn led to radical changes in the field of psychology. The Russian Pavlov described conditioned reflexes.

6. **D.** The Austrian Sigmund Freud investigated the subconscious mind and began to develop the techniques of psychoanalysis.

7. **B.** In 1905, Albert Einstein invented his theory of relativity. Einstein demonstrated that time and space are not absolutes, but that they are relative to the observer. He worked out a fundamental equation ($E = mc^2$), which stated the relationship between matter and energy. His findings, comparable in importance to Newton's discoveries more than two centuries earlier, were of fundamental significance not merely for pure physics, but also for astronomy and new insights into the structure of the universe.

8. **B.** Probing into the last recesses of the soul, into feelings of anxiety, fear, and guilt, writers such as Kafka *(Metamorphosis)* and Proust *(Remembrance of Things Past)* attempted a new approach in what came to be known as the "surrealist" manner. It was not appreciated for at least a generation. Newspapers and journals came to exercise, through their art and literary criticism, a growing influence on public taste, in addition to that on political and social attitudes.

# CHAPTER 19
# The Road to World War I (1890-1914)

**1898** Germany builds large navy, Fashoda crisis
**1899** Outbreak of Boer War
**1900** Boxer Rising in China
**1901** Planck, quantum theory
**1902** British-Japanese alliance
**1903** Panama independence established
Trans-Siberian Railway completed
First airplane flown (Wright brothers)
Shaw, *Man and Superman*
**1904** Entente Cordiale of France and England
Outbreak of Russo-Japanese War
**1905** Peace of Portsmouth
Revolution in St. Petersburg; a Duma introduced
Independence of Norway established
Einstein, relativity theory
**1907** Anglo-Russian treaty over Persia
Triple Entente completed
**1908** First Congress of Psychoanalysis (Freud)
Young Turk revolt
**1909** Expressionist school of painting started
**1911** Italy annexes Turkish Tripoli
Amundsen discovers South Pole
**1912** Outbreak of First Balkan War
**1913** Second Balkan War
Atomic structure described by Niels Bohr
**1914** Panama Canal opened
Clayton (antitrust) Act in United States
Outbreak of First World War

*When Bismarck retired from the political scene in 1890, the Western world entered a new stage in international relations. Prophets of supernationalism had long been at work. In Britain, the writer Carlyle, the journalist Bagehot, and the statesman Joseph Chamberlain had been fervent advocates of Britain's imperialistic role. The historian Lecky stated, "real liberty is for supermen and opposed to* democracy." France, stung by defeat in the 1870-71 Franco-Prussian war, inflamed to reassert national pride by men such as General Boulanger, Delcasse and Poincare, and even Renan, author of the Life of Jesus.

In Germany, national passions and a longing for national glory were incited by historians such as Treitschke and Droysen, military men such as Bernhardi, and even Wagner, master of a new style in opera. In Russia, Pan-Slavists agitated for a great Slavic empire under Russian leadership; many extolled a future messianic role for "Holy Russia." Italy nursed her Irredentist dreams. Polish chauvinists demanded the restoration of their medieval multinational dominion. In the United States, too, repercussions of nationalism were felt; the Spanish-American War and the policy of "walking softly and carrying a big stick" in foreign affairs, as expressed by President Theodore Roosevelt, were evidences of the all-encompassing trend.

Unfortunately for the peace of the world, the West possessed not only the spirit but, with its science and technology, also the means to make its nationalistic creeds an instrument of international policy and expansion. Competition among the nationalist Western powers led to new alliances and, eventually, to conflict and war.

## ■ INTERNATIONAL REALIGNMENTS

The first ominous step in the direction of war came at the expiration of the German-Russian Reinsurance Treaty. The lapse of the treaty in 1890 enabled France to end its isolation and to conclude a political and subsequently military alliance with Russia. In this way, the large Bismarckian coalition system in Europe was gradually replaced by two competitive and opposed alliance systems: the "Triple Alliance" of Germany-Austria-Italy, and the "Triple Entente" of France-England-Russia.

Bismarck, who was dismissed in 1890, watched these developments with growing concern. He died eight years after his dismissal, embittered over the ingratitude of his emperor. Actually, the dismissal was not only due to disagreements over certain external and internal policies, but also to the gulf between old and new, and to the changing temper and ambitions of succeeding generations.

### New Course

The "New Course," which brought about the change, resulted in part from a shift in economic conditions and in part from personal influences. Bismarck's successors and Emperor William II believed that Germany's friendship with Austria was indispensable, but that it was incompatible with an alliance with Russia. They therefore risked giving up Russia; they hoped to compensate for the broken Russian alliance by establishing closer ties with Britain. William was the beloved grandson of Queen Victoria, and both Britain and Germany had already made overtures toward each other signaling the desire for closer cooperation. They had, however, overlooked numerous adverse factors: differences of political systems and ideologies, German military buildup, personal animosities, commercial rivalries, colonial disputes, and lack of popular support for common policies. They also overlooked the fact that the British parliamentary system did not lend itself easily to the making of a binding alliance. Moreover, the Germans trusted injudiciously in the idea that Britain would never reconcile its divergent interests—especially in colonial matters—with France and Russia. They, therefore, overestimated Britain's desire to ally herself with Germany. They risked offending Britain in a most sensitive spot: its domination of the seas. Ambitious to play a leading role on the sea, Germany started a large navy-building program during the 1890s under the able leadership of Admiral Tirpitz. This led to bitter competition that was costly to the taxpayer, a burden to strategists, and an impediment to friendship.

### Dual Entente and Entente Cordiale

Its resulting coolness toward Germany encouraged Britain, at the turn of the century, to lend a favorable ear to French suggestions for renewed amity. By then, France was already strengthened through its new alliance with Russia. France and Britain had exchanged courtesy visits of statesmen and military units. They made a number of agreements, concluded an offensive and defensive alliance disclosed as early as 1894, and, most important, negotiated huge French loans to Russia.

Now France, under the direction of foreign minister Delcasse, began to court Britain. In 1898, a clash between France and Britain occurred in the Sudan, which Britain coveted in order to build its African north-south connections from Cairo to the Cape. France wanted to occupy it for the purpose of building its west-east connections from the Atlantic to the Red Sea. Troops bent on their respective missions collided at Fashoda. Delcasse shrewdly used the occasion for a friendly settlement. He had the French troops called back. In exchange for renouncing plans in the Sudan, he settled for a free hand in Morocco.

This led to further rapprochement. When Edward, Prince of Wales, became king of England, he paid a visit to Paris; other state visits were exchanged. These events brought understanding and political agreements regarding North Africa, East Asia, and Newfoundland. Finally, an "Entente Cordiale" emerged. Without constituting a firm alliance, it laid the basis for frequent consultation and occasional exchanges of military plans. It is worth noting that the 1904-05 Russo-Japanese war could have increased tension between England and France, as Russia's ally, France, should have aided Russia and Japan's ally, England, should have aided Japan. Instead, both England and France found, through mutual discussions, ways to shirk their diplomatic responsibilities in favor of close alliance.

## Triple Entente

Franco-British relations remained insecure so long as France wanted to preserve an alliance with Russia in spite of British-Russian competition. (Such had previously been the dilemma of Germany in the face of Austrian-Russian rivalry.) Circumstances, however, favored France. In 1905, Russia was defeated by Japan and weakened by revolution at home. This paved the way for a settlement of Anglo-Russian misunderstandings. Russia's reverses forced it to give up its plans of expansion in the Far East and in the

*Figure 19-1 Europe's Alliance Systems on the eve of World War I*

direction of the English lifelines through the Mediterranean. The reverses also changed the psychological climate. Revolution in Russia brought a parliamentary system, though relatively weak, to the great satisfaction of British public opinion. No more than one area of possible conflict now remained—Persia. Conflict there was smoothed over by a peace agreement in 1907. The agreement allowed the British a free hand in Afghanistan; it divided Persia into spheres of influence, with the northern part reserved for Russia and the southern part for Britain.

With the Russo-English feud thus settled, France could proceed with its alliance system. Political and military missions were exchanged among all three countries. The Dual Entente grew gradually into the Triple Entente of France-England-Russia. Germany, limited to its Triple Alliance with weak Austria and unreliable Italy, no longer possessed the position of strength it had enjoyed in Bismarck's times.

## ■ NATIONAL READJUSTMENTS

In most countries, questions related to foreign affairs were given priority over domestic problems. All the Western nations experienced economic growth and, with it, an increase in social problems. All of them developed democratic and humanitarian institutions, albeit with the handicaps of burdensome bureaucracies and, frequently, powerful military groups that gained undue influence in the shaping of national policies. The extent and the speed of these changes varied in the different countries; subtle shifts in the strength of the nations were to have grave consequences for the individual citizen, as well as for the peace of the world. Yet people in positions of responsibility and authority seldom appreciated this aspect of modern society involving the relationships between domestic and foreign affairs.

### The Continental Countries

Among the European nations, Germany was the first to reform its domestic economic and social policies to meet the challenges of a modern society. Within limits imposed by size and population, the Scandinavian countries, Holland, and Switzerland followed. The Southern European countries adapted themselves more slowly to the Industrial Age. In political matters, however, adjustment did not proceed from north to south, as in the case of economic and social change, but rather from west to east and southeast. The Atlantic nations were ahead of the central European powers on the path of democracy; in turn, the central Europeans were ahead of the Eastern and Balkan nations.

### *Germany*

During the 25 years before the outbreak of World War I, few additional improvements were made in Germany's political institutions. Notwithstanding attempts by socialists to inaugurate radical changes and efforts by liberals to democratize government, widespread complacency persisted. Little was done to broaden constitutional rights, reduce military influences, extend secondary education despite school reform efforts, or improve the procedures of the efficient and honest, but sometimes harsh and overbearing, government officials.

Class stratification remained strong. The northern and eastern landholding nobility retained its hold on many offices. Simultaneously, it opposed land reforms that might have given agriculture the same basis for stability and progress that industry enjoyed. On the other hand, the country gained rapidly in strength as exporter, financier, and importer. Its role in international affairs steadily increased. Social insurance legislation was greatly improved.

### *France*

A similar conservatism prevailed in large areas of France, especially in the provinces, where many people owned small landed properties, had adequate savings, and led a quiet and comparatively easy life.

The leaders of industry were also conservative and did not progressively improve their plants. Investments with safe returns were still preferred to the speculative financing of new enterprises that the times demanded. But among the inhabitants of the towns, radicalism and unrest were strong. Various issues and incidents kept political reform movements alive and prevented complacency.

First, there was the memory of military defeat, which stirred up nationalistic movements affecting political alignments. Second was the religious issue. Positivist groups following the ideas of Auguste Comte and atheists carried on a constant struggle against the Catholic majority. This conflict led to the suppression of monastic orders in 1903, and after a quarrel with the Vatican over France's political relations with Italy, to the separation of church and state in 1905. Third was the issue of socialism. Social legislation had followed the German model. But dissatisfaction persisted among the industrial workers, especially in the foundries of northern France and in the textile mills. Numerous strikes occurred. These were suppressed on several occasions with the help of the army. But the socialist movement grew. Even though radical syndicalism, which favored direct action of labor unions through general strikes, eventually receded, the socialist faction steadily gained influence in parliament and challenged the conservative forces.

Fourth was the emerging of a more progressive political culture. This was sparked in 1894 by an anti-Semitic outbreak. Anti-Semitism was found not only in France, but also in most of the West. In France, it led to a crisis when a Jewish army captain, Dreyfus, was falsely accused of treason. After an unfair trial, he was condemned to exile on Devil's Island; it took twelve years and the fervent protests of such patriots as the famous writer Zola and the politician Clemenceau to secure a reversal of the judgment and public amends to Dreyfus. The "Dreyfus Affair" deeply stirred French emotions and eventually brought a purge of a corrupt militaristic clique. It also contributed to the rise of modern Jewish nationalism, Zionism. It further led to improved legal procedures and, indirectly, to the strengthening of national security. Last was the issue of foreign policy, involving the alliance with Russia, the entente with England, the penetration into Morocco, the enlargement of the African empire in regions adjoining the Sahara, and the conquest of Madagascar. Liberals and socialists pointed out the inherent dangers of France's expansionist policy and the unfitness of France's agreements with autocratic, backward tsarist Russia; yet, the nation as a whole approved.

### *Italy*

During the 25 years preceding World War I, Italy gained in stability and prestige. In the north of the country, important textile and machine industries were founded. Railway and shipbuilding programs progressed. Educational standards were improved. Legislation helped to mitigate at least some of the worst social inequities. Both the national government and the local political representatives gained in administrative experience. Notwithstanding a number of financial scandals involving members of the government, corruption diminished; slowly, an adequate bureaucracy was trained.

After 1900, the political situation improved. Anarchistic activities, which in that year led to the assassination of the king, Humbert I, abated. Dire poverty continued to prevail, and class differences remained, not only in urban but also in rural areas and between the northern and southern parts of the country. Still, Marxist and other socialistic movements gradually took on the same peaceful, constitutional forms as in other European countries. Moreover, Italy's foreign and colonial policies were conducted wisely. Ventures like the ill-fated expedition of 1896 for the conquest of Ethiopia were not repeated; instead, feasible aims were pursued. The conquest of Tripoli in 1911 helped to satisfy the nationalistic ambitions of the people.

### *The Smaller Northern Countries*

Similar political and social problems beset large and small powers alike. In Austria-Hungary, tensions were sharp between the various nationalities composing the empire. They often centered around

Hungary, dominated by large landholders, and around Hungarian influence on the empire's policies. Much anti-Semitism existed, despite the integration of the Jewish upper class into their German surroundings. Moreover, worker dissatisfaction grew, although the country was less industrialized than the West.

Solutions varied with geographic factors, traditions, and available leaders. Democratic, political and social institutions developed in Scandinavian countries and in Holland, Belgium, and Switzerland. Military ambitions in all these nations continued to be negligible, except in perusing colonial possessions, particularly in the case of Belgium's ambitions in Africa. International agreements guaranteed a neutral status to Switzerland and Belgium. A peaceful settlement solved one of the thorniest problems—the fight of the Norwegians for national independence. At the Congress of Vienna, control over Norway had been granted to the Swedish king, but Norway had never reconciled itself to this arrangement. In 1905, Sweden voluntarily recognized Norway's independence.

Intellectual activities flourished, especially in Scandinavia, where writers such as Ibsen, Strindberg, Hans Christian Andersen, and Lagerlof, the literary critic Brandes, and the composer Grieg gained fame, and where excellent school systems were built up. Progress was made in the development of industries wherever natural resources were available: iron and lumber in Sweden, electricity in Switzerland, coal in Belgium, colonial products in Holland. On the other hand, the major social debates of the age—socialistic movements and clericalism—brought strife to many small countries. As elsewhere, these problems were eventually settled. Cooperative institutions were created in Scandinavia and, making up for a large part of the national economy, contributed to economic peace and stability.

### Southern and Eastern European Countries

Less promising was the development of the "second-rate powers"—Spain and Ottoman Turkey and the new Balkan nations. They possessed few of the economic and social resources needed for modernization. They showed little initiative or progressive thought. Wealthy landlords, who often controlled political and economic affairs, were opposed to modern trends. Industrial development lagged. Colonial expansion was not a solution available to any of these nations except Spain; trade was insignificant. Agriculture continued under antiquated methods and under feudal institutions. Yet, nationalistic ambitions were often manifest. Spain and Ottoman Turkey had memories of past grandeur. Some Balkan states, such as Serbia, espoused a Pan-Slavic national goal and dreamed of future grandeur. But most of these states included national minorities within their borders and were plagued by disorders created by them. This also caused difficult frontier problems.

Spain, with a large part of the population living in abject poverty, was the victim of repeated revolutionary activity. Monarchical and republican forms alternated; parliamentary and democratic institutions proved futile. Governments ruled with the help of army and Church. In Ottoman Turkey, not even the recognition of the independence of Serbia and Rumania, nor the subsequent establishment of Bulgaria, solved the nationality question. Revolts within the ruling elite surrounding the Ottoman sultanate contributed to a state of permanent political disorder. The aim of abolishing the despotic powers of the sultan and rejuvenating the state apparatus was not attained until after the end of World War I.

### England and the British Empire

Under capable statesmen—the aged Gladstone and, after him, Salisbury, Balfour, Joseph Chamberlain, Asquith, and Lloyd George—Britain continued along its established lines. It lost its position as the leading industrial power to Germany and the United States; it also lost some of the markets in Latin America and elsewhere that it had dominated in previous decades. Still, economic conditions remained favorable, and the population looked with satisfaction upon the material progress of the country.

Numerous political and social improvements were made. The judiciary was reorganized. Special, so-called "board" schools were formed to improve lagging educational standards and, by 1891, free elementary schooling was finally introduced. Social insurance was broadened to cover unemployment. A reform in the agricultural system, advocated by Gladstone, was eventually carried out.

The House of Lords demonstrated its lack of understanding of modern conditions by opposing such legislation and by advocating the use of force to break up labor strikes. In 1911, it was deprived of much of its power. Its right to veto legislation was sharply restricted. The working class gained steadily in influence. A Parliamentary Salary Act was passed to enable men without private means to become representatives in Parliament.

Yet, the laws providing voting rights for men still contained a number of special requirements that actually deprived some of the population of the possibility of exercising that right. Nor did women gain any political rights. As a result, women (suffragettes) started a vigorous agitation for the extension of voting rights to women—an agitation that occasionally led to violence.

The British Empire itself was kept intact, even though Britain's relations to some of the larger and more important colonies had to be restructured. In 1900, 1907, and 1910, the "dominion status" introduced earlier for Canada was granted successively to Australia, New Zealand, and South Africa. However, no timely solution was found for India. Despite vigorous protests, the Indians did not succeed in ending their colonial status. Nor was adequate progress made in the Irish question. Despite legislation providing for improvement in the status of the Irish peasants, Irish resistance under the gifted leadership of Charles S. Parnell was resolute. Even when violence broke out, the Parliament in Britain refused to permit the Irish the desired "home rule," and the issue remained unsolved.

## Russia

While the Continental European nations and England saw progress in constitutional development between 1890 and 1914, a combination of internal and external forces worked revolutionary changes in Russia. Existing institutions were negatively affected by pressure from domestic radical groups and penetration of Western thought.

### Industrialization After 1870

For at least two decades prior to 1890, it had been clear that Russia, if it wanted to maintain its power and independence, would have to build modern industries. Around 1870, Russia initiated a large railroad-building program. After 1890, the process of industrial and technical modernization was speeded by the efforts of Count Witte; he had started his public career as minister of railways, and then became minister of finance, and, finally, Russia's first prime minister. It was Witte who secured loans from abroad, especially from politically interested France. During the period 1891 to 1903, many new industrial enterprises were founded in western Russia, in St. Petersburg and Moscow, in the Don River region, and in the Urals; a Trans-Siberian railroad to Vladivostok was built and a Trans-Caspian and a Trans-Caucasian railroad were started. Witte also introduced protective tariffs, furthered social legislation, and established the gold standard.

### Revolutionary Activity

Russia was well on the way to improved living conditions and industrial greatness. But, for lack of corresponding political changes, the total situation deteriorated; the gulf between rulers and subjects widened. Although, as elsewhere, anarchist violence diminished while the cooperative movement and moderate socialism gained strength, the revolutionary temper grew and was intensified by the continued lack of representative and constitutional government. The revolutionary spirit was shown not only by workers and peasants, but also by the increasingly important bourgeoisie and by the intellectuals—scientists, professors, writers, and artists, all of whom were highly responsive to Western influence.

The situation became more critical still when, after 1900, an unfavorable business cycle in Europe affected Russia. Disturbances once more spread in the industrial centers and among the peasantry. A new move toward radicalism occurred. The extremists among the socialists rejected the slow path of peaceful evolution by means of education, propaganda, and constitutional procedures. Insisting on revolutionary means, they gained new adherents and won a majority at a congress that Russian socialists and their émigré comrades held in London in 1903. Hence they called themselves "Bolsheviks" (the "larger," the "majority") as opposed to "Mensheviks" (the "lesser," the "minority").

### Russo-Japanese War (1904-1905)

At this crucial moment, the government became involved in a dangerous foreign enterprise. Stimulated by the imperialistic policies of other European nations, the Russians had already entered the race for colonies; they were especially eager to obtain concessions in China. Following the repression of a Chinese independence movement, the so-called "Boxer Rebellion," Russia had demanded a lease on the Chinese harbor of Port Arthur and had occupied Manchuria. Britain and Japan, both coveting economic and military predominance in China for themselves, had reacted to this advance by concluding an alliance in 1902. Thus backed, Japan attacked Russia in 1904. Unprepared industrially, Russia suffered severe defeats on land near Mukden and on the sea near Tsushima. In 1905, it sued for peace. A peace treaty, brokered by President Theodore Roosevelt of the United States, was concluded that year at Portsmouth, New Hampshire. Russia ceded Port Arthur and half of Sakhalin to Japan and recognized Korea as a Japanese sphere of interest.

### Revolution of 1905

In the meantime, revolution had broken out at home. For years, the Russian government had played a dangerous double game. Through its police and spies, it had often cooperated with the rebellious labor class. It hoped that by supporting economic demands and even strikes against capitalists, it might deflect attention from the political shortcomings of the regime. But it had succeeded only in forfeiting the support of the bourgeoisie without gaining that of the workers. And when led by one of the dupes of this system, the priest Gapon, workers of a large munitions factory in St. Petersburg used the wartime opportunity to press their demands for political rights; their illusion about the government quickly came to an end. Singing hymns and marching upon the imperial palace to submit a petition, the workers were violently attacked. "Bloody Sunday" of January 1905 ended with thousands of victims dead or wounded.

This incident welded the antigovernmental forces into one. In vain, the tsar attempted to calm the opposition by halfhearted promises. Peasant uprisings spread. Strikes occurred in all industries. The various subjected nationalities prepared for a final blow. Patriots, outraged by the military loss to Japan, failed to rally around the throne. In October, a general strike was called, and violence in the countryside forced the government to make radical concessions. A "manifesto" was published, by which the tsar issued a constitution and granted autonomy to the Finns. Thus, autocracy in Russia finally ended; it was to be replaced by constitutional government.

### The Beginnings of Constitutional Government

The manifesto instituted the Duma, a nationwide representative body with legislative powers that was to be elected by the various classes of the population. Financial and military decisions remained in the hands of the tsar. Political parties became legal: Conservatives; Cadets, or Constitutional Democrats; Social Revolutionaries, or right-wing socialists less committed to revolution; Mensheviks; and Bolsheviks.

By its concessions, the tsarist government split the revolutionary opposition, as had been done in France in 1848. The liberal bourgeoisie, relying on the Duma to press for further reforms, abandoned their alliance with the working class and the socialists. These struck once more in December 1905. The uprising was brutally suppressed, and the tsarist government proceeded with its reform plans. Actually, it went back twice on its promises to the liberals, twice dissolved the Duma, and arbitrarily changed the constitution.

Without consulting the Duma, it also wrote, on its own initiative, the final chapter of peasant emancipation. At the suggestion of Prime Minister Stolypin, it annulled all remaining restrictions on the peasants and abolished the *mir*. Peasants from then on were no longer bound to village communities, but gained personal property rights to their lands, which they could now sell and leave at will. But once all this had been accomplished, a Third Duma was convened. With it began a real measure of constitutional government.

## The United States

The year 1900 did not mark any drastic break in American history, such as that which had occurred in European history. Social progress was steadily but slowly achieved. To many, however, the administrations of Theodore Roosevelt and Woodrow Wilson seemed to represent the dawn of a new era for the Western Hemisphere as well.

### *Industrialism and Social Legislation*

Economically, the United States continued to benefit from the work in fundamental sciences carried on in Europe. Thousands of its citizens went there to study philosophy, mathematics, natural sciences, and medicine. But technological application of scientific discoveries, owing to the inventive genius of men like Thomas Edison, was more rapid than in Europe. Deriving the necessary supply of laborers from the flow of immigrants, industries grew at an astounding pace. Early standardization of tools and parts made mass production possible. The small business owners were often unable to compete with entrepreneurs such as Morgan, Rockefeller, and Ford, who built huge industrial empires. Not even antitrust legislation could check their power. Nevertheless, socialism did not gain as in Europe. Threatened by depressions and unemployment, workers fought for better conditions and wages, organized strikes, and formed unions; however, they did not adopt the concept of the "class struggle." A socialist party under Eugene Debs did not attract enough voters to gain representation. In agriculture, the recurrence of major depressions did not lead to political radicalism among the farmers. Unlike Europe, there was still enough land available for extensive, rather than merely intensive, cultivation of the soil. The farmers benefited, moreover, from the rapid growth of the national economy.

Democratic institutions made the government and the two main political parties sensitive to popular needs. The challenge of third (reform) parties, such as the Greenback and the Populist parties, contributed to the timely passage of progressive social legislation. During the administrations of Theodore Roosevelt and Woodrow Wilson, many such laws were passed. Effective programs for the conservation of natural resources were instituted. The women's rights movement made some gains; in various states, women were granted voting rights.

### *Imperialism*

If socialist doctrine and various other economic and political problems of Europe were of less significance for the United States, the issue of imperialism did not remain alien to America. British interference in Venezuelan affairs released violent emotions and forced the British to submit the question to arbitration in 1899. The United States went to war against Spain, later annexing Puerto Rico and the Philippines and sponsoring Cuba as an independent state subject to American economic imperialism and political protection. The United States annexed Hawaii in 1898 and established naval stations in that area. Colombia was forced to renounce part of her territories, namely Panama. An American Zone was established where the Panama Canal was dug across the Isthmus. It was finished in 1914. The United States participated in the international action against China during the Boxer Rebellion and insisted on a subsequent economic "open-door" policy in the Far East. The Monroe Doctrine was reinterpreted to allow for possible United States interference in Latin American affairs. "Dollar diplomacy" supplemented military measures in the pursuit of U.S. imperialism.

# ■ PEACE AND WAR

Social institutions and aspirations, which had prevailed ever since Napoleonic times and had been accepted as typifying the entire 19th century, came to an end in 1914 when World War I broke out. With our knowledge, gained in retrospect, that war did come in 1914, we are inclined to see in the nationalistic developments before 1914 a path inexorably leading to this conflict and to violence. But the forces against war were also strong. The view cannot be maintained that war was the only means of solving the existing international problems.

## International Movements to Prevent War

One of the major aspects of the 19th-century liberal creed was its humanitarianism—a heritage from the Age of Enlightenment. And one of the most important humanitarian aims was the abolition of war. As technology created ever more deadly weapons, and as the spirit of the peoples was steadily poisoned by nationalistic propaganda and rivalry, the forces seeking to preserve permanent peace became increasingly active. Numerous steps were proposed, and some taken, to avoid a catastrophe.

### *Private Initiatives for the Organization of Peace*

Most of the peace movements were initiated and promoted by private individuals, not by governments. Some of these individuals advocated Christian precepts rejecting violence. Others adhered to Marxist views rejecting nationalism. Some were pacifists, others in search of an international legal order. Some wished for peace in order to conserve existing conditions, others wanted it in order to reform society. The means by which the workers for peace proposed to maintain peace were also diverse: political alliances, international law, arbitration, congresses, disarmament, and education. They founded organizations to investigate the causes of war and explore the possibilities of avoiding it. Some of them tried to influence political leaders and electorates in the direction of peace by emphasizing the dangers and all-embracing character of modern warfare. Prizes were offered to men who contributed to the promotion of peace: benefactors established such funds as the Nobel Peace Prize and the Carnegie Peace Endowment.

In numerous countries, vigorous propaganda against military service was carried out. Socialists held their own "Internationals," congresses at which nationalistic competition was denounced; they were, however, also used to coordinate various Marxist movements. At home, they voted in parliaments against military appropriations. Businessmen and bankers set up trusts and cartels whose profits depended upon peace, for they ignored national boundaries, divided up markets, and made foreign loans and investments.

### *Official International and Peace Organizations*

Governments could not afford to disregard the demands for peace put forward by so many segments of the populations. One of the first official organizations created before 1914 for the promotion of international cooperation, understanding, and peace was the International Postal Union. A Red Cross convention was signed that led to the creation of national Red Cross organizations subject to international rules. A number of disputes regarding borders and the interpretation of treaties were arbitrated, often involving major powers such as the United States, Britain, Germany, and Spain. International congresses were held.

In 1899, a Peace Conference convened at The Hague in the Netherlands. While it failed in many respects, it did succeed in founding a Permanent Court of Arbitration. In the Western Hemisphere, the Pan-American Union was established. An international sports organization was formed to provide opportunities for friendly competition among the youth of several nations; and, in 1896, the first modern Olympic Games were held in Athens.

## International Crises Leading to War

Notwithstanding these peacemaking efforts, war came. It was ushered in by a long series of crises.

### The Far East

Although the situation in the Far East appeared to be dangerous, it was not there that the real threat lay. In fact, the Western colonizing nations had, without resorting to war, divided the various Pacific islands among themselves, and international rivalry in China had abated. Before the end of the century, Germany had seized Tsingtao; Russia, Port Arthur; Britain, Weihaiwei; and France, Kwangchowan. The United States had secured economic advantages through its open-door policy. Even Japan had gained concessions. In 1895, after a successful war, Japan had deprived China of the Korean peninsula and the island of Formosa; it had also received economic privileges in China itself. A few years later, Japan had concluded an anti-Russian alliance with Britain and had then secured from Russia some Chinese spoils. Yet, international rivalry stopped it from extending too far. Thus, the tensions in the Far East were relieved. After 1910, a reform party emerged in China, the old dynasty deposed, and under the leadership of Sun Yat-sen, first steps were taken toward the building of a modern state that prevented a further spoliation of the country.

### Africa

More threatening were the developments in Africa. Toward the end of the century, Italy invaded Ethiopia, where it was defeated; France and Britain clashed in the Sudan at Fashoda. The Egyptians and Sudanese under the forces of the Muhammad Ahmed al-Mahdi staged a desperate revolt against the British. The revolt cost the brutal British general Charles Gordon his life and subjected the British to a damaging defeat at Khartoum. Not until 1898 was the al-Mahdi defeated at Omdurman and native resistance ended. Finally, the French began to penetrate into Morocco. Each of these events had serious repercussions among the Western nations and caused conflict. Then, a critical situation arose in South Africa. Subsequent to the discovery of gold in the Dutch territories of Transvaal, an unofficial English expedition, which was backed by the imperialistic British prime minister of the Cape Colony, Cecil Rhodes, tried to gain control over the area. This "Jameson Raid" failed, but it led to war between Britain and the Dutch settlers, the Boers. The outbreak of the Boer War shocked not only Holland, but also all other European nations. Yet, it was vigorously pursued, quickly demonstrating the inherent dangers of all colonial issues for the peace of the West. Ill will between Britain and Germany was provoked when the German emperor congratulated Kruger, leader of the Boers, for his valiant defense. The war itself continued until Boer resistance was crushed. A moderate peace was made, and in 1910 the creation of the Dominion of South Africa gave, indirectly, a measure of autonomy to the Boers. However, animosity persisted, not only between Britain and the Boers, but also among the European powers.

### Berlin-Baghdad Railway

Another crisis arose, in connection with a German railroad project. Railroads served both economic and strategic purposes everywhere. The Russians built their famous Trans-Siberian Railway; the British planned a railroad from the Cape through the length of Africa to Cairo; and the Germans proposed one connecting Berlin with Baghdad via Constantinople. Lacking the capital needed for this enterprise,

Germany suggested international participation, but Britain and, subsequently, France refused cooperation. The British feared for their Middle Eastern connections and did not wish to see Germany penetrate into any areas near India; the French sided with their newly won British allies.

The German proposal also antagonized the Russians. They had envisioned their own domination over Ottoman Turkey and, ever since Bismarck's dismissal, had watched German policies with distrust. A rapprochement, attempted in 1905 in a conference between Emperor William II and Tsar Nicholas II, was not meaningful. Because of existing alliances, neither party ratified the settled-upon agreement. Eventually, the Germans appeased Russian apprehensions, but they never reconciled Britain to the Baghdad railroad plan. Nor were Russian and British fears lessened when closer German-Turkish collaboration was established, with increased German naval support to rebuild Ottoman's navy by appointing a German general to be the sultan's military adviser—a position parallel to that of his British naval adviser. But the real tension that existed between Britain and Germany concerned their naval arms race. What concerned Britain most was Germany's determination to build a powerful naval force. The British feared that this could interfere with British international trade or even blockade the British Isles. Germany's naval program was the single most important reason that Britain moved closer first to France and then to Russia.

### Morocco

The Fashoda crisis had brought an agreement between France and Britain that favored French expansion in Morocco. It disregarded possible interests of other nations. As a result, Morocco faced considerable difficulty. Morocco was rich in lands well suited to agriculture and grazing; it was also a valuable strategic asset. In 1905, the Germans demanded concessions in Morocco and began to support nationalists opposed to French rule. William II paid a provocative visit to the Moroccan ruler at Tangier. This Moroccan development led to a serious crisis that was only, with difficulty, settled by an international conference at Algeciras (1906). There, France's Entente Cordiale with England brought its fruits; France was almost unanimously supported. Germany, which had undiplomatically provoked the issue, had to be satisfied with insignificant gains. Five years later, Germany reopened the issue through an equally undiplomatic act, sending a naval unit to the Moroccan port of Agadir. This time a settlement was reached only with still greater difficulty. The international atmosphere was further heightened with tension.

### Bosnia

Despite the gravity of all these colonial disputes and the dangers of war that they involved, it was ultimately the situation in the Balkans that led to an irreparable crisis. Next to the issue of Alsace-Lorraine, Bismarck had always most feared the dangers of Balkan nationalism because of its implications for all Europe. All great powers collided there. Russia wanted to win the straits and dominate its Slavic sister nations; Germany and Austria wanted to expand southeastward; France wanted to preserve long-standing economic and cultural investments; Britain wanted to keep the other great powers away from the eastern Mediterranean, its chief link to India. In addition, Turkey sought to retain the rest of its European possessions. The various Balkan nations (Serbia, Romania, and Bulgaria—excited by their recently won independence—as well as Montenegro and Greece) were pitted against Ottoman Turkey, against Austria, and against one another. No arrangement since the Congress of Berlin had achieved more than a temporary respite.

Early in the 20th century, a national revival occurred in Ottoman Turkey. The Young Turks, a nationalist reform party, introduced a constitutional monarchy under Sultan Abdul-Hamid II. Had their reform succeeded, the great European powers would have lost the influence they were accustomed to exercising in the Balkans. In view of such a prospect, the two nations most affected decided to act: in 1908, the foreign ministers of Russia and Austria met at Buchlau. Following a program that had been outlined in the 1870s, the Russians agreed not to interfere with an Austrian occupation of Bosnia, and the Austrians not to interfere with Russian plans regarding the straits. The Austrians promptly helped themselves to their share of the bargain. But Russia, faced by other nations with vital interests in the region assigned to it, found itself stalled. There developed an extremely bitter resentment at what Russia considered Austrian duplicity. Serbia, with claims of its own on Bosnia, was not less incensed. What had been intended as a compromise turned into an additional controversy that brought Europe to the brink of war.

### *Balkan Wars*

A major disaster was temporarily avoided, but the crisis hastened a local upheaval in the Balkans. In 1912, Italy's annexation of Turkish Tripolitana had demonstrated the continued military weakness of the Turkish Empire. The Balkan nations deemed the moment ripe for rebellion against the sultan. The war was fought in two sections. First, Bulgarians, Serbs, Montenegrins, and Greeks invaded Turkey; they forced Ottoman Turkey to make a peace depriving it of all European possessions except Constantinople. Second, these victorious rebels, plus Romania, went to war with one another. As one result, Bulgaria lost most of its spoils.

The Balkan wars foreshadowed future patterns of warfare. International law was violated by every belligerent; terrible devastations and massacres occurred. Peace brought only additional sources of misery: It forced migration of peoples and population exchanges, subjection of people to alien rule, economic disruption, and general impoverishment. Nothing was settled. Indeed, yet another splinter nation—Albania—was created. Dissatisfaction was general; a festering wound was to poison areas far beyond the Balkans.

### *Sarajevo and the Outbreak of World War I*

In June 1914, the final crisis occurred. In Sarajevo, Bosnia, a Serbian nationalist assassinated the successor to the Austrian throne, Archduke Francis Ferdinand. The Austrians, enraged at the involvement of some members of the Serbian government and at the encouragement given by Russian Pan-Slavists to Serbian nationalists, sent an ultimatum to Serbia that would have put a virtual end to Serbian independence. Assured that Russia could not and would not desert it as before, Serbia refused full compliance. Austria, counting on German support, lacked the desire to modify the conditions of its ultimatum. In vain some of the great powers increased their diplomatic effort at the last moment to stop an outbreak that, because of treaty obligations, was bound to bring France into the war as an ally of Russia, and that was likely as well to engulf Britain, Italy, and, once more, most of the Balkan nations. On August 1, 1914, World War I broke out.

### **Internal Factors**

It is often forgotten that internal political and party considerations in major countries sharpen international crises. The internal difficulties at this time were not insurmountable. But in order to maintain themselves in power, governments had to make concessions to right-wing forces everywhere: Britain to the anti-Irish, imperialists, and capitalists; Germany to agrarian reactionaries and industrialists; France to chauvinist politicians and army officers; Austria-Hungary to the nobility and the enemies of Slavic national aspirations; Russia to those bent on maintaining the dated social structure. In the United States, as well, party considerations eventually contributed to war policies.

### **Perspective**

*Following Bismarck's dismissal, the European international system that he had maintained to guarantee peace gradually dissolved. A steadily growing nationalism and colonialism increased tensions, and two opposing alliance systems were formed by the major European powers. Economic rivalry between the nations and internal social struggles contributed to the difficulties. Social-democratic and labor parties—in Russia, partly of a revolutionary nature—gained in strength despite legislation passed in all countries to improve social conditions. In the United States, unrestricted capitalism reached an apex. Both the wealth and influence of leading entrepreneurs and enterprises increased.*

*Numerous conflicts between great and small nations raised the specter of war. Russia's war against Japan led to revolution at home. Clashes between European nations in Africa, as well as among the Balkan peoples, added to the danger. Pacifist organizations failed in their efforts to prevent war. The period of peace came to an end and World War I broke out.*

## Selected Readings

Fieldhouse, D. K. *Colonialism, 1870-1945: An Introduction* (New York: St. Martin's Press, 1983).
Robert, J. M. *Europe, 1880–1914* (New York: Longman 1989).
Lichtheim, George. *Imperialism* (New York: Praeger, 1971).
Gulick, Edward V. *Europe's Classical Balance of Power* (Ithaca: Cornell University Press, 1955).
Hale, Oron J. *The Great Illusion, 1900-1914* (New York: Harper & Row, 1971).
Khon, Hans. Pan-Slavism: Its History and Ideology (New York: Vintage Books, 1960).
Langer, William L. *European Alliances and Alignments* (New York: Knopf, 1962).
Morris, Richard B. and Morris, Jeffrey B. *Encyclopedia of American History* (New York: HarperCollins Publishers, 1996).

## Test Yourself

1. The Triple Alliance preceding World War I was composed of_____.
   A. Germany, Austria-Hungary, and Italy
   B. Britain, France, and Russia
   C. Russia, Germany, and the Ottoman Empire
   D. Germany, France, and Britain

2. The Triple Entente prior to World War I was composed of_____.
   A. Germany, Austria-Hungary, and Bulgaria
   B. France, England, and Russia
   C. France, Germany and England
   D. France, Bulgaria, and Austria-Hungary

3. The Russo-Japanese War in 1904-1905 was settled with the signing of the Treaty of_____.
   A. Portsmouth
   B. Versailles
   C. Paris
   D. Frankfurt

4. In June 1914, Archduke Franz-Ferdinand of Austria-Hungary was assassinated in the city of_____.
   A. Paris
   B. Berlin
   C. Sarajevo
   D. Moscow

5. A Parliamentary salary act was passed in Great Britain in 1911 in order to_____.
   A. Enable the poor to make a minimum wage
   B. Enable men without private means to become ministers of parliament
   C. Extend social security to all men
   D. Extend credit to poor workers

6. Anti-Semitism in France was sparked by_____.
   A. The Balfour Declaration
   B. The French Mandate
   C. The Triple Entente
   D. The Dreyfus Affair

7. Early in the 20th century, the "Young Turks" introduced a constitutional monarchy under the reign of_____.
   A. Mustafa Kemal
   B. Sultan Abdul Hamid II
   C. Sultan Mahmud II
   D. None of the above

8. World War I broke out on _____.
   A. August 1, 1914
   B. July 23, 1914
   C. December 7, 1914
   D. November 11, 1914

## Answers and Explanations

1. **A.** The first ominous step in the direction of war came at the expiration of the German-Russian Reinsurance Treaty. The lapse of the treaty in 1890 enabled France to end its isolation and to conclude a political, and subsequently a military, alliance with Russia. The "Triple Alliance" of Germany-Austria-Italy began prior to the First World War.

2. **B.** The large Bismarckian coalition system in Europe was gradually replaced by two competitive and opposed alliance systems: the "Triple Alliance" of Germany-Austria-Italy, and the "Triple Entente" of France-England-Russia.

3. **A.** Unprepared industrially, Russia suffered severe defeats on land near Mukden and on the sea near Tsushima. In 1905, it sued for peace. A peace treaty, brokered by President Theodore Roosevelt of the United States, was concluded that year at Portsmouth, New Hampshire. Russia ceded Port Arthur and half of Sakhalin to Japan and recognized Korea as a Japanese sphere of interest.

4. **C.** In June 1914, the final crisis occurred. In Sarajevo, Bosnia, a Serbian nationalist assassinated the successor to the Austrian throne, Archduke Francis Ferdinand. The Austrians, enraged at the involvement of some members of the Serbian government and at the encouragement given by Russian Pan-Slavists to Serbian nationalists, sent an ultimatum to Serbia that would have put a virtual end to Serbian independence.

5. **B.** The House of Lords demonstrated its lack of understanding of modern conditions by opposing such legislation and by advocating the use of force to break up strikes. In 1911, it was deprived of much of its power. Its right to veto legislation was sharply restricted. The working class gained steadily in influence. A Parliamentary Salary Act was passed to enable men without private means to become representatives in Parliament.

6. **D.** Anti-Semitism was found, not only in France, but also in most of the West. In France, it led to a crisis when a Jewish army captain, Dreyfus, was falsely accused of treason. After an unfair trial, he was condemned to exile on Devil's Island; it took twelve years and the fervent protests of such patriots as the famous writer Zola and the politician, Clemenceau, to secure a reversal of the judgment and public amends to Dreyfus.

7. **B.** Early in the 20th century, a national revival occurred in Ottoman Turkey. The Young Turks, a nationalist reform party, introduced a constitutional monarchy under Sultan Abdul-Hamid II. Had their reform succeeded, the great European powers would have lost the influence they were accustomed to exercise in the Balkans.

8. **A.** The First World War broke out on August 1, 1914 when Germany invaded Belgium.

# CHAPTER 20

# War, Peace, and Revolution (1914-1919)

**1914** First Battle of the Marne
**1916** Battle of Verdun
**1917** Abdication of Russian tsar: February Revolution
October Revolution in Russia: Bolsheviks (Lenin) establish communism
**1918** German-Russian Peace of Brest-Litovsk
Armistice concludes First World War
Revolution in Germany, Austria, and Turkey: republics declared
**1919** Allied intervention in Russia; civil war in Russia
Treaty of Versailles; League of Nations

*The years 1914 to 1919 brought such deep and clear changes that someday the period surrounding World War I may well be considered a no less decisive turning point in history than that of the Reformation years 1517 to 1521. During the first quarter of the twentieth century, new points of view concerning nature and society transformed science, religion, and the arts, and led to the evolution of new social and political structures.*

*Three fundamental changes are discernible: (1) The European state system, completed with the Peace of Westphalia in 1648 and modified in 1815 and 1870, broke down without being replaced by a new tenable system. Instead, the nationalistic objectives of every nation were acknowledged, with the consequence that instability prevailed throughout the world. (2) The European balance of power, established around 1713 (when the wars of Louis XIV ended), was destroyed. A regrouping took place, requiring the participation of an additional power—the United States of America—to assume the function of balancing the divergent groups. (3) The dominant influence of liberalism, which had been the aim of the most progressive forces of society since the Enlightenment, came to an end. Collectivism gained everywhere, and in one area—Russia—it achieved complete victory in its extreme socialistic form.*

## ■ WORLD WAR I

The conflict that broke out on August 1, 1914, brought "total" warfare such as previous ages had not known. Other wars had affected all aspects of life, had engulfed military and civilian populations, and had inflicted "total" destruction. Such were the War of Liberation of the Netherlands, the Thirty Years' War, and the American Civil War. But "total" destruction applied only to those localities in which armies actually operated.

By the time of the First World War, division of labor and use of modem communications had increased the interdependence of large areas so much that the effects of war touched ever-widening areas. War embraced nations in their entirety. Mobilization meant the mustering of all productive forces at home, as well as of armies. The destruction of the enemy's industries, manpower, and morale became essential objectives. Thus, the blockade of Germany brought untold suffering to its civilian population. Only fundamental discoveries (such as Haber's discovery of the process of synthesizing ammonia and producing fertilizer artificially) enabled the country to continue the war. German submarine warfare had a comparable effect upon the English people. The war stimulated the inventive powers of nations. Many new weapons and techniques were devised or perfected, such as combat planes, armored tanks, poison gases, flame-throwers, and air bombing.

## Origins of World War I

Historical events and processes are too complex to allow an enumeration of "causes." At the most, a few tentative conclusions can be drawn. In the case of World War I, a number of basic contributing factors merit consideration. (1) The force of nationalism led to numerous crises involving overseas lands as well as European territories. (2) The existing system of competing alliances, less the result of aggressive intentions than of fear, pitted nations against one another. (3) The secrecy of diplomatic intercourse made the various nations suspect that sinister agreements were being made against their interests. Secrecy brought universal distrust and was therefore a threat to peace. (4) The absence of a "balance of power" proved as much a danger to peace as formerly the existence of such a balance had proved to be. The old system was not replaced by international cooperation, but rather by an anarchical state of international affairs rooted in nineteenth-century liberalism. (5) The feeling of the "unavoidability" of war prevailed, partly brought about by irresponsible sensationalistic journalism. (6) The instability of the economic system caused business cycles of booms and depressions and made large segments of the population lose their sense of security. Thus dissatisfaction with the existing economic order was heightened. (7) The scientific spirit and scientific inventions upset sociological patterns and mores. In addition, they changed the economic balance between nations and led to new jealousies. (8) The lack of foresighted leadership contributed to instability. Some statesmen, politicians, military men, and educators prepared for an armed conflict; others, with equal determination, devoted their lives to avoiding one. But the majority of leaders, though well-meaning, were weak and vacillating. The foremost statesmen lacked originality as well as independent judgment. They allowed themselves to be swayed by irresponsible advisers, political parties, the mob, or simply the general course of events. Thus, as Lloyd George once said, the nations "backed into war."

## War Preparations

The world situation and historical trends pointed in the direction of war. Yet, the actual outbreak of World War I was made possible only by the maintenance of large military establishments on land and on sea and by the development of careful strategic plans.

### *Armaments*

Compulsory military service was in effect in most Continental countries. Everywhere military budgets were extremely burdensome. France was most heavily armed, with almost two percent of its population in its land forces. Germany had proportionately a smaller, but more efficient army and an increasingly well trained and equipped naval force. England had a small army, a large navy. Russia had the greatest number of battalions, the poorest equipment. Austria had enough troops, but the diversity of their national origins detracted from their dependability.

### Strategy

Germany's position in the center of Europe was the most precarious, in view of the possibility of attack from two sides—a constant threat that developed after the destruction of Bismarck's carefully built system of alliances. Consequently, its strategic preparations were the most elaborate. For allies, Germany could count only on the Austrians. Italy, although temporarily committed to Germany, eventually joined the other side in 1915.

### Schlieffen Plan

The Germans had therefore worked out the Schlieffen plan (named after the German chief of staff Alfred Schlieffen and introduced in 1905) according to which, in case of attack from two sides, a holding action in the east against Russia was to be undertaken while efforts were to be made to reach a quick decision in the west against France. Troops were to march through neutral Belgium in order to attack the French from the north, occupy the coastline, cut off possible help from England, and force Paris to surrender, then race back on rails to fight the slower mobilizing Russians.

### Entente Plans

This plan was not unknown to the Triple Entente of France, Russia, and Britain. The British had not yet promised unconditional adherence to the Entente, but they participated in military preparations that included strategic talks with "neutral" Belgium. Entente plans called for a Russian thrust, first into Austria, then into East Prussia, and a French attack along the Rhine.

### War Guilt

Analysis of the events that led to World War I shows that it would be unjust to conclude that the conflict was instigated by any one of the belligerents. The victorious nations later required Germany to acknowledge responsibility. Such one-sided accusation was made in order to gain practical advantages, although these ultimately did not materialize. An objective appraisal indicated that all the participants shared in the responsibility. Austria-Hungary and France were guilty because they followed policies of expansion and of revenge, respectively. Russia fostered a war atmosphere, nurtured Pan-Slavism, and allowed too much latitude to ambitious statesmen. England and Germany were animated by the generally prevailing imperialistic spirit. They could have refused to participate in such a war and thereby made it impossible, but they failed to do so. Further, Germany's famous blank check in support of Austria and not discouraging its aggression *vis-à-vis* Serbia added to the heightened tension. Among the German (as among the French) military and political circles were many who were not averse to the idea of a war. Germany's extensive navy-building program had contributed much to the tension and to ultimate disaster.

### The Course of the War

The first two years of the war witnessed startling victories by Germany. As a result, almost the entire war was fought on the soil of Belgium, France, northern Italy, and Polish Russia. (Minor action took place in the German colonies.) The war was fought mostly on land by armies consisting of millions of conscripts on each side. Naval and air engagements were of comparatively little significance. Germany won many important battles, but failed to turn these into a decisive victory.

As the struggle continued, Japan, Italy, Romania, and various small nations joined the Allies, while the Central Powers gained the support of Turkey and Bulgaria. Participation by the United States ultimately decided the issue. Then not even the collapse of Russia (which relieved Germany of the necessity

Figure 20–1 World War I: Trench warfare and the Western Front

to fight on two fronts) could prevent the defeat of the Central Powers. In November 1918, they asked for an armistice.

## Campaigns of 1914 to 1916

In a sense, the first three months of the war were the most critical. According to plan, Germany invaded Belgium, whereupon England promptly declared war on Germany. Nevertheless, the Germans conquered Belgium and pushed deep into France. But the Schlieffen plan was not consummated, for they did not gain control of the English Channel coast, and therefore could not prevent British aid from reaching France, nor did they take Paris.

At the end of August, apprehensive of Russian penetration into Germany, the Germans reduced their forces on the Western front and sent them to the East. They succeeded in decisively defeating and repelling the Russian forces in the great battle of Tannenberg and Masurian Lakes. But a consequence was that early in September their advance in the West was stopped short at the Marne River (First Battle of the Marne). What was planned as a short, lightning war turned into an interminably grim one. Throughout the year 1915, millions of soldiers faced one another in trenches, unable to strike a decisive blow. In 1916, the Germans attempted to break the deadlock. Two terrible battles were fought, one at Verdun, the other on the Somme River, bringing unprecedented losses to both sides. An important naval engagement took place off the shores of Jutland. But the situation was not changed. Only in the East, where the fronts were mobile, was a decision reached. The Russian armies were pushed out of German territory. Soon Austria, too, was liberated. By 1916, the Germans had penetrated deep into Russian territory.

### Campaign of 1917

The year 1917 began with no change in sight. Yet, that year proved to be decisive, for two major events completely altered the situation. The first event was the Russian Revolution, which overthrew the tsarist government and established a liberal democratic regime (the "Provisional Government") in February 1917. Although Russia remained in the war for a time, and even staged a mighty summer offensive, the failure of this effort merely hastened the disintegration of the Russian army.

The second event was the entry of the United States into the war. Strong pro-English leanings, democratic idealism, American investments in Allied countries, effective English propaganda (coupled with the interruption of news reports from German sources), and, finally, Germany's unrestricted submarine warfare, which cost the United States heavily in lives and goods—all these factors contributed to abandonment of American neutrality. Active participation by United States armed forces (comparatively few of whom saw action in battle) did help the Allies and gave them renewed hope. However, American reserves in manpower and weapons, economic resources, and food supplies were far more decisive in swinging the tide of war against the Central Powers. American aid did not actually make itself fully felt before a second phase of the Russian Revolution occurred. In October 1917 (November according to the Western calendar), the Provisional Government was overthrown by the Bolsheviks, who promptly concluded an armistice with Germany.

### End of World War I (1918)

Early in 1918, the armistice between Russia and Germany was supplemented by a peace treaty, which was concluded at Brest-Litovsk. Germany insisted on the separation of Livonia, Poland, the Ukraine, and other territories from Russia; it posed as an advocate of self-determination for all peoples but actually hoped to impose its own control upon these areas. But Germany's victory in the East could not make up for the increased danger threatening her from the West. In the course of the spring and summer of 1918, the German armies were forced to retreat, and by September, it had become evident that, despite Brest-Litovsk, the war was lost for Germany. Her military position had become untenable, there were sailors' mutinies that spread Soviet style revolution throughout, and internal unrest was brewing. To avert trouble at home, various steps were undertaken to democratize the country, such as granting universal, equal suffrage in Prussia. But this failed to placate Germany's enemies (bent on a complete overhauling of the German government) and Germany's own liberals and socialists. Desperately, in the fall of 1918, the imperial government offered to negotiate peace along lines laid down in "Fourteen Points" proposed by President Woodrow Wilson. Germany's allies (Bulgaria, Turkey, and Austria-Hungary) also sued for peace, and their rulers abdicated. Although Britain and France held numerous reservations regarding Wilson's war aims, the German government could hold out no longer, and an armistice was concluded in November.

### The Home Front

Contributing to Germany's defeat were the difficult circumstances behind the front. Just as with sieges of towns during the Middle Ages, now whole countries were besieged and faced starvation. In most countries, therefore, much depended upon the organization of the home front and its resources. Industries had to be reoriented, raw materials provided, and food supplies secured. The courage of the population had to be maintained and their support guaranteed.

Russia and Germany suffered most. In Germany, the emergency had led to a mighty effort to organize a war economy. It was efficient, but with outlets to the world largely cut off (which made it also impossible to counter the enemy's propaganda or, in turn, to reach the enemy's populations), no effort was adequate. Nor was the attempt to put England in a similar predicament by means of unrestricted submarine warfare a successful one. The conviction in Germany that the war could be won vastly diminished. Together with the military defeats of the army, collapse could, after four years, no longer be avoided.

*Figure 20–2 Europe after World War I*

### Abdication of German Emperor

By this time, revolution had broken out in Germany. The emperor had fled to Holland and, like other kings and princes of the individual German states had given up his throne. A republic was instituted. There was street fighting in Berlin and elsewhere, soldiers and sailors deserted, and communists attempted to seize power. But the socialists, supported by the liberal democratic parties, took over the government. Thus, simultaneously with the end of the war, Bismarck's imperial structure fell to pieces. Democrats and socialists had to assume the heritage under difficult circumstances.

## ■ PEACE AT VERSAILLES (1919)

About one hundred years intervened between the Congress of Vienna and the Treaty of Versailles. During this period, the temper of the times had changed fundamentally. At Vienna, the defeated nation had taken part in the settlement, but at Versailles the voice of the vanquished was rarely heard. The prompt return of the defeated to the community of nations had been the aim of the victors in 1815, but the postponement of such a result was the objective of the victors in 1919. A balance of power was sought after Napoleon's downfall, whereas a permanent weakening of the Central Powers was desired by the Allies at Versailles. Statesmen at Vienna drew frontiers in conformity to historic dynastic rights and interests, whereas the spirit of nationalism and revenge dictated boundary arrangements in 1919. Moreover, for the first time, a non-European power, the United States, played a leading part in a European peace settlement, while Russia, which had been so prominent in the negotiations of 1815, did not even participate.

## Terms of the Treaties

The decisions made at Versailles (spelled out in the treaty with Germany and, subsequently, in separate treaties with Austria, Bulgaria, and Turkey) were the result of numerous compromises. Early on, it became clear that the victors were pursuing divergent aims. Although President Wilson was a leading figure in the negotiations, his Fourteen Points were brushed aside whenever they seemed favorable to the interests of the defeated nations. Wilson's principles called for freedom of the seas, removal of economic barriers, disarmament, impartial distribution of colonies, evacuation by Germany of all territories occupied during the war, self-determination of subjected peoples, and the establishment of a League of Nations. Instead, the ideas of Premier Clemenceau of France, who presided at sessions of the peace congress, prevailed. He advocated such harsh terms that, as he intended and openly avowed, they could not be fulfilled and Germany would be kept in permanent submission. Generally, he was supported by Prime Minister Lloyd George of Britain.

### Terms for Germany

The final treaty stipulated that Germany surrender all its colonies and special rights overseas, cede Alsace-Lorraine to France, and give France the right to control and exploit for a period of fifteen years the rich industrial area of the Saar. Germany was forced to give up its fleet—some units of which were scuttled by the crews—and a large part of its merchant marine. It had to cede territories in the west to Belgium, in the east to newly formed Poland, and, after a plebiscite, some lands in the north to Denmark. Danzig was made a free state, and a Polish corridor, separating German East Prussia from the main territory of the German republic, was created.

Germany's army was reduced to one hundred thousand men; conscription was prohibited. The production of many types of armament was either forbidden or limited. Germany had to accede to occupation of its western lands and agree not to maintain military forces in the Rhineland. In addition, it was ordered to pay, as reparations, a war indemnity the amount of which was left open; yet, payments were to begin immediately. Finally, it was forced to sign a clause acknowledging that it had caused the war.

### Terms for Other Defeated Countries

Separate treaties were concluded with Bulgaria, Turkey, and Austria-Hungary. Bulgaria lost Thrace, had to limit its armaments, and, like Germany, was ordered to pay reparations. Turkey lost practically all its non-Turkish empire in Asia and Africa. Most of this area either was taken over by France and England or, wherever separate states were created, was brought within the orbit of French or British influence. Turkey also agreed to the freedom and demilitarization of the straits of Dardanelles and Bosporus.

Austria-Hungary was split into pieces, a decision that disrupted the economic unity that had been slowly forming in the middle Danube area. The territory was allocated to five nations as follows: to Austria, the German-speaking areas (except some which were handed over to Italy, Hungary, or Czechoslovakia); to Yugoslavia (newly formed out of Serbia), Bosnia and other provinces; to Poland, Krakow and parts of Austrian Galicia; to Czechoslovakia (formerly Bohemia), Moravia and parts of Galicia; and to Hungary, the Magyar areas, except Transylvania, which was ceded to Romania.

### Founding of the League of Nations

In a world torn by hatreds generated during the war and radically changed by its outcome, a just and durable peace settlement could hardly be expected. Bitterness remained everywhere. Aware of this difficulty, President Wilson hoped for necessary peaceful adjustments through a League of Nations, which he had advocated in his Fourteen Points. France and England did not favor such a league, but agreed to it (just as Metternich had once agreed to the Holy Alliance), in the expectation that it might serve as a conservative influence.

The league was endowed with neither executive nor legislative power. It was to serve essentially as an open forum for international discussions. An International Court of Justice was connected with it, as well as various agencies concerned with humanitarian questions, health problems, labor conditions, the slave trade, and educational matters. The league was charged with administering the former German colonies, but all of them were surrendered either outright or as "mandates" to the victors. From the beginning, the organization was handicapped by the fact that three of the five great powers were not members: the United States because of domestic opposition, party politics, and demands for reservations with regard to some obligations under the league's authority; Germany because of its defeat; and Russia because of its communistic form of government.

## Political and Economic Effects

The Peace of Versailles was signed in June 1919. It reflected the profound changes that nationalism, liberalism, and socialism had already initiated.

### The International Scene

There were fifteen states in the Europe of 1815; now there were twenty-seven fully independent nations. These included the Balkan countries and Hungary, Czechoslovakia, Poland, Finland, and the three Baltic states—Lithuania, Latvia, and Estonia. The last great multinational empires of Europe—Austria, Russia, Turkey—were shrunken or destroyed. The war affected Russia the most through the re-creation of Poland. Moreover, Western Europe offered little opportunity to advance self-determination, though promised, was put into practice only where it affected adversely the defeated Central Powers. It was not accorded to the peoples of colonial nations, such as India. Nor was it granted to Austrians who had voted to join Germany, to Germans who were transferred to Italy, to Yugoslavs who were likewise incorporated into Italy, or to Alsatians, the Irish, Macedonians, Slovaks, and other minorities. It was totally disregarded in Eastern Europe.

With the help of France, and notwithstanding a decision by an international group fixing Poland's eastern boundary along a so-called "Curzon Line," the Poles invaded Russia and annexed western lands of Russia—White Russia. They invaded Lithuania and incorporated the capital, Vilna. They also seized most of Germany's industrial Upper Silesia, after the people, in a plebiscite, had decided 14 to 9 against them. Because the principle of self-determination was disregarded, minority problems also persisted in Turkey, Greece, Czechoslovakia, and elsewhere. They poisoned international relations even in cases where population exchanges were undertaken.

### Political Trends Within Nations

The war experience and outcome had the effect of swinging public opinion and political institutions sharply to the left. Few of the European monarchies survived. Nearly all the new states were established as republics; the defeated countries were so reestablished. The republics had either democratic or socialist governments. Socialists were the dominant minority in various central European countries. They also gained many votes and constituted strong opposition parties in many Western and Eastern nations. Communists ruled Russia.

### The World Economic Picture

As in politics, so in economics, World War I upset the status quo. Capitalism had to adapt itself to new conditions. War had imposed many restrictions on capitalism; nowhere in Europe did it regain its former strength. One of the Fourteen Points had called for removal of economic barriers. While many ignored this point, Germany was forced to open its borders to imports. Many European countries placed higher barriers against the free exchange of goods than those existing before the war. Russia, under the Bolsheviks, almost entirely shut itself off economically from the Western world.

Everywhere, trends toward independence from foreign supplies increased. There was a shift in financial strength. London lost its leading financial position to New York, and the United States changed from a debtor to a creditor nation. European currencies depreciated. War reparations upset the international balance of payments and necessitated redoubled export efforts on the part of Germany; this hurt other exporting nations. Russia repudiated the debts contracted by tsarist governments, thus rejecting all repayments. Having granted Russia huge loans, France was the chief victim of repudiation, but Britain, Belgium, and the United States also lost substantial investments. Moreover, a sharp line of demarcation was drawn between the capitalistic and the communistic worlds. Some of the new nations in Eastern Europe were built up by the Western nations as a guard, *a cordon sanitaire,* against Bolshevism because of its anti-capitalistic organization. On the whole, the first steps in building a "world safe for democracy" seemed none too promising.

## ■ THE RUSSIAN REVOLUTION

While the Western nations were busy rearranging the political map of Europe, the attention of the Russians was directed toward constructing an entirely new social order. The significance of the Russian Revolution far surpasses the effect it had on the outcome of World War I. It was the first revolution in Western history to give the industrial workers political power and leadership in a major nation, and to introduce a socialistic system. It constituted a substantial defeat of the bourgeoisie and of the liberal-democratic system for which the middle classes generally stood. It generated forces that became world-wide in scope.

### February Revolution (1917)

Radicalism in Russia had decreased and terrorist activities had ceased ever since the Revolution of 1905 and Stolypin's agrarian reform. Within its narrow limits, the Duma had come to gain influence and had started to build a constitutional system. The chief leaders of the radicals, notably Lenin, lived in exile; the times appeared unfavorable to them. But after 1910, and especially after the outbreak of war, the situation changed.

Inasmuch as social progress had been slow, the strain of war proved disastrous. Moreover, the war governments were managed by reactionaries, the court was filled with intriguers, and the tsar, Nicholas II, was personally incapable as a ruler. He and his wife, Alexandra, fell under the spell of Rasputin, a monk who with apparent success had administered to their ill son. The very fact of the influence of this greedy and dissipated man, even if he possessed rare common sense, indicated the corruption of the whole tsaristic system. Military defeats, manpower losses, widespread famine, and political graft hastened its disintegration.

Revolutionary activities were resumed. In the winter of 1916, Rasputin was murdered. In January 1917, strikes broke out, and mutinies occurred in the army and navy. The moderate parties in the Duma thereupon asked the tsar to yield wider powers to the parliament and to dismiss his government. Instead, the tsar dissolved the Duma. Thereupon, the liberal parties joined the socialists in the demand for his abdication. More strikes broke out. Soldiers deserted. Threatened from all sides, Nicholas II abdicated. The monarchy fell with him, and in February (March, according to the Western calendar) 1917, a Provisional Government was instituted by the Duma.

### Provisional Government (1917)

The new government was administered mainly by representatives of the liberal parties. It established freedom of religion, women's rights, and the legal equality of all citizens. It attacked the disturbing nationality problem by starting the Poles on the road to independence and by helping other national groups make a beginning in self-government. It passed laws to provide for social welfare, and it promised the peasants redistribution of the land along lines to be decided by a popular assembly after the end of the war.

But in all its actions, the government was hindered by continuing World War I and by "soviets" (or councils) of workers and soldiers, which the socialists had set up and in which the communists dominated. The Soviet of Petrograd (as St. Petersburg had been renamed in nationalistic fervor) actually, if not legally, came to constitute a second governmental agency in the country; it interfered with the decisions of the regular government by supervising, countersigning, or rejecting its acts.

In April 1917, Lenin returned from exile, followed soon thereafter by Trotsky. Under their leadership, the strength of the socialist opposition grew rapidly. Lenin's simple, easily understood slogan of "Peace, Land, and Bread" appealed to the war-tired, hungry population—especially to the peasantry. Radicalism spread. Ever-widening circles demanded the establishment of the dictatorship of the proletariat. Soon, the more moderate members of the government resigned. A new offensive against the Germans collapsed. Then, in July, a Bolshevik uprising occurred; it was crushed, but only with difficulty. The liberal government was replaced by one under the Social-Revolutionary leaders Kerensky. He, too, was unwilling to accept the primary demand of the soviets—to end the war.

The situation thereupon deteriorated further. It led to a coup by one of the generals, who hoped to replace Kerensky's government with a military dictatorship. Kerensky was obliged to turn for help to the soviets, to free their leaders who had been arrested after the July revolts, and to call a "pre-Parliament."

### October Revolution (1917) and Introduction of Communism

But it was too late. In October, Lenin, who had fled to Finland in July, returned and called for another armed uprising. The soldiers followed his lead. At the end of October (November in the West), the Provisional Government was driven out. Kerensky fled and most of his colleagues were arrested. Thus began the rule of the communists.

### *Bolshevik Leaders*

The new government was formed by Lenin. Lenin was the son of a superintendent of schools who belonged to the lower nobility. Out of idealism, Lenin had engaged early in revolutionary activities. Single-mindedly, he had devoted his great intellectual and organizing abilities solely to the preparation and implementation of the revolution. He had spent most of his life in exile, had edited various communist newspapers, had published books and pamphlets, and had welded the nucleus of the Russian Bolshevik party into a centralized, efficient, and devoted group. His most important collaborator after the overturn of the tsarist government was Leon Trotsky, of a fairly well-to-do Jewish family. Trotsky was a man as fervent in his idealism and as willing to sacrifice as Lenin himself. But he was more erratic and more individualistic. Trotsky had been one of the leaders of the 1905 revolution. He had suffered years in prison and banishment. Not until May 1917 had he been able to return to Russia from exile in America. He became Lenin's commissar for foreign affairs.

Figure 20–3 Revolution and Civil War in Russia, 1914–1920

Notable among other members of the new Bolshevik government was Stalin, a revolutionary from Georgia, whose parents were a shoemaker and a washerwoman. He studied at an Orthodox seminary, from which he ran away to devote himself to the Bolshevik cause. Less intellectual than either Lenin or Trotsky, he proved himself an efficient, ruthless, and practical revolutionary. By 1912, he had become editor of *Pravda,* the Bolshevik newspaper in St. Petersburg. Stalin was subsequently exiled to Siberia and did not return until 1917. Lenin made him commissar for nationality questions.

### *Initial Bolshevik Reconstruction of Russia*

Lenin's government did not hesitate to carry out the Bolshevik program. Without regard for international consequences, Lenin fulfilled his promise of peace. Russia's allies refused to recognize the necessity for Russia to leave its allies and end the war; they rejected the Bolshevik proposal of a peace without annexation and reparations, and sought to force Russia to continue the war. However, Lenin began negotiations with the Germans. Within a month, he concluded an armistice; in March 1918, the Peace of Brest-Litovsk was negotiated.

With equal determination, Lenin initiated the work of socialist reconstruction. Private property and church property were confiscated. Banks and bank accounts were nationalized. Factories were handed over to the workers (and later nationalized). The lands of the nobility and the rich were seized by the peasants.

All trading activities, except those of small businesses owned and operated by individuals, were taken over by the state. The employment of one person by another was forbidden. A new police force of ardent Bolsheviks was organized. Control over the army was assumed by party commissars. Every citizen was instructed to go to work for the new government. The peasants were ordered to deliver fixed quotas of their crops. As to Russia's international role, Lenin paid little attention to traditional values. He based his policies on the expectation of world revolution, which he envisioned as the inevitable result of the war. In the meantime, he concentrated on one task only: the maintenance of communist rule in Russia.

## Perspective

The war which began in August 1914 had its origin in an atmosphere of nationalism and economic rivalry. The leaders in the various countries fail to seek diplomatic means for settling the differences peacefully. All prepared for war.

Germany scored initial victories, but they were not decisive. Hopes for a short war faded: long, drawn-out trench warfare followed. Gradually, the geographic location of the Central Powers made itself disastrously felt. Lack of food and resources, added to heavy losses in manpower, undermined their strength. In 1917, the United States, with all its vast reserves, openly entered the conflict on the side of the Allies. A year later, Germany was forced to sue for peace. Thus, the end came in November 1918.

The Treaty of Versailles deprived Germany of territories in all border regions, regardless of the promised principles of self-determination for all peoples. The treaty also imposed degrading stipulations and demanded unlimited reparation payments. The Austrian-Hungarian Empire was divided up. A League of Nations, advocated by the United States, was founded but not endowed with power to act decisively on the international scene. It failed to become an efficient agent for peace.

In the meantime, a two-stage revolution occurred in Russia. It put an end to tsardom and autocracy, and ushered in, first a liberal-democratic, then a socialist (communist), regime.

## Selected Readings

Jenkins, Phillip. *A History of the United States* (New York: Palgrave Macmillan, 2003).

Carr, Edward H. *1917: Before and After* (London: Macmillan, 1969).

Fromkin, David. *Europe's Last Summer: Who Started the Great War in 1914?* (New York: Knopf, 2004).

Martel, Gordon. *The Origins of the World War* (London: Longman, 1996).

Remarque, Erich Maria. *All Quiet on the Western Front* (Boston: Little, Brown, 1930).

Strachan, Hew, ed., *The Oxford Illustrated History of the First World War* (Oxford: Oxford University Press, 1998).

Ropp, Theodore. *War in the Modern World* (1966).

Trotsky, Leon. *History of the Russian Revolution* (New York: Doubleday, Doran & Co., 1937).

Ulam, Adam B. *The Bolshevik: the Intellectual and Political History of the Triumph of Communism in Russia* (New York: Macmillan, 1965).

## Test Yourself

1. Before the start of World War I, the German war plan was also known as_____.
   A. The Schlieffen Plan
   B. The Bismarck Plan
   C. The Prussian Plan
   D. The Berlin Plan

2. When the war started in 1914, the Ottoman Empire took the position of_____.
   A. Supporting the Germans
   B. Neutrality
   C. Supporting the English
   D. None of the Above

3. The two first years of World War I witnessed startling victories by_____.
   A. France
   B. England
   C. Italy
   D. Germany

4. American intervention in World War I took place in _____.
   A. April 1914
   B. April 1916
   C. April 1917
   D. April 1918

5. World War I officially ended with the signing in 1919 of the treaty of_____.
   A. Paris
   B. Portsmouth
   C. Versailles
   D. Berlin

6. One of the key results of World War I was the establishment of_____.
   A. a Workers League
   B. a Socialist League
   C. a European League
   D. a League of Nations

7. The Russian Revolution of October 1917 was led by_____.
   A. Trotsky
   B. Lenin
   C. Kerensky
   D. Stalin

8. When Russia decided to withdraw from World War I, it was the result of Lenin's negotiations with the Germans that culminated in the signing of the Peace of _____.
   A. Brest-Litovsk
   B. Moscow
   C. Berlin
   D. St. Petersburg

## Answers and Explanations

1. **A.** The German was plan was known as the Schlieffen Plan which was designed by General Alfred Schlieffen in 1913.

2. **B.** The Ottoman Empire was neutral at the start of the war on August 1, 1914; however, the Ottomans broke that neutrality by joining the German alliance in November.

3. **D.** The first two years of the war witnessed startling victories by the Germans; as a result, almost the entire war was fought on the soils of Belgium, France and Russia.

4. **C.** The American Congress authorized President Wilson to declare war on Germany in April 1917 in order to assist American allies in Britain and France.

5. **C.** The warring parties gathered in Paris in early 1919 to negotiate final settlements to bring the war to an end; one of those settlements was the Treaty of Versailles.

6. **D.** In a world torn by hatreds generated during the war and radically changed by its outcome, a just and durable peace settlement could hardly be expected. Bitterness remained everywhere. Aware of this difficulty, President Wilson hoped for necessary peaceful adjustments through a League of Nations, which he had advocated in his Fourteen Points. France and England did not favor such a league, but agreed to it (just as Metternich had once agreed to the Holy Alliance), in the expectation that it might serve as a conservative influence.

7. **B.** In October, Lenin, who had fled to Finland in July, returned and called for another armed uprising. The soldiers followed his lead. At the end of October (November in the West), the Provisional Government was driven out. Kerensky fled and most of his colleagues were arrested. Thus began the rule of the communists.

8. **A.** Lenin began negotiations with the Germans. Within a month, he concluded an armistice; in March, 1918, the Peace of Brest-Litovsk was negotiated.

**CHAPTER 21**

# The Twilight of Liberalism (1921-1929)

**1920** Polish-Russian war
**1921** Disarmament conference held in Washington
NEP established in Soviet-Russia
**1922** German–Russian treaty of Rapallo
Mussolini establishes Fascist regime in Italy
Sinclair Lewis, *Babbitt*
James Joyce, *Ulysses*
**1923** French invade the Ruhr
USSR established
Stabilization of German currency
**1924** Dawes plan for German reparations adopted
Death of Lenin
**1925** Locarno Treaty
**1926** Nationalization of oil industry in Mexico
**1928** Briand-Kellogg Peace Pact
First Five-Year Plan initiated in USSR
**1929** Stalin's dictatorship established; Trotsky banished
Italy-Papacy concordat: Vatican City becomes sovereign Papal State
Crash of New York Stock Exchange

*With war and devastation, any widespread feelings of security and complacency faded, but this very fading made possible the blossoming of vigorous new intellectual activity in Western culture. During the 1920s, scientific and technological endeavors broadened in scope and significance. Literature, painting, and architecture flourished, bringing to maturity the revolutionary concepts of art that had been in their pioneer stages before the war. Political experiments in democracy, socialism, and communism generated much idealism. The New World, having come of age, now contributed to the cultural accomplishments of the West in the same manner as had the European nations.*

## ■ CULTURAL TRENDS

Western countries became more and more focused upon technology and the social sciences. Scientific advances continued, and scientific methods of research and experimentation were applied to the new disciplines of psychology and sociology. Science affected the work of philosophers, historians, and economists. It stimulated education. A new approach to the study of the process of learning was sought, and experiments in new types of schools were undertaken. It influenced literature, which became less concerned with the character, ideas, and behavior of the exceptional individual and more concerned with the average person and the collective behavior of the masses. Its effects can be traced in painting, architecture, and music, all of which gave expression to modern psychological and sociological trends. Even religious thought came to be increasingly reconciled to modern science.

### Science and Technology

The war had accelerated scientific work and the search for new technologies. The work of 20th-century scientists increased people's realization of the complexities of the cosmos. In most scientific fields, further specialization became necessary.

### *Physical Sciences*

The most spectacular advances were made in the physical sciences, particularly in research involving the world of the atom. Physicists such as Ernest Rutherford, Niels Bohr, and Erwin Schroddinger achieved fundamental progress in understanding the structure and the processes operating within the atom. Werner Heisenberg proposed the uncertainty principle, which postulated final limits on human possibilities of observation, thus restricting, on the atomic level, the area in which scientific verification is possible. This led to further advances in quantum mechanics. Astronomers developed the idea of a constantly expanding universe to explain many puzzling phenomena in this field. Albert Einstein elaborated his theory of relativity and began work on a formula that would be as all-inclusive in explaining the relationship of natural forces as Newton's gravitational laws had once seemed to be.

### *Technology*

Inventions that had been created in preceding decades found practical applications and altered the average person's lifestyle. The automobile, now made more affordable through the work of Henry Ford in the United States, became increasingly important for commercial uses and in private family life. It also affected national policies by creating a need for highway construction and a demand for oil, which greatly influenced international policies in the second half of the 20th century. The airplane, whose development had been rapidly furthered during the war, came into commercial use. Priority was given to speed, not only in transportation, but in almost all areas of modern life. In 1927, Charles Lindbergh accomplished the first nonstop transatlantic flight from New York to Paris. Radio was developed, bringing music and other programs to the average household of which it became a part, just like the telephone. Television had its first tryouts, and the moving-picture industry changed with the introduction of sound. Manufacturing processes were modernized. In the late 19th century, his stopwatch in hand, the American, F. W. Taylor, had identified every movement that a worker was required to make at a given job, and the worker was thus strictly bound to a schedule. After the First World War, the conveyor belt and the moving assembly line, children of Taylorism, dominated the actions of the factory worker, who was reduced to functioning like a component in a machine. Although wages were generally higher because of wartime labor shortages, resentment grew, work-related ailments increased, and bitter opposition in the form of trade unionism resulted.

*Figure 21-1 Henry Ford, 1863-1947*

*Figure 21-2 Charles Lindbergh made the first nonstop solo flight in 1927*

## Chemistry

New information about the molecular structure of matter enabled chemists to broaden their efforts to produce synthetic materials. This meant that rare or expensive natural products, such as rubber and silk, could be increasingly replaced by artificial materials. The development of synthetics also went beyond the realm of science by affecting economic, social, and political life. New products changed the habits and work of the average person and simultaneously redirected the policies of whole nations. They reduced the dependence of great powers upon their colonies for raw materials and led to the creation of new industries. This, in turn, eased some international tensions, generated others, encouraged nationalism, affected independence movements among colonial peoples, and eventually contributed to recurring shifts in the balance of power.

### Biology and Medicine

Aside from physics and chemistry, notable advances were also made in most other areas of science. Biologists made fundamental advances in the study of cell physiology and heredity, including the phenomenon of mutations. New therapies for a wide variety of diseases were developed. Vitamins were identified by Frederick Hopkins, and penicillin was discovered by Alexander Fleming in 1928. Hormones and antibiotics were added to the physician's arsenal.

Progress in public health brought new methods for combating epidemics caused by mosquitoes, lice, rats, and other carriers of disease. Improved sanitary practices also contributed to better health and a longer life for millions of people. This resulted in growing populations, which led to crowded urban locations and rapidly growing suburban areas. Nevertheless, material standards of living were improving because science—particularly advances in chemistry, plant pathology, veterinary medicine, and agronomy—made possible a vast increase in agricultural production, and the food supply was more ample than ever before.

### Psychology and Sociology

Finally, the two new fields of scientific psychology and sociology made rapid progress. Psychologists applied the theories expounded by Freud and his disciples. They evolved new ideas in normal and abnormal psychology. Sociologists applied the research techniques of psychologists and arrived at interesting, though necessarily tentative, conclusions regarding collective behavior—conclusions that had considerable influence in the fields of philosophy, political science, and history.

### Philosophy and Economic Theory

In a world dominated by scientific endeavors, philosophy continued to occupy itself largely with rational, materialistic, and social questions, rather than with transcendental or metaphysical problems. Such outstanding thinkers as Bertrand Russell, Alfred North Whitehead, John Dewey, and Ludwig Wittgenstein were interested in science and its methods, as well as in the effects of science on human society. Pragmatic tendencies were strong, and the theories of symbolic logic and logical positivism were developed. Logical positivism followed the example of 19th-century positivists like Auguste Comte in excluding metaphysical and transcendental concerns from the domain of philosophy. They went even further by devoting themselves to the technical analysis of language and to the belief that the meaning of any statement lies in its method of verification. The unification of all the sciences through a common logical language was the ultimate goal. The question and meaning of "progress" was reexamined. In line with evolutionary theories, the facts of history and experience, rather than abstract concepts, were adopted as the basis for most interpretations of the evolution of human society.

Some philosophers, such as Oswald Spengler in his *Decline of the West* (1918-1922), came to view human history as a biological process subject to natural laws. They insisted that every culture passes through a cycle of youth, maturity, and old age with its resulting deterioration. In this philosophy, we can see the disillusionment that resulted from the First World War and the tremendous blow inflicted by the conflict upon the idealism and boundless confidence with which the generation entered the 20th century.

Scientific and historical approaches also marked the work of economists. In the 19th century, Karl Marx had turned to history in order to understand economic developments. Many 20th-century economists, among them John Maynard Keynes and Joseph Schumpeter, adopted the same method. After studying the evolutionary social process in history, they reviewed and criticized the propositions of the classical economic theorists. In general, they came to reject all idealistic and utopian views, and like many philosophers, they accepted "utility" as their standard. Some economists concluded that utility governed "value" and thereby, the major phases of the economic process within the changing historical setting. They developed extensive statistical methods and, with the help of statistics, investigated business cycles, price movements, and all the other characteristics of capitalism.

A special place of importance belongs to the German Max Weber (1864-1920), an influential sociologist who helped create the constitution of the postwar Weimar Republic. His studies concerning the relationship between society and the individual were embodied in his most famous work, *The Protestant Ethic and the Spirit of Capitalism* (1904). This work explored the effects of the Protestant Reformation on the growth of capitalism and, by extension, modern Western society, particularly, the new perception of wealth and its accumulation. Weber's ideas helped to counter the influence exercised at the time by certain Marxist thinkers.

## Education

Growing attention was paid to mass education in order to prepare Western schoolchildren and adults for the increasingly complex tasks facing them in the modern world, including how to handle machinery and how to live alongside it, how to exercise newly won civil rights, how to use a constantly expanding leisure time. In the decade after World War I, therefore, while literacy was becoming nearly universal and spreading to the most remote regions of the United States and Soviet-Russia, educational goals experienced a radical transformation. Study of the classics—a foundation of modern civilization—was curtailed in order to allow more time for study of the natural sciences. Instruction emphasized experience and practice rather than memorization, which had long been regarded as an indispensable tool of knowledge. Discipline was relaxed, and students were given greater freedom to achieve "self-expression."

With mass education, a leveling process began whereby uniformity in thinking habits was promoted. Numerous experimental schools were founded. Social adjustment to the mechanized modern world was considered a major task for "democratic" education. To be sure, opposition arose against the new trends in education. Critics of the idea of "progressive education" believed that lack of rigid intellectual training and discipline would lead to a resurgence of barbarism. Even in communist Soviet Russia, a foremost advocate of progressive education, a reaction occurred during the 1930s.

## Literature and the Fine Arts

The 1920s stand out as a time particularly rich in writers and artists of ability and significant accomplishment. It was during this period that the trends developed under the leadership of the Expressionists during the last decade and a half before World War I came into full flowering. With the upheavals of war, revolution, and postwar adjustment, many of the former restraints broke down. Writers and artists of genius could follow their inclinations more freely and proceed with important experimental work. Today, there is little doubt about the broad historical and social significance of their works.

### Literature

The novel continued to offer an artistic frame that seemed most appropriate to the temper of the time. It lent itself to realistic description and to criticism of the social scene. Among the leading writers of fiction were the Frenchmen Romain Rolland, Andre Gide, and Andre Malraux; the Englishmen Thomas Hardy, also famous for his poetry, John Galsworthy, and D. H. Lawrence; and the Russians Maxim Gorky, Alexei Tolstoy, and Vladimir Mayakovsky, all of whom were actually products of the pre-revolutionary days. *Remembrance of Things Past* (1913-1927) by Marcel Proust, and *Ulysses* (1922), by the Irishman James Joyce, became foremost examples of the type of psychological study and penetrating observation of human instincts and behavior that have since become known as "stream-of-consciousness" writing. Unusually vigorous and important literary talents emerged in the United States with Sinclair, Lewis, F. Scott Fitzgerald, Theodore Dreiser, John Dos Passos, Upton Sinclair, and Ernest Hemingway; and in Germany with Heinrich and Thomas Mann, Franz Werfel, and Hermann Hesse.

Compared to prose, creative work in drama and poetry was of lesser importance. The American Eugene O'Neill, who rejected 19th-century farce for symbolic expressionism, and the Englishman

George Bernard Shaw, who, despite advancing age, still remained one of the most productive authors and critics, excelled in drama. In lyric poetry, the most prominent writers were the Irishman William Butler Yeats, the American T. S. Eliot, the Frenchman Paul Valery, and the Germans Stefan George and Rainer Maria Rilke. Of course, the largest audiences were not reached by these great writers, but by newspapers, journals, magazines, and sensational novels.

Just as literacy was rapidly advancing everywhere in the West, means of communication were being invented that dispensed with the written word. Radio, cinema, photographs, cartoons, and illustrated advertisements (i.e., audiovisual media) were used to disseminate information, entertainment, and propaganda on an unprecedented scale. Though they often contributed to the corruption of people's tastes, they also contributed to their education and elevation. The film, in particular, with a number of outstanding productions and excellent actors, such as Charles Chaplin and Greta Garbo, gained a major place in the cultural scene.

### *Painting and Sculpture*

In the fine arts, Expressionism reached its climax and brought forth a movement known as Surrealism. Many outstanding painters and sculptors concentrated on human psychology rather than on visual imagery. They sought to express an inner reality: a view of 20th-century men and women as being torn by the multiplicity of modern problems that they had to face without the confidence that a feeling of harmony with either nature or a world spirit had given individuals in other times. Artists were concerned with the social patterns of their age, and they sought to explain or criticize them.

Outstanding contributors were the painters Pablo Picasso, who began a new phase of creativity in his life, and Diego Rivera, who was influenced by Communist ideology, as well as the Swiss Paul Klee; and the sculptors Sir Jacob Epstein, Ivan Mestrovic, Aristide Maillol, and Henry Moore. Since these painters and sculptors often preferred an abstract type of expression, it was difficult for the average person to understand their works. Most people were drawn to other, more conservative artists who favored a simpler, more direct language. Especially in countries ruled by Communist and Fascist regimes, intellectualized, abstract trends were ridiculed and rejected, whereas artistic creations rooted in national folklore and serving, if possible, the ideologies of the regimes were promoted.

### *Architecture*

Vigorous and artistically meaningful developments also occurred in the field of architecture. Functionalism, which had begun to dominate building styles during the period before World War I, now spread rapidly. It emphasized simplicity, the utmost restraint in ornamentation, and clear, geometric lines. It sought to bring aesthetic values into harmony with the practical demands of life in an industrial age. City planning and apartment, factory, and office building projects engaged the attention of architects. Social needs guided their creative endeavors. The Bauhaus in Dessau, Germany, a school of painters and architects, became a center for modern concepts in building. Similarly, in the Netherlands, France, and the United States, the functional style with its characteristic aesthetic values made rapid progress. Owing to masters such as Walter Gropius, Ludwig Mies van der Rohe, Frank Lloyd Wright, and Le Corbusier, town landscapes in Europe and America began to change. Uncluttered lines and a variety of color began to give many of them an impression of beauty that most 19th-century towns, in their grayness, imitative styles, over-ornamentation, and slums, had sadly lacked.

### *Music*

In music, traditional harmonic concepts survived in most of the popular compositions, and folklore continued to inspire composers. Composers such as Arnold Schonberg, Igor Stravinsky, Paul Hindemith, and the older Finnish composer, Jean Sibelius, continued their experimental works. Some of them were involved with the creation of atonal music. Like expressionist painting, atonal music failed to have an immediate appeal for the uninitiated; nevertheless, it attracted a growing audience of intellectuals. The Soviet Union produced Sergei Prokofiev and Dmitri Shostakovich. America's chief contribution consisted of popular and often "intellectualized" jazz. Jazz originated with black musicians, inspired broad audiences, and influenced many leading composers. Also in the United States a special type of musical theater, the so-called "musical," originated, but few operas of importance were written. Classical and modern concert music were enjoyed by ever-widening audiences. Many excellent orchestras were founded, especially in America. Improved radio reception and better phonographs contributed to an unprecedented awareness of the great musical heritage of the West.

Considerable attention was paid to the Czech composers, Smetana and Dvorak, who had worked in the 19th century, and to the younger Janacek. However, unlike the German masters whom they admired and whose appeal was universal, they emphasized, in a sign of the pervasiveness of nationalistic feelings, special national values. Janacek expressly admonished his students "to compose in the national style."

### Religion

It is significant that the rapid progress of science, technology, and secular education did not intensify the conflict between science and religion, which dated back to the preceding century. Scientists began to appreciate the limitations and relativity of their knowledge, while most churches allowed a larger place for science in the minds of rational people. Atheism no longer claimed converts as in preceding decades, except in Russia, where Marxist aims called for a condemnation of all religion as a form of superstition. The challenge of science caused the churches to reassess their teachings and ultimately to strengthen their spiritual forces. Even in Russia, the church gained rather than lost by this challenge and by the withdrawal of many who had adhered to religion only out of convention.

Relations between church and state became more peaceful. With the separation of church and state, governments exercised less control over religious institutions. A spiritual revival, especially among Protestants, led to a Neo-Orthodoxy, which had its roots in ideas expounded by the 19th-century Danish theologian, Soren Kierkegaard. Neo-Orthodoxy asked for a reaffirmation of the Christian doctrine and a resolute acceptance of the fundamental tenets of Christianity. These demanded a "painful abandonment" to faith by the individual. The Catholic, Jacques Maritain, and the Protestant, Karl Barth, were the two outstanding theologians who adhered to this position. Both insisted, with equal fervor, on the obligation of the faithful to perform their duty in promoting human concerns in daily life and politics.

## ■ INTERNATIONAL TRENDS

Like most wars, World War I created more problems than it resolved. The international arrangements made at Versailles were quickly shattered. The League of Nations proved ineffective. The gulf widened between the views of capitalist countries and those of Russia, as well as between the interests of colonial powers and those of their dependencies. Few politicians understood the fact that mechanized civilization, with its numerous pressures, required new attitudes.

### Major International Problems

The two problems most disturbing to international relationships after World War I were Communism and reparations. At first, the Western powers sought to solve these problems by force. They attempted to suppress Communism with armed might and to collect reparations using threats. When this method failed, they slowly settled down to the task of making compromises. Unfortunately for the peace of the West, they delayed too long.

## Communism

At the end of the war, communism seemed to be only weakly established in Russia. Hoping, therefore, to be able to restore a capitalistic, liberal-democratic regime, four powers—America, Britain, France, and Japan—decided to crush the Bolsheviks. They invaded Russia in 1918 in order to force the country back into the war against Germany. When the World War ended, they continued to support the old tsarist forces in order to oust the Bolshevik government. This "intervention" led to catastrophe. After two bitter years, foreign troops were forced to quit Russian soil. Simultaneously, Russian monarchists and anti-Communists, led by Anton Denikin, Pyotr Wrangel, Aleksandr Kolchak, and other tsarist officers, either surrendered or fled the country. By 1922, the Bolsheviks were in full control of most of Russia. Regions that had attempted to establish independent regimes, such as Siberia, parts of the Caucasus, and parts of the Ukraine, were reunited with Russia proper and became components of the Soviet Union.

Thus, within four years, Communist power had firmly established itself. From then on, it became an ever-greater force in the world. Even when absent from international conferences, the Soviet Union had to be considered in all political settlements. It secured recognition from most European nations and gradually expanded its influence abroad through the *Comintern, the Third* (Communistic) *International,* which Lenin had sponsored in 1919.

## Reparations

Some of the French leaders at Versailles had insisted upon the imposition of extremely burdensome reparations. They hoped that reparation payments would not only help in the reconstruction of war-damaged France, but would also make possible the permanent subjugation of Germany. These expectations were not realized. It quickly became clear that reparations were a two-edged weapon. By forcing Germany to increase its industrial capacity and to bend its efforts toward exports in order to earn the means for making reparations payments, the insistence on reparations caused a major disturbance for the Western economy. German currency became inflated to a degree never before experienced; at one point, the German paper mark was quoted in Berlin at two and a half trillion to the American dollar (the prewar exchange rate had been 4.2 marks to the dollar). The victors thus made it possible for the German government to pay its internal debt in inflated currency and gain strength, while other countries experienced unemployment and a limited inflation. Moreover, unemployment and inflation led to a new radicalism everywhere. Mortgage holders, bondholders, and other creditors suffered, retired people were impoverished, and millions of people lost interest in the preservation of the capitalistic system. Finally, a wedge was driven between the Allies themselves, especially between France and England, which desired economic stability, and between the United States and its European partners, who refused to pay war debts to the United States so long as they could not collect from Germany. In 1927, an economic conference was called to find a solution to the problem, but it failed to achieve its purpose. Thus, reparations served neither the Allied interests nor the cause of world peace and reconstruction.

## International Solutions

As time went on, the task of finding a basis, different from the Versailles Treaty, for rebuilding the Western community of nations became more urgent; but a solution was delayed as long as the aims of the Western states remained at variance. France desired domination on the European continent and therefore insisted on strict fulfillment of the stipulations of Versailles. Simultaneously, by entering into bilateral arrangements with Poland, Czechoslovakia, and Yugoslavia, it sought to build up in eastern-central Europe an alliance system that would serve the double purpose of erecting a *cordon sanitaire* against Communist Russia and a counterweight against German might. England, however, wanted the reestablishment of a balance of power. Not only should France be prevented from becoming a menace to England, but Communism should also be held in check. The United States, which refused to become a party to the Versailles Treaty, followed a policy of isolationism wherever possible. Germany sought a revision of the treaty and the reestablishment of its prewar position. Russia, which ranked fifth among the great powers and, like the United States, was not a signatory to the Versailles Treaty, detached itself completely from the West. Russia saw as its aims the consolidation of a socialist society at home and the spread of Communism abroad.

### *Rapallo (1922)*
The divergent aims of the great powers foreshadowed a long period of negotiation. Since the League of Nations failed to fulfill its intended role, conference after conference had to be called. Various meetings took place in 1920. In 1921, a naval conference was held in Washington for the purpose of promoting disarmament. The only thing achieved, however, was a redistribution of naval strength. The arrangement was significant, inasmuch as England, formerly the greatest power on the seas, had to accept a place of equality with the United States; Japan ranked third, while Italy and France shared fourth and fifth places.

A year later, a more important conference was held in Genoa, to which both Germany and the Soviet-Russia were invited. It led to a German-Russian treaty. This treaty, negotiated in nearby Rapallo, changed the existing distribution of power as much as the Franco-Russian alliance had in 1890. Germany and Soviet Russia, both isolated and weak since the war, agreed upon formal political recognition and economic cooperation and, thereby, became powerful actors on the international stage. France reacted bitterly. In the following year, 1923, France used Germany's inability to pay reparations as an excuse for occupying the great German industrial region of the Ruhr River valley. Both the United States and England refused to associate themselves with such a punitive measure and even withdrew their occupation troops. As a result, the French invasion of the Ruhr gained little and further complicated the international situation.

### *Locarno (1925)*
Under the circumstances, the need for a realistic attack upon Western economic and political problems became more urgent. Steps were finally taken at the urging of the United States. In 1924, the realization of the close relationship between political and economic problems prompted the creation of a program to address the reparations (the Dawes plan). It fixed German reparations at a sum commensurate with Germany's ability to pay; American loans were put at Germany's disposal so that Germany might provide for its new obligations.

Once adopted, the Dawes plan opened the way for a settlement of political disputes. This was achieved by a conference held in Locarno in 1925. Owing to the efforts of the French and German foreign ministers, Aristide Briand and Gustav Stresemann, respectively, an agreement concerning the disputed Franco-German border was reached. The agreement guaranteed that Germany's western boundaries as established by the Versailles Treaty would be maintained. In the following year, Germany joined the League of Nations. Simultaneously, military supervision of Germany was ended.

### **Briand-Kellogg Pact (1928)**
Further steps toward the preservation of peace were taken in the next year. Inequalities in military strength continued to threaten world peace, and regional meetings and disarmament conferences among the victors had accomplished little. Therefore the American secretary of state, Frank Kellogg, proposed a pact providing for the compulsory arbitration of future political differences. The pact was signed by the United States and the leading European powers in 1928.

### **Solutions to Colonial Problems**
World War I marked the end of an era of Western civilization, not only in Europe, but also in the European colonies. Under pressure of world opinion humanitarian views, and socialist propaganda,

European political domination began to recede. Meanwhile, national movements led by native, upper classes gained in strength. Germany and Russia dropped out of the colonial picture altogether. Germany, by virtue of the Versailles Treaty, had lost its colonies everywhere. Russia, in line with communist ideology, voluntarily renounced treaty advantages secured by tsarist governments in China, Afghanistan, Persia, and Turkey.

Other nations also had to modify their relations with colonial areas. The United States eased its controls in Central America and reformed the government of the Philippines. France, Japan, and Britain, although attempting to preserve their empires and even to enlarge them, also had to make concessions. France was obliged to give up some control in the Near East and to liberalize its policies in North Africa. Japanese troops were forced to leave Siberia, where they had made territorial acquisitions during the anti-Bolshevik intervention of 1918-1920.

Britain, the largest colonial power, had to make the broadest concessions. In 1923, it gave its dominions the right to make independent treaties with foreign powers. Between 1926 and 1931, it created the British Commonwealth, which provided for the equal status of dominions and the parent country within the empire. It also allowed for independent management of internal and external affairs. In 1931, Britain confirmed the new status of the colonies by means of the Statute of Westminster. Britain resigned its protectorate over Egypt in 1922 and broadened that country's independence in 1936. In order to safeguard British investments and the supply of oil, however, it insisted on continued control of the Arab states, Palestine, Transjordan, and Iraq which were once controlled by the dissolved Ottoman Empire. It also refused to withdraw from India. As a result, Britain became involved in a desperate struggle against Indian nationalists led by Mahatma Gandhi, who advocated passive resistance to all English authority and defiance of Western civilization. Although Gandhi's economic precepts, which were based upon a reliance on traditional Indian production methods, could not survive in an industrialized world, his moral stand gained wide recognition and laid the foundation for India's future independence. This objective was achieved in 1947, after his death.

All Western countries lost their privileged status and their extraterritorial rights in China. Further colonialism there was forestalled by the continued reform work of Sun Yat-sen and his party, the Kuomintang. In most colonies where European political power had to withdraw, European techniques were assumed by native forces.

## ■ NATIONAL TRENDS

Internal political developments in the Western nations after World War I were marked by the progressive introduction of democratic institutions and social legislation. Women came to take an increasingly important part in national affairs, but the process of democratization failed to alleviate social tensions. As occurred after the French Revolution, conflicts increased between rich and poor, between those who willingly accepted changing conditions and others who looked back longingly at former "better times." In many countries, bad feelings existed between those who had served on the front lines during the war and those who had stayed at home. Some of the latter were accused of being war profiteers. The demands of the Versailles Treaty and the triumph of Communism now added fuel to internal conflicts in the West.

### Britain

Reform of its empire, loss of its place as the leading financial power, and the redoubled competition of the United States and a recovering Germany, forced Britain to make numerous internal adjustments. The Liberal party declined. For three years after 1919, Britain's wartime leader, Lloyd George, continued to preside over a coalition cabinet, but an economic recession following the end of hostilities and a return to peacetime production restored the Conservatives to power. Thereafter, the Liberal party was eclipsed by the Labor party, and in 1924, the first Labor cabinet in British history was formed. It lasted only a few months, during which time Britain formally recognized the Soviet Union, and then had to yield again to the Conservatives.

Under Liberal leadership, England benefited from the general revival that began after the reparations problem had been responsibly resolved through the Dawes plan, and the political climate improved through the Locamo agreements. Its trade balance and financial position improved. The government enacted social legislation to alleviate the plight of the unemployed. England modernized its industries. It achieved further political democratization in 1928 by granting equal suffrage to women. However, grave problems remained, including persistent unemployment, distress in some industries, and numerous acrimonious strikes, especially of coal miners, which climaxed with a general strike. The Irish were dissatisfied with England's wartime promises. They received only dominion status in 1922 and particularly resented the separation of Ulster from the Irish Free State. They fought desperately for complete independence, but all of these issues were overshadowed when, in 1929, a worldwide economic crisis interrupted what progress had been achieved. Combined with the loosening of ties with the dominions through the Statute of Westminster, it opened a new phase in England's history.

## France

Another victor of 1918, France, faced problems of a very different kind. As the literary critic, Andre Siegfried, had observed before 1914, its people still led a more contented life than its progressive and dynamic neighbors. Favored by tradition, character, and resources, life in France had not changed as it had in the highly industrialized countries. Its economy was more balanced and self-sufficient. Its political position satisfied the nationalists after the victory of 1918. In addition, its prosperity was aided by German reparations and American debt cancellations.

Under the surface, however, French conditions were precarious. The prewar trend of stagnating population growth figures remained. Politically, the individualism of the French reasserted itself, split the parties into numerous groups, and impeded nationwide cooperation. Constant changes in government prevented the passing of the timely legislation needed to adapt the economic structure to modern requirements. Inflation haunted the country and increased instability. Initiative was lacking, and corruption and scandals were frequent. In contrast to the situation in other great nations, the right of women to vote was withheld, living standards of the poor were little improved, and class differences remained intact. Thus, despite the military victory, prospects for the nation to retain its international position were substantially diminished.

## Germany

Having been defeated in war, shaken by the revolution that had brought the imperial government to an end, and deprived of valuable industrial regions in its east and west, Germany faced the future under grave handicaps. At Weimar, in central Germany, a democratic constitution for the new German republic, which later became known as the Weimar Republic, was drawn up in 1919 by bourgeois and socialist liberals. It provided for parliamentary government, ministerial responsibility to the parliament, equal suffrage of all citizens (including women), and guarantees of other civil rights. A socialist, Friedrich Ebert, became its first president, but the new political organization received little support or respect. Bitter partisan recriminations divided the country. The Bolshevists under the leadership of the so-called Spartacists hoped to turn it into a Communist state, while reactionaries sought to reestablish the old monarchical forms. As in France, individualism led to a large number of splinter parties, which hindered the formation of effective governments and necessitated constantly changing coalitions. Although the civil service remained intact, and government officials worked faithfully and honestly, civil war marked the political scene.

A terrible and prolonged inflation resulted from the reparations demanded at Versailles, hurting even the victors themselves. It primarily ruined the middle class in Germany, which would have been the force to build a sound democratic society. As a result, the middle class listened to demagogic promises of the extreme right or the extreme left. Resentment was kept alive by the Peace of Versailles and its frontier stipulations, reparations, and war-guilt clauses. Political disorders were common. On one hand, disappointed war youths, assisted by officers of the old army clique, tried to overthrow the democratic government. In 1920, they staged the Kapp Putsch, an uprising that ultimately failed, but several ministers and party leaders were assassinated. In Bavaria in 1923, a small, ultranationalist group, led by an Austrian, Adolf Hitler, undertook the Bierhall Putsch, which, like the Kapp Putsch, was promptly put down.

On the other hand, leftist parties sought the destruction of the government by organizing strikes and several armed rebellions. With the help of the army, these were put down. The Treaty of Rapallo with Russia did not ensure internal stability, though it did restore Germany to its former place as a great power. It was then that inflation reached its worst form. The reparations payments could not be made, and, thereupon, the French and Belgians marched into the Ruhr district.

Hopes for constructive progress were reawakened only after the currency was stabilized in 1923. Reparations were reduced by the Dawes plan, a successful foreign policy was initiated by Stresemann, and foreign occupation troops were withdrawn. The Locarno Treaty brought a measure of reconciliation with the West. Even then, however, difficulties remained, and nationalist extremists as well as Bolshevists exploited them by pointing to the weakness of the national economy and to the restrictions imposed at Versailles. Thus was widespread disrespect kept alive for a government that was trying to be liberal and to adapt itself to democratic forms. As long as economic conditions improved, these extremists had little chance; but when depression came in 1929, the nihilistic forces triumphed.

## Russia

While England, France, Germany, and other Western countries adhered to moderately liberal democratic (and occasionally mildly socialistic) institutions, Russia set about building a Communist society.

### Period of War Communism (1919-1921)

The Soviet constitution of 1918 established a dictatorship of the proletariat, and all parties except the Communist disappeared. The former ruling classes were disfranchised. The nobility, capitalists, rich peasants, priests, and non-Communist intelligentsia were persecuted, exiled, or condemned to death. The government was put into the hands of a Central Committee of Soviets, and its executive organ, the Politburo. It was supported by a new, well-trained "Red Army" and a new Bolshevik police force, which was ruthless in its use of terrorist methods. The state took control of all banks, industries, large businesses, and foreign trade, and thus combined political with economic power to a degree unparalleled in any Western country.

### Period of the Nep (1921-1927)

Nevertheless, owing to foreign war, civil strife, famine, and dissatisfaction among the peasants, who, unlike the industrial workers, had gained little influence in the government, Communism might not have survived in Russia had Lenin not changed his tactics in 1921. A serious crisis had developed. The peasants refused to fulfill their quotas for the delivery of foodstuffs. Production came to a standstill. A contingent of sailors revolted. Faced by these problems, Lenin reintroduced, despite opposition from within his own ranks, a number of capitalistic institutions. Small-scale private enterprise in trade and agriculture was once again allowed. The policy of food levies was replaced by taxation of peasants. The terror was reduced. Aid from capitalistic countries was accepted, and a stable currency was restored. Schools were reopened, and pre-Revolutionary scientists were reemployed. Also, a compromise with the Orthodox Church was arranged. Lenin's new policy, known as the NEP (New Economic Policy), brought internal improvements at the very time that Russia gained external prestige through the Rapallo Treaty and won formal recognition from the leading European powers.

### Period of First Five-Year Plan (1928-1932)

In July 1923, a new constitution was published. It established the Union of Socialist Soviet Republics (USSR), composed of Great Russia, Siberia, the Ukraine, and the Caucasus. Shortly thereafter, Lenin died, but his work survived in spite of a bitter struggle for party leadership between his two chief co-workers, Leon Trotsky and Joseph Stalin. With the help of the Party apparatus that he controlled, Stalin, the great organizer, triumphed over Trotsky. Stalin held the view that Communism had to be built on firm ground in Russia before it could be spread abroad. He rejected the individualistic tendencies of Trotsky and insisted on strict Party discipline and central direction. Ideologically, he steered a middle road. Under him, the NEP, which had served well as a temporary expedient, was eliminated, and Communist planning was resumed. The first of a series of Five-Year Plans, published in 1928, provided for the central direction of all economic activities by government and Party. It stipulated production quotas for all sectors of the economy: factories, agriculture, and individual workers. It aimed at developing the resources of the country and at improving backward regions, especially the arctic areas of Siberia. It coordinated the activities of the various industries and controlled channels of domestic and foreign distribution. Prices and wages were fixed.

The Plan promoted the collective farm, called *kolkhoz,* or "large farm." The land would belong to the state, but its activities would be managed autonomously in accordance with the Plan. Its cultivation would be performed in common by its members, and its products sold by state or *kolkhoz* stores. Individuals retained for themselves no more than a house and garden, but shared according to their work in a possible surplus of the collective. Mechanical help was rendered by government-run tractor stations.

The Plan was, in many respects, a success. It also provided for public education, theaters, and other cultural activities and led to a rapid increase in Russia's production capabilities. However, its rigorous

*Figure 21–3 Joseph Stalin: 1878–1953*

enforcement caused the population untold suffering. Particularly in rural areas, the *kulaks* (prosperous peasants with individual holdings), whose activity had been allowed during the NEP, were sacrificed to Communistic aims. Hundreds of thousands of them perished either from starvation or as the result of exile and persecution.

Under a dictatorship of the Soviets, the state police were given almost unlimited power. The government exercised strict censorship of books and publications. It persecuted all who voiced critical or anti-Communist opinions and undertook a continuous, all-embracing propaganda campaign. Contacts of Soviet citizens with foreign countries became almost impossible, News from the outside world rarely reached them, and no one felt safe. Labor camps were constructed and filled with both innocent and guilty citizens. Emigration was halted, while immigrants from the West—enthusiasts who hoped for the better society offered by communism and who intended to help build the country under the Five-Year Plan—were admitted. Living standards improved, but much was sacrificed to the aim of building a Communist society.

## The United States

In the United States, World War I had left less destruction, fewer losses, and less of an imprint than in Europe. Consequently, social change was less extreme. A Republican administration, which replaced the Democrats in 1921, adopted many of the policies of political and economic liberalism. The nation prospered as business expanded, national production increased rapidly, and standards of living improved. There was substantial progress in education, science, literature, and the arts. Indications of such progress included the large number of foreign students attracted to American universities, the development of inventions and technology, the organization of excellent orchestras, the founding of numerous museums, and the great variety of works of literature that gained worldwide attention. In foreign affairs, the United States, despite popular isolationist sentiments, took a more active role than ever before in contributing to the solution of world problems. A rash of political corruption and crime incidents accompanied the "noble experiment" of national Prohibition, a constitutional amendment that outlawed alcoholic beverages. Such corruption, however, failed to impede the economic and cultural progress of the nation.

While the position of U.S. economic strength was maintained, serious social problems were ignored. Little attention was given to warnings about the difficulties of the farmers and the overextension of credit. Not until the stock market crash of 1929, which marked the end of the era of prosperity, did the government begin to work on solutions for some of the fundamental problems confronting the United States and other Western nations.

## Other Western Countries

The smaller countries of the West, with the exception of Italy, did not suffer as much as the major powers from either the war or the difficulties created in its aftermath by revolutions, inflation, impoverishment, and social disorganiation. None adapted Communism. Most of them made considerable progress in the development of industrial production, educational standards, and political democracy. In some countries, such as Poland and Hungary, feudalistic institutions that favored the owners of large landed estates continued to prevail. In others, dictatorships prospered, as in Latin America.

In most Western nations, nationalism persisted as a dominant influence. Poland led armed aggression against its neighbors. In Czechoslovakia, Italy, and various Balkan nations, attempts at building national industries were motivated primarily by nationalistic aspirations. Latin America struggled against foreign economic domination. Mexico nationalized the oil companies owned by business interests in the United States. When the worldwide depression began in the late 1920s, the nationalistic trends reflected by these events created problems among the smaller nations similar to those confronting the major powers of the Western world.

## Perspective

*Instead of creating a postwar period of stability, the Versailles Treaty led to hostility, fear, and undue hardship. Moreover, the rise of Communism in Russia, and civil war, which was worsened by Allied intervention, hunger, and disorder, had a devastating effect on developments not only in the Soviet Union, but in the entire West. The establishment of a dictatorship in Soviet-Russia and the government's experiments there with Five-Year Plans challenged economic and political institutions in the West. Far from finding its own new order, the West saw inflation of an unknown order, labor disputes, and strikes, as well as a steady weakening of the middle class. Attempts to modify the consequences of the Versailles Treaty in conferences held in Genoa, Rapallo, and Locarno, and the reduction of reparations payments proved insufficient. Failing to promote democracy, the Versailles Treaty actually hindered it. Nationalism flared up everywhere. Colonial regions attacked their masters. Ireland and other dominions demanded full independence from England.*

*The shocks of war and the postwar period acted as a stimulus to intellectual developments, as witnessed by the arts, film, architecture, and education. In the field of religion, both atheistic movements and Neo-Orthodox tendencies increased. In philosophy, pragmatism dominated. The natural sciences moved into the center of Western intellectual activity. Scholars in many countries contributed new theories and made important discoveries. This led to technical achievements in such areas as transportation and communications, which altered living conditions for rich and poor alike.*

## Selected Readings

Bendiner, Elmer. A *Time for Angels: The Tragicomic History of the League of Nations* (New York: Knopf, 1975).

Cipolla, Carlo M., ed., *The Fontana Economic History of Europe,* 6 vols. (New York: Barnes & Noble, 1977).

Craig, Gordon A. *Europe Since 1914* (Hinsdale, ILL.: The Dryden Press, 1972).

de Jone, Alex. *The Weimar Chronicle: Prelude to Hitler* (New York: Paddington Press, 1978).

Fussell, Paul. *The Great War and Modern Memory* (New York: Oxford University Press, 1975).

Gerhardie, William. *God's Fifth Column: A Biography of the Age, 1890–1940* (1981).

Fitzpatrick, Sheila, *The Russian Revolution, 1917-1932* (Oxford: Oxford University Press, 1994).

Joll, J. *Europe Since 1870: An International History* (London: Weidenfeld and Nicolson, 1973).

Keynes, John Maynard. *The Economic Consequences of the Peace* (New York: St. Martin's Press, 1971).

McNeill, William H. *The Pursuit of Power: Technology, Armed Force and Society Since* A.D. *1000* (Chicago: The University of Chicago Press, 1982).

Roth, Jack J., ed., *World War I: A Turning Point in Modern History* (New York: Knopf, 1967).

Smith, Page *Redeeming the Time: A People's History of the 1920s and the New Deal* (New York: Penguin Books, 1991).

Walters, F. P. *A History of the League of Nations,* 2 v. (Oxford: Oxford University Press, 1960).

## Test Yourself

1. In 1927, Charles Lindburgh accomplished_____.
   A. The first flight in an airplane
   B. The first transatlantic flight
   C. The first transpacific flight
   D. None of the above

2. Oswald Spengler in his *Decline of the West* (1918-1922) came to view human history as_____.
   A. A scientific process subject to divine laws
   B. A matter of divine intervention
   C. A biological process subject to natural laws
   D. None of the above

3. The work titled *The Protestant Ethic and the Spirit of Capitalism* was published in 1904 by_____.
   A. Sigmund Freud
   B. Karl Marx
   C. Frederick Engels
   D. Max Weber

4. Right before his death, Lenin recognized the importance of capitalist investment in the Russian economy and consequently agreed to_____.
   A. A new socialist policy (NSP)
   B. A new communist policy (NCP)
   C. A new democratic policy (NDP)
   D. Institute a new economic policy (NEP)

5. When Lenin died in 1923, he was succeeded by _____.
   A. Trotsky
   B. Stalin
   C. Khrushchev
   D. None of the above

6. When World War I ended, the Ottoman Empire collapsed and the bulk of its Arab domain came under the control of _____.
   A. Britain
   B. Germany
   C. Italy
   D. None of the above

7. The Briand-Kellogg Pact of 1928 addressed among other things_____.
   A. Inequalities of economies among nations
   B. Inequalities of military strength among nations
   C. Compulsory arbitration of future political differences among nations
   D. Both B and C

8. The Treaty of Locarno, which settled political disputes among European powers, was signed in _____.
   A. 1928
   B. 1925
   C. 1927
   D. 1930

## Answers and Explanations

1. **B.** In 1927, Charles Lindbergh accomplished the first nonstop, transatlantic flight from New York to Paris.

2. **C.** Some philosophers, such as Oswald Spengler in his *Decline of the West* (1918-1922), came to view human history as a biological process subject to natural laws. They insisted that every culture passes through a cycle of youth, maturity, and old age, with its resulting deterioration. In this philosophy, we can see the disillusionment that resulted from the First World War and the tremendous blow inflicted by the conflict upon the idealism and boundless confidence with which the generation entered the 20th century.

3. **D.** A special place of importance belongs to the German, Max Weber (1864-1920), an influential sociologist who helped create the constitution of the postwar Weimar Republic. His studies concerning the relationship between society and the individual were embodied in his most famous work, *The Protestant Ethic and the Spirit of Capitalism* (1904). This work explored the effects of the Protestant Reformation, particularly, the new perception of wealth and its accumulation on the growth of capitalism and, by extension, modern Western society. Weber's ideas helped to counter the influence exercised at the time by certain Marxist thinkers.

4. **D.** Faced by these problems, Lenin reintroduced, notwithstanding opposition within his own ranks, a number of capitalistic institutions. Small-scale private enterprise in trade and agriculture was once again allowed. The policy of food levies was replaced by taxation of peasants. The terror was reduced. Aid from capitalistic countries was accepted, and a stable currency was restored. Schools were reopened and pre-Revolutionary scientists were reemployed. Also, a compromise with the Orthodox Church was arranged. Lenin's new policy, known as the NEP (New Economic Policy), brought internal improvements at the very time that Russia gained external prestige through the Rapallo Treaty and won formal recognition from the leading European powers.

5. **B.** In July 1923, a new constitution was published. It established the Union of Socialist Soviet Republics (USSR), composed of Great Russia, Siberia, the Ukraine, and the Caucasus. Shortly thereafter, Lenin died, but his work survived, despite a bitter struggle for party leadership between his two chief co-workers, Leon Trotsky and Joseph Stalin. With the help of the Party apparatus that he controlled, Stalin, the great organizer, triumphed over Trotsky. Stalin held the view that Communism had to be built on firm ground in Russia before it could be spread abroad. He rejected the individualistic tendencies of Trotsky and insisted on strict Party discipline and central direction. Ideologically, he steered a middle road. Under him, the NEP, which had served well as a temporary expedient, was eliminated, and Communist planning was resumed.

6. **A.** In order to safeguard British investments and the supply of oil, however, Britain insisted on continued control of the Arab states, Palestine, Transjordan, and Iraq which were once controlled by the dissolved Ottoman Empire.

7. **D.** Inequalities in military strength continued to endanger world peace; regional meetings and disarmament conferences among the victors had accomplished little. Thereupon, the American Secretary of State, Frank Kellogg, proposed a pact that provided for compulsory arbitration of future political differences. The pact was signed by the United States and the leading European powers in 1928.

8. B. Under the circumstances, the need for a realistic attack upon Western economic and political problems became more urgent. Steps were finally taken at the initiative of the United States. In 1924, with the realization of the close relationship between political and economic problems, a reparations plan (the Dawes plan) was worked out. It fixed German reparations at a sum commensurate with Germany's ability to pay, and American loans were put at Germany's disposal so that Germany might provide for its new obligations. Once adopted, the Dawes plan opened the way for a settlement of political disputes. This was achieved by a conference held in Locarno in 1925. Owing to the efforts of the French and German foreign ministers, Aristide Briand and Gustav Stresemann, respectively, an agreement concerning the disputed Franco-German border was reached. The agreement guaranteed that Germany's western boundaries as established by the Versailles Treaty would be maintained. In the following year, Germany joined the League of Nations. Simultaneously, the military supervision of Germany was ended.

# CHAPTER 22
# Depression, Fascism, and War (1929-1945)

**1927** Heisenberg's indeterminacy theory
**1930** Young Plan for reparations adopted
Passive resistance against England in India (Gandhi)
**1931** England gives up gold standard
England promulgates Statute of Westminster
Austrian Kreditanstalt collapses
**1932** Lausanne Reparation Conference
Britain introduces protective tariffs
Japanese expansion in Chinese territory
**1933** Hitler becomes German chancellor
F. D. Roosevelt becomes U. S. president
U.S.A. gives up gold standard
**1934** Russia enters League of Nations
**1935** Social security acts passed in U.S.A.
**1936** Purges in Russia; Stalin constitution passed
Italy annexes Abyssinia; Rome-Berlin Axis
Outbreak of civil war in Spain
Germany reintroduces conscription and reoccupies the Rhineland
**1937** Constitution for Ireland (Eire)
**1938** Austria united with Germany
Munich Conference ("appeasement")
Incorporation of Sudetenland into Germany
**1939** Collapse of Czechoslovakia
Italy invades Albania
Soviet-Nazi Pact
Outbreak of World War II
Partition of Poland between Germany and Russia
Russia attacks Finland

**1940** Germany occupies Norway, Denmark, Holland, and Belgium
Incorporation of Estonia, Latvia, and Lithuania into USSR
Collapse of France
**1941** Germany invades Russia
Attack on Pearl Harbor by Japan; U.S.A. enters war
**1942** Allied landing in Africa
**1943** German defeat at Stalingrad
**1944** Allied landing in Normandy, France
**1945** Yalta Conference
Surrender of Germany and Japan
United Nations established
First atomic bomb (dropped by U.S.A. on Japan)

*The three words—depression, Fascism, and war— indicate a causal relationship, but they do not suffice to explain the pattern of major historical events in the 1930s. The decline of liberalism, the growing strength of nationalism, the achievements in science and technology, the failures of education, the short-sightedness of politicians and economists, the weakness of people in responsible positions, and the contradictions within human nature, all contributed to the complex events of this period. In retrospect, however, the consideration of three forces—depression, fascism, and war—to which might be added a fourth, Bolshevism, may serve as an adequate guide to analysis of the major developments.*

## ■ DEPRESSION

According to some economists, cycles of prosperity and depression are inevitable in a capitalistic society. A cycle of this kind occurred after World War I. The war boom lasted until 1919. There was a brief depression in 1920, which was followed by a long period of prosperity from which all countries, neutrals as well as those directly involved in the war, benefited. The universal prosperity engendered overconfidence in both political and in economic affairs. Excessive optimism and speculation resulted in the production of more goods than the market could absorb. From 1925 to 1929, the gap was bridged through an expansion of credit, but when debts reached dangerous levels, banks became reluctant to make more loans. Prices dropped, production fell, and confidence was undermined.

### The Crash (1929)

By 1929, a depression had begun to develop in the Western economy. New industries were created, but older ones declined in importance. Ensuing unemployment brought a chain of reactions, since even reduced production could no longer be absorbed. Unemployment increased. In October of 1929, the so-called "crash" of the New York Stock Exchange occurred, ruining many leading business enterprises. The close relationship between domestic business and foreign trade meant that a depression in any one country, especially the United States, inevitably affected all others—not excluding Communist Russia, which was compelled to accept reduced prices for its exports. In 1931, the collapse of one of the great international banks, the Kreditanstalt in Vienna, intensified the downward turn of business in all countries. Most countries gave up the gold standard. Insecurity replaced complacency.

### Social Consequences of Depression

The consequences of economic disaster were felt in all areas of public and private life. Many people who had considered themselves financially secure lost their means of livelihood. Farmers, unable to find a market for their products, lost their land. Millions of factory workers were idle. Unemployment figures climbed to incredible heights in the leading industrial countries, such as the United States, Germany, and England. Even in Russia, the only large Western country that did not have an unemployment problem, the depression prevented any substantial improvement of living standards. Insecurity, demoralization, and impoverishment changed people's outlook and, in a world that seemed to be disintegrating, made them ready everywhere to seek salvation in radical corrective measures.

## Political Consequences

Naturally, Western governments tried to take remedial action, but in so doing, they contributed to a further weakening of liberal, laissez-faire institutions. In the United States, the Republican president, Herbert Hoover, introduced several farm-relief measures. He also advocated new forms of social legislation. In 1933, during the Democrat Franklin Roosevelt's first term, the United States devalued the dollar and instituted a program of social security insurance. The governments of all European countries began providing subsidies for manufacturers and exporters and found it necessary to establish extensive controls over business. Tariff rates were raised and the exchange of currency was restricted. The export of gold and other funds was forbidden.

In 1931, England gave up the gold standard. As in previous emergencies, it had recourse to a national coalition cabinet, which was under a Labor party minister this time. In 1932, the country abandoned its free-trade policy, introducing new protective tariffs while providing "preference tariffs" for members of the empire.

In Germany, meanwhile, the government claimed almost dictatorial powers under an emergency clause of the constitution. Then, backed only by a minority against the position of a large but ideologically divided majority, it followed the example of other Western governments in enacting laws to relieve economic distress. However, also like the others, it found itself unable to solve the basic unemployment problem.

The effects of the depression were less severe in France and Italy, which were not so dependent upon highly developed industries, and in the agricultural countries of the East. Nevertheless, even in these countries, suffering was widespread, and long-established political systems were imperiled as the radical parties of right or left gained adherents. Repercussions also developed in the Far East wherever European economic methods and influence had made headway. Japan, in particular, experienced reverses owing to the loss of its foreign markets and was tempted to utilize the drastic remedies of war and territorial expansion.

## International Consequences

The undermining of national economies destroyed the international balance of power, and statesmen sought in vain to restore it. The League of Nations, which, notwithstanding adverse criticisms then and since, had succeeded in settling numerous, though minor, international disputes and in arranging various international contracts, proved unfit for such a major task. Again, the world had to rely on traditional diplomacy.

Diplomats first turned their attention to the reparations problem. As early as 1929, a new plan, which was named after the American industrialist Owen D. Young, had been drafted, which unlike the 1924 plan drafted by Young and Charles G. Dewes, reduced German reparations to approximately $26 billion, one-third the amount originally assessed in 1921. Payments were spread out over fifty-eight years, ending in 1988, and were to be made to the new Bank for International Settlements. The Young plan also called for the dissolution of the Reparations Commission and an end to Allied occupation of the Rhineland. The German government quickly agreed to these terms by setting German reparations at levels pegged to the country's ability to pay, had substantially reduced the remaining balance. In 1932, the remaining reparations debts were essentially canceled. Next, the former Allies held a disarmament conference in a futile attempt to economize by reducing military expenditures. Furthermore, to improve the international economic situation, Germany and Austria proposed a customs union, whereby a free central European trading area would have been created. However, the plan, which had political implications, was vetoed by the victorious nations. Finally, in 1933, a general World Economic Conference was held in London to discuss concerted remedial actions. By that time, however, the various nations had initiated individual programs to deal with the crisis, and none of them was ready to accept international measures that might impede domestic relief programs. The United States, in particular, was reluctant to agree to proposed international economic ties, and the conference ended in failure. In 1934, another disarmament conference revealed a further disintegration of the international community, owing to the triumph of the Fascist form of government in Germany.

## Fascism

As a political ideology, fascism had a comparatively long history before the 1930s. Its roots lay in the economic developments and nationalistic trends of the late 19th and early 20th centuries. Like socialism, fascism embraced a variety of ideas, objectives, and programs, differing in radicalism. In some of its aspects, fascism was heralded by writers hostile to the major political developments of the liberal age. Among these were sociologists such as the Italian Vilfredo Pareto, who felt that contemporary social thought was based mainly on the rational views derived from the Age of Enlightenment and that it neglected the irrational element in human behavior. With the onset of a worldwide depression, which many people attributed to the inefficiency of the democratic and capitalistic systems, fascism gained millions of adherents. Fascism appeared to offer an alternative to those who rejected democracy, but could not accept the Bolshevik doctrines of the international Communist community. Demagogues would prevail over responsible political behavior. The political and economic implications of fascism made it a decisive influence in countries such as Germany and Italy, which, as a consequence of World War I, had to endure, in addition to economic difficulties, the frustration of their national ambitions.

## Characteristics of Fascism

Fascism was consistent with the trend of opposition to 19th-century liberalism, but its opposition was far more radical than that of any other political movement except Communism. The type of fascism that developed in the 1920s and 1930s relegated the individual to a minor role in society. It subordinated people entirely to the state, which was extolled as an all-embracing source of authority. The state was to become the ultimate judge of right and wrong, "right" being defined as whatever served the state's interests. In Fascist countries, no party but that of the Fascists was allowed, and parliamentary activity was reduced to a mere formality. Instead of freely elected governments, fascism would provide a single leader to whom all allegiance was primarily owed and who would have such authority as despots had exercised in earlier centuries. It would countenance no other loyalties. The Fascists claimed the right to regulate or direct economic activities. They sought to free their country from dependence upon other countries, economically as well as politically, and they appealed to conservatives and industrialists. They undertook to restrict civil liberties and to censor the radio, books, the cinema, and newspapers, suppressing any opinions that might encourage opposition to the leader of the nation. It was their aim to control the work of scholars and artists, whose endeavors were to be judged on the basis of utility to the nation.

In most cases, Fascism conflicted with religion and promoted atheism. Inasmuch as it wanted to avoid any double allegiance, it sought to reduce Church influence. Its moral creed was generally opposed to Christian beliefs and to many ethical concepts developed in the West during its 2,000 years of historical development. It sought to gain support from the masses by emphasizing the socialistic aspects of its creed—support that it needed in view of its illegitimate origin. Extolling the role of laborer and peasant, the Fascists promised to introduce social improvements, provide work through public projects, and raise wages. They would not permit independent labor organizations, but they would safeguard private property rights and protect the business "leader." They considered it the task of the government to form public opinion by using its most potent weapon, propaganda, and would not hesitate to twist facts, present half-truths, and blame the ills of preceding eras on minority groups such as Communists, Jews, and others. Eventually, having roused chauvinistic ambitions, Fascists embarked upon an expansionist foreign policy. In general, Fascists were "men of action, not doctrinaires."

## Spread of Fascism (1922–1940)

The first country to adopt Fascism and the one that named the movement was Italy. The Fascist leader Benito Mussolini established his regime in 1922. In 1923, Turkey under Mustafa Kemal, later called Ataturk, instituted a government exhibiting Fascist traits. In 1926, Joseph Pilsudski seized power in Poland and imposed a total military dictatorship with slight Fascist overtones until his death in 1935. In 1928, Antonio Salazar seized the government in Portugal, and he established a dictatorship there in 1933. Everywhere, Fascism sought the support of the military and usually obtained it. During the period from 1929 to 1935, the Baltic states—Latvia, Estonia, and Lithuania—adopted some features of the Fascist state. In 1929, King Alexander arbitrarily converted the parliamentary government of Yugoslavia into a personal dictatorship. Hungary introduced a Fascist system under Gyula Gombos in 1932 and 1933. Adolf Hitler established his regime in Germany in 1933. In Greece, Ioannis Metaxas abolished democratic institutions in 1936, and three years later, Francisco Franco triumphed in Spain. These dictators permitted no opposition. Their orders had to be obeyed, and their policy of aggressive nationalism prevailed. During World War II, Fascist governments, usually with the help of native groups, were imposed upon several additional countries.

## Fascism in Action

The regime established in Italy served as a model for other Fascist states until Hitler's Germany was accepted as a model in the late 1930s.

### Italy

In Italy, Fascism began in 1919 with the formation of a political party by Mussolini who, early in his career, had been a newspaperman and Socialist. He opposed the liberal trend, but promised his followers social improvements along non-Communistic lines. He assured them that he would put an end to social strife, establish order, and reestablish the prestige of Italy, which, he insisted, had fared badly at the hands of the Allies at Versailles. He gained support from workers, from industrialists who were afraid of Communism, from ex-soldiers who were disappointed with postwar conditions, and from small businessmen. Leading a number of armed bands, the "Black Shirts," he marched on the government in Rome in 1922, whereupon King Victor Emmanuel III assigned him the task of forming a new government, rather than risk civil war. Having gained control, Mussolini abolished all parties except his own, assembled a new parliament consisting of representatives of the various economic groups instead of representatives of political parties, and thus introduced what came to be known as a corporate state. Direction of policy was vested in the hands of the leader (*Il Duce*). All forms of social strife, particularly strikes, were outlawed. The opposition was brutally suppressed, and some of its leaders were murdered. Employers and workers were called upon to work for the new order through "patriotic cooperation." The army was reorganized; programs to drain the swamps and to implement the reforestation of the denuded mountain areas were begun. Improvements were made to public services. In 1929, Mussolini signed a concordat with the papacy, which provided for the recognition of Vatican City as a sovereign state, compensation for the territorial losses of the Church, and designation of Catholicism as the official religion of Italy. On the whole, the population felt invigorated and hopeful. It tolerated the injustices and brutality committed by the regime and applauded Mussolini's plans for national aggrandizement. Some social legislation strengthened the regime, but it promised more than it delivered, especially with regard to the impoverished south.

### Germany

The pattern set by Fascism in Italy was perfected in Germany. The movement there was known as National Socialism, indicating its twofold objective. A political party supported by armed bands of Brown Shirts was organized by Hitler. After a vain attempt at a *putsch*, or takeover, in 1923, he applied his oratorical skills and personal magnetism to gain a following. By 1932, the Nazi party had become the largest in the country, and its armed organizations were a threat to internal peace.

### Seizure of Power

In 1933, after repressive constitutional measures against the Nazis had proved to be useless, Hitler was entrusted with the formation of a government. He thus achieved power "legally." With the approval and assistance of some industrialists and the demoralized segments of the middle class and the proletariat, who had suffered the consequences of Germany's defeat in 1918 and had been impoverished by inflation and depression, he substituted an authoritarian system for the national constitution. The Western powers had come too late with their support of democracy in the Weimar republic, their abolition of the worst consequences of Versailles, and the cancellation of the reparation payments. He suppressed, first, the Communist Party, then all other parties, and sent his political enemies into concentration camps or had them murdered. Hitler then established himself as dictator and *Fuehrer*. Abandoning the left-wing tendencies apparent in the early stages of the party, he turned the resentment of the masses against the Jews, whom he presented as the instigators of existing political and economic evils. He preached a rabid racial doctrine that was designed to appeal to the frustrated population. All activities in art, science, and business had to be coordinated with party doctrines, and the "leadership principle" was extended to all areas of national life.

### Legislation

Hitler attacked the unemployment problem, first, by initiating public-works projects and a compulsory national labor service, then by building an armaments industry in violation of the Versailles agreement and, finally, by reintroducing compulsory military service. Simultaneously, he inaugurated measures to assist farmers, relieving them of their mortgage burdens and protecting inherited farms against continued indebtedness. These measures helped to revive economic life and to get the millions of disoriented unemployed off the streets. Private enterprises benefited from these measures and reemployed the people. Within a few years, unemployment had been replaced with a labor shortage, which forced wages to rise. A four-year plan was initiated, which mobilized all the economic forces in the country. Its financing was helped by the confiscation of property owned by Jews (and by many non-Jews, as well), who were expelled from public life and business. Steps were taken to make Germany less dependent upon foreign imports and to develop new internal resources instead; for example, many new oil wells were dug, and artificial rubber production was undertaken on a large scale. The resulting national revival—accompanied by such institutions as extra vacations through the "Strength and Joy" organization, through film festivals and sports events, including the Olympic games of 1936—impressed both Germans and foreigners to such an extent that the injustices of the system and its neglect of the concepts embodied in Western laws and ethics were too readily overlooked. Whatever feeble opposition could be offered—by individuals, by conservative groups, by long-time staff officials of the bureaucracy, by army officers or clergymen—was defeated by defamatory propaganda and, when necessary, by violence.

### Spain

Spain became the third great center of Fascism. Unlike Germany and Italy, Spain refrained from imperialistic enterprises, primarily because of its internal weaknesses, and again, unlike the two others, it did not combat traditional religious forces, but augmented party strength through an alliance with the Catholic Church. As early as 1923, a dictatorship had been established in Spain under Miguel Primo de

Rivera. He had not succeeded in resolving factional strife in the country, however. Old problems persisted, including the domineering influence of a small landowning class faced by an impoverished peasantry; the division of interests between the industrialized north and the agricultural south; the aggressiveness of both clerics and of large atheistic groups; the imposition of censorship; the agitation of monarchists opposed to fervent republicans; and the weakness of a moderating and mediating middle class.

Having failed to solve either social or political problems, Rivera resigned in 1930. In the following year, the king, potentially an effective unifying influence for the country, was forced into exile. An election put a republican government into office. At first, it was moderately liberal, but later, it became strongly socialistic. It aroused the bitter resistance of the conservatives by passing extensive anticlerical and anticapitalistic legislation. As a result, civil war broke out in 1936.

It was perhaps unequaled by any other modern war in its brutality. Foreign interventionists soon participated—Communists, Fascists, and volunteers from democratic countries. For years, the triangular struggle raged among these three groups, until in 1939, Franco, leader of the Falange, as the Spanish Fascists came to be known, emerged victorious. He achieved internal peace by rewarding his adherents and by crushing all opponents. His personal dictatorship solved few of Spain's domestic problems, however.

## Democracies versus Fascism

Fascist doctrines and their apparent successes, particularly in the economic sphere, as in dealing with unemployment, won many adherents in the traditionally democratic countries of the West. Since these countries had not experienced the frustration of national ambitions, most people remained loyal to their well-established governments and avoided Fascist experiments regardless of economic difficulties and social tensions, unrest and strikes.

### *Europe*

France, most of all, was in great danger. Fascists gained much ground there. In 1937, a popular-front government, which had been trying to save the country both from the rightist and equally strong leftist extremists, was upset. The traditional forces succeeded in meeting the threat and preserving most of the democratic institutions. In Holland, Norway, and other nations, Fascist parties also gained influence. Yet there, too, established institutions prevailed. The small Fascist party in England had even fewer opportunities to make headway, for the government gradually introduced measures to improve social conditions, modernize its foreign-trade policy, and adjust its methods of administration to contemporary needs. The English electorate, meanwhile, proved its traditional aversion to radical changes. A crisis, such as that associated with the abdication of King Edward VIII, could be settled without disturbing the political structure. In the member nations of the Commonwealth, especially in Australia and New Zealand, the governments, opposed to all radicalism and prepared to preserve capitalism, prevented the triumph of Fascism by far-reaching social legislation in the interests of the workers.

### *The United States*

The influence of Fascist groups in the United States was kept at a negligible level as social and economic changes similar to those in Europe were inaugurated during the New Deal administrations of Franklin D. Roosevelt. Social security laws were passed, such as those providing for old-age and unemployment insurance and minimum wages in industry. The gold standard was abandoned; debtors were granted a moratorium; huge government projects, e.g., the electrification of the Tennessee Valley were undertaken; and some national planning was also attempted. Private enterprise and banking were brought under partial regulation by government, and thus a system of subsidies was used to influence the farmer's decisions about the types of crops and the acreage to be planted. Agriculture began to recover. To be sure, more radical attempts at regimentation, such as Roosevelt's proposal for "packing" (adding new judges to) the United States Supreme Court, were defeated, but even in the United States, emphasis was placed upon "leadership," and a bureaucracy dependent upon a strong central government grew rapidly. Public confidence was eventually restored, and, although a great deal of unemployment persisted, the American economy recuperated. The automobile industry again saw growth, and the standards of living of the masses improved.

Internal recovery was reflected in United States foreign policies. Despite the continued opposition of isolationists, interest and participation in European affairs increased. The Roosevelt government formally recognized the Bolshevik government in Russia, promoted closer cooperation with non-Fascist nations, adopted a conciliatory attitude toward Latin American nations, proclaimed a good-neighbor policy, and settled long-standing quarrels. Through the Pan-American Union, it advanced political and economic collaboration. Thus, owing to timely action, Fascism was given no chance to develop in the United States.

## Communism versus Fascism

While Fascism was making headway in central Europe, and while a modified liberal-democratic system was being introduced in the western areas of the continent, Communism increased its hold in Russia and made the appearance of any other ideology impossible.

### Russian Planning

By 1930, the first Five-Year Plan, which was to lay the economic foundation for the new society, was well on its way toward successful completion. Production in heavy industries began to surpass the levels of tsarist Russia. The transportation system was repaired and grew rapidly, with such vast undertakings as the railway connection between Turkistan and Siberia (Turksib Railroad) and the improvement of inland waterways. Domestic commerce and foreign trade could again be expanded. The prices of consumer goods were reduced. Stability returned to the lives of the ordinary workers, and collective farming became the dominant system in agriculture. The threat of external interference receded with the strengthening of the armed forces. In 1932, a second Five-Year Plan provided for the continuation of the same domestic policies. Collectivization was continued until most private farms had disappeared, and heavy industries were given preference over those producing consumer goods.

### Russian Government

In 1936, a new constitution was adopted for the Soviet Union. By then the nation consisted of 13 republics, each enjoying local autonomy, but subject to central political direction and central economic planning. The executive power remained in the hands of the Politburo, with Stalin at its head. Civil rights were formally extended to all Russians. Thus after twenty years of discrimination, constitutional inequities directed against various "bourgeois" groups of the population were abolished. As before, only one party, the Communist, was allowed to exist and function. However, Communist practice differed from theory. The Party and its functionaries exercised strict supervision over all economic and social enterprises. Promised civil rights were disregarded, dissenting voices were silenced, and hundreds of thousands, possibly millions, of citizens were banished to Siberia. Workers and peasants, despite the existence of labor unions and collective-farm councils, had little chance to make their voices heard. Freedom of movement was sharply restricted. Scholars, physicians, authors, teachers, and artists who tried to act independently found their works censored and their lives imperiled. Labor camps were filled with political prisoners. One wave of purges followed another. The struggle for supreme power that had begun with Stalin and Trotsky soon engulfed all supporters of Trotsky, who had been banished in 1929. In 1940, he was assassinated in Mexico by a Soviet agent. His adherents were brought to trial for treason and exiled or executed. By 1938, Stalin was defending himself against "right" and "left" opposition and had disposed of most of the leading Bolshevists. The terror also embraced the supreme command of the army, whose chief of staff and other high-ranking officers were executed. Purges of political opponents became an integral part of the Bolshevik system.

### *Russian Society*

Despite sacrifices, the ideal communist society promised by the regime was slow in developing. A continual move toward the formation of new classes and elites became apparent as those who had constituted the upper classes in pre-Revolutionary times and those who had risen with the Revolution were overthrown. The Party hierarchy and officials in the state bureaucracy enjoyed numerous privileges and maintained a living standard far higher than that of the masses. In addition, intellectuals loyal to the Stalinist system and an elite group of workers rose above the level of the masses. In order to speed up production, the government offered special rewards and prizes to workers who surpassed the productivity the norms demanded of them. In industry, such workers were known as *Stakhanovites*, in honor of Aleksei Stakhanov, a miner who had shown extraordinary inventiveness and efficiency in raising production. Nevertheless, although industrial output increased rapidly, the intensive system eventually aroused dissatisfaction among ordinary workers. The recipients of the high wages were not greatly served because investment possibilities were lacking, and the costs of luxuries were fixed so as to quickly channel any extra income back into the state treasury.

### *Culture in the Soviet Union*

The Soviet government paid much attention to education. Illiteracy was practically wiped out. The emphasis was put on discipline in the schools. Training in the natural sciences, aside from political instruction in Marxism, was emphasized. As long as citizens conformed to the political demands, theater, film, music, and literature were encouraged, and some outstanding work was achieved.

## ■WORLD WAR II

With three vigorous ideologies—Fascism, remodeled democracy, and Bolshevism—competing during the 1930s, suspicion and hatred spread throughout the world. Sharpened by continued economic difficulties, they led to a rapid worsening of international relations. This happened despite the fact that the pressures of the Versailles settlement had been reduced, and treaties based on equality had been made. Eventually, Germany rearmed itself and laid claim to adjoining territories. Germany's actions met with appeasement until its demands, increasing with every success, imperiled the western European powers, and they decided to take up arms again. In 1939, World War II broke out.

### International Tension

The first significant step on the road to war came with the withdrawal, in 1933, of Hitler's Germany from the League of Nations. In itself, this action had no great effect upon the international scene. The League had only recently demonstrated its political impotence anew when it was unable to cope effectively with the Japanese invasion of Chinese territory and the subsequent establishment of Manchuria as a separate state subject to Japanese influence. Hitler's exit was a psychological shock, however, because it emphasized the League's weaknesses and demonstrated the rebirth of extreme nationalism. His action was answered by the initiation of a policy of "collective security." Cooperative agreements similar to those made among the Allies prior to 1914 were negotiated.

In 1935, France concluded a special defensive agreement with Russia. The Soviet Union was drawn into the League of Nations, and pacts were made among Russia, France, and some of the smaller East European countries, such as Czechoslovakia and Rumania. England assumed a friendlier attitude toward Russia. These moves were used by Germany to justify its own military preparations. Denouncing the prohibitory stipulations of the Versailles Treaty, Hitler began the full-scale rearmament of Germany in 1935 and the reintroduction of compulsory military service, pacifying England by a naval agreement that guaranteed British superiority on the seas. He then proceeded to send troops into the demilitarized Rhineland without encountering serious opposition from the Allies, who realized that Germany would eventually have to be granted its full sovereign rights.

The Allies were divided in their political aims and in their assessment of Hitler in the role of a counterweight to Bolshevik power. Moreover, the Allies had become involved in another difficulty. In 1935, Fascist Italy invaded Ethiopia, and the League of Nations decreed a number of economic sanctions. Britain and France did not wish to offend the Italian dictator whom they regarded as a potential opponent to Hitler's expansionist schemes. They also did not apply the sanctions vigorously. In this way, they failed to stop Mussolini and succeeded only in alienating him. In turn, Mussolini turned to Hitler, with whom he concluded the Rome-Berlin Axis alliance in 1936. This was supplemented by the Anti-Comintern Pact between Germany and Japan. Thus, the West was once again split into two camps. The United States remained outside both camps and in a position to swing the balance of power in either direction.

## Appeasement (1938)

Faced with increasing Fascist aggression, the democratic countries of the West were at a disadvantage. Relying on slow parliamentary procedures, they were faced with ruthless and determined men, whose arbitrary will could, at any moment, be transformed into deeds. So long as they were militarily weak, Western diplomats were compelled to appease their Fascist opponents and, while trying to come to terms with them, seek support from enemies of Fascism outside the democratic camp. However, they failed to pursue wholeheartedly the negotiations they had initiated with the only nation able to give them powerful support: the Soviet Union.

Consequently, Hitler was free to resume his expansionist schemes. Early in 1938, he united Austria and Germany—a union that Austrians and Germans had long desired. Austria had voted for the *Anschluss*, inclusion of Austria into greater Germany, soon after the end of World War I, but had been forbidden to take such action. An objective hitherto denied to Germany's democratic governments was now granted to the Nazis. Encouraged by this achievement, Hitler next demanded the incorporation of the Sudetenland, a region of western Czechoslovakia settled largely by Germans. Again, a pretext for the Nazi claim was offered: the idea that the Germans in that area had the right of self-determination. Unprepared for war, even though the Spanish Civil War had served as a proving ground for weapons, the Western powers agreed to a series of conferences. At Munich in 1938, they handed the Sudetenland over to Hitler. The Soviet Union, though affected by whatever position France and England would take, had not even been invited, and the French alliance system in the east thus collapsed.

## Outbreak of War (1939)

Peace was not promoted by appeasement, for, contrary to his assertion, Hitler annexed the rest of Czechoslovakia in the following year. This time, not even the incorporation of German populations desirous of joining the Reich could be used as an argument, inasmuch as it was an alien Czech population, proud of its independence and achievements that was forced under Nazi domination. The Western powers refused to give their sanction to this annexation and quickened their military preparations. They also revived the moribund political negotiations with Soviet Russia.

It was too late. In April 1939, Italy invaded and subjugated Albania. Germany forced Lithuania to surrender Memel and reclaimed Danzig, two areas that had been separated from Germany by the Treaty of Versailles. Next, Poland was asked to return other former German possessions, but with the backing of the Western countries, refused to do so. This time the Western powers were unwilling to make any compromises. They had become convinced of Hitler's untrustworthiness, but, more important, they had also witnessed the growing radicalism of Nazi ideology and its social implications. The extreme brutality of the Nazis was apparent in their treatment of opponents, especially the Jews, who were plundered, tortured, forced into exile, imprisoned in labor camps, and murdered.

This state-sponsored persecution was radically and perhaps prophetically demonstrated to the liberal democracies of the West in November of 1938 during the widespread rioting of *Kristallnacht* ("The Night of Broken Glass"), during which Jews were arrested, beaten and murdered and their shops and homes looted. Joseph Goebbels, Hitler's minister of propaganda, assured the world that the episode was a spontaneous uprising. Up until this time, emigration of the Jews from the Reich had been the official Nazi objective, but *Kristallnacht* seemed to usher in a new and more horrendous phase in the persecution.

The policy of appeasement was discarded, and no additional concessions were promised to Hitler—not even when, in August, the conclusion of a trade and nonaggression pact between Germany and the Soviet Union was suddenly announced, and the pro-Western diplomat, Maxim Litvinov, was replaced by the anti-Western Vyacheslav Molotov as Soviet foreign minister. The pact ended all hopes for collective security. In September, German armies marched into Poland. World War II had begun.

## Early Campaigns (1939-1941)

Cavalrymen were no match for armored Panzer units and dive-bombing aircraft, and Polish resistance collapsed within a few weeks. Just before the end came, Russian armies from the east marched into the country, and Poland experienced its fourth partition in modern history. This development was followed by a half-year lull (the "Phony War") on the Western front. Russia, however, continued its military actions, first by attacking Finland, then by incorporating and "sovietizing" the Baltic states. The Finns put up a surprisingly long and successful resistance, but eventually, they had to submit and cede some of their eastern territories.

The Finnish-Russian campaign had scarcely ended when hostilities were resumed in the West. In April 1940, German forces attacked neutral Norway, Denmark, Holland, and Belgium. Aided by native Fascists, the "quislings," named after the chief Fascist in Norway, they quickly forced these countries to surrender. Hitler then turned on France, whose government was weakened by indecision, confusion, and corruption, and whose general staff were overconfident about France's main defense system along the western border, the Maginot Line. This Maginot defense system of massive concrete bunkers and static gun emplacements had been built on the basis of experiences in World War I, but it proved inadequate to cope with new techniques of mobile warfare and aerial support. It was bypassed in the north and collapsed within a few days. The Nazis overran the entire northern coastal area of France, as well as Paris, and on June 5, 1940, France capitulated. The British auxiliary corps narrowly escaped to England.

France's catastrophe was the signal for Mussolini to enter the war: He promptly seized areas in southern France that had once been under Italian rule. A pro-German French government led by World War I hero, Marshal Henri Petain, was soon organized at Vichy. Despite the collapse of France, however, England did not yield. Under the leadership of a new prime minister, Winston Churchill, the British took effective defensive measures and continued the desperate struggle. Neither prolonged Nazi air attacks nor intensive submarine warfare could soften the island nation's resolve nor prepare the ground for invasion.

Consequently, the Germans shifted their attention southeastward in the direction of Egypt and the Suez Canal. Joined by the Italians, they opened a new front in Africa. Still another area was engulfed by war when in October 1940 Mussolini failed in an attack upon Greece, and the Germans rushed to his aid. By the end of May 1941, all the Balkan countries had either surrendered or made alliances with the Axis powers after installing Fascist governments.

*Figure 22–1 World War II in Europe*

## Global War (1941-1943)

The remaining months of 1941 proved to be a turning point in the war. The first decisive event occurred in June, when Hitler, after negotiations that had shown steadily deteriorating relations by November 1940, turned upon his Russian ally and invaded the Soviet Union. This move radically changed the balance of power, for what the negotiations of England and her allies had failed to achieve, Hitler's megalomania brought about: a common front for the Bolshevik and democratic nations and a two-front war for Germany. Both sides were fully armed. At first, the Germans enjoyed great successes against the Soviet forces. Within a few months, they reached the outskirts of Leningrad, Moscow, and Sevastopol, and they conquered the industrially valuable Don River basin and the rich agricultural lands of the Ukraine. However, they failed to capture Moscow and heavy losses and severe winter weather forced them to retreat. Then, the second decisive event took place.

Japanese imperial ambitions had consistently been thwarted by England and the United States in the Far East and the Pacific region. Both these nations were firmly established in the area. Negotiations to resolve their differences accomplished nothing, and Japan decided to seize the initiative with a lightning

*Figure 22–1 World War II in the Pacific*

and daring move. On December 7, 1941, the American naval base at Pearl Harbor in the Hawaiian Islands was attacked by Japanese aircraft. Concerted ground, air, and naval assaults upon a number of American and British island possessions followed.

Although not specifically bound by any treaty agreements with Japan, Hitler promptly declared war on the United States, thus committing the enormous physical resources of the self-proclaimed "arsenal of democracy" to the conflict in Europe.

From the beginning, the American people had been on the side of the Allies. Disregarding strict neutrality, they had supported England, and supplies and arms had been shipped across the Atlantic under a lend-lease plan. Moreover, the United States had introduced peacetime conscription, which paved the way for eventual military intervention. Hatred of Hitler's Germany became more and more inflamed as the Nazis disregarded all international treaties and moral precepts, attacked neutral nations, impressed labor from conquered countries into their war industries, looted art depositories, established their concentration camps for political opponents everywhere, and began a fearful extermination campaign against Jews, homosexuals and gypsies on the Continent.

In the course of Hitler's "Final Solution" to the Jewish "problem," millions of Jews perished in gas chambers and camps that sprang up throughout occupied Europe, particularly in the east. Massacres had occurred before in modern history. For example, the Armenians in the Turkish Empire were slaughtered in 1915, and Stalin's collectivization program during the 1930s was responsible for uncounted masses of victims. The Holocaust remains unique, however, for the number of victims and for the systematic application of science and technology to the task of mass genocide. Also unique was the ideological obsession that accompanied the destruction of European Jewry. The full details of the Holocaust only became evident after the liberation of Europe.

When America became an active belligerent on the Anglo-Russian side, the fate of the Axis powers was sealed. Japan conquered much of the Chinese coast, overwhelmed French Indochina and "impregnable" British Singapore, invaded Burma and Dutch Indonesia, and drove the Americans out of the Philippines. Germany penetrated still deeper into Russia, reached the Caucasus and Volga, took an enormous toll on Allied shipping with its submarines, and, together with Italy, conquered North Africa to the Egyptian border. However, the ultimate goal of winning the war was not achieved.

## Defeat of Italy, Germany, and Japan (1943-1945)

Early in 1943, Germany's military reversals began. At Stalingrad, the Nazis suffered a terrible defeat as an entire army surrendered to the Russians. In Africa, the Germans and Italians had to retreat before invading Allied armies, and by May 1943, all Axis forces had been either driven out of Africa or captured. The submarine menace had been overcome through the speedy production of replacement ships in America and the development of new defensive devices. Continuous heavy bombardment of German cities brought ruin to that country, which had previously been almost untouched by direct action. Japan's unchecked drive was halted. In July 1943, the Allies invaded Italy. Mussolini's government fell, and thus the first Fascist regime disappeared. Italy was accepted as an additional ally.

In June 1944, the long-planned invasion of Hitler's "Fortress Europe," which the Soviets had long demanded, but which had always been delayed, began as American and Allied troops landed in Normandy and quickly drove the German forces back. By September, they had reached the frontier and begun their invasion of the German homeland itself. Rather than submit to the Allied demand for unconditional surrender, and notwithstanding a last attempt by determined German resistance fighters to get rid of Hitler, German soldiers obeyed the order of the Nazi leaders to fight to the bitter end. The most desperate resistance was put up against the Russians, who, having liberated their own and neighboring countries from the Nazis, had crossed the German borders from the east. Only when American and Russian troops had joined in the center of Germany and Berlin was in flames did Hitler take his own life, only then did the country capitulate.

The Allies promptly turned their full force against Japan. The Japanese had already lost most of their previous conquests and been forced into a steady retreat on land and sea. Their fate was sealed when, in August 1945, the Americans dropped an atomic bomb, the first one ever used in war, on Hiroshima, destroying the town. Shortly thereafter, the Americans launched another such attack on Nagasaki. Simultaneously, the Russians entered the war against Japan, and the country was forced to surrender.

## End of World War II

No peace treaty was signed at the end of the war because the disagreements among the Allies multiplied during the last year of hostilities. In fact, they agreed unanimously on only one point: to destroy the power of Germany and Japan.

### *Occupation and Conferences*

Germany and Japan were occupied and governed by the victors. In Japan, this procedure was comparatively easy, for, though deprived of all overseas possessions, Japan's home territory was left intact, and the United States took charge of the administration. The situation was different in Germany, which was divided into four zones of occupation. Millions of inhabitants were driven out of their homes, and countless people perished. Workers were abducted, factories were dismantled, and production was brought to an almost complete standstill. A terrible famine resulted, and a cold winter added to the misery. Moral laws were ignored on all sides. No constructive plans for Germany's future existed, since the victors (Russia, England, and the United States) had failed to provide for them. In a conference at Teheran, in 1943, they had been concerned mainly with the conduct of the war. Early in 1945, when victory was in sight, they had planned, in a second conference held at Yalta, the division and occupation of Germany and a drastic reduction in its economic, industrial, and military power. During the summer of 1945, after Germany's capitulation, when a third conference was held at Potsdam, the task of determining a common future peace policy should have been undertaken. However, the Potsdam meeting disclosed fundamental disagreements between the democratic West and the Communist East. Russia had quickly established a Communist regime in eastern Germany, such as had already been established in Poland, Hungary, Rumania—in fact, wherever Soviet Russia maintained occupation troops. On the other hand, the Western Allies sought liberal-democratic forms of government, such as had been reestablished in Italy and in France, where General de Gaulle took over the reins of government. During the war, he had proved to be an unflinching leader of the resistance movement from outside of France, and he was a staunch defender of French independence *vis-à-vis* the Allies.

### The United Nations

The founding of a new world organization, the United Nations, was equally unable to foster cooperation. The United Nations was created to provide an international forum comparable to the defunct League of Nations and to organize humanitarian agencies concerned with economics, agriculture, health, and education. Like the League, however, it received no military or police force. Control over the organization was vested in a Security Council and a General Assembly, but the three principal victors in the war—England, Russia, and the United States—as well as France and China, were each given a veto power over decisions in the Council, a power that was subsequently often used.

### New Beginnings

The two world wars differed fundamentally in their causes, conduct, and consequences. In 1914, nations had been trapped in their diplomatic efforts and had backed into the war. World War II had been unilaterally provoked by the Fascist countries. Ideological differences had been slight before World War I, but they played a major role in the World War II era. Warfare was much more savage during the later conflict than the earlier one. Women and children of the victors and the vanquished alike were engulfed by the holocaust. Civilians and soldiers were equally involved, and little mercy was shown to prisoners by either side. Whole population groups were murdered. After the war, many statesmen, industrialists, military leaders, and other citizens in the defeated countries, those who were helpless tools as well as those who had willingly perpetrated atrocities, were tried and punished as criminals, as were large numbers of collaborators in France and other allied countries.

Nevertheless, World War II did not constitute so sharp a break in the course of history. The war of 1914 shattered the social and cultural patterns of the 19th century, a society based upon the ideas of enlightenment and dedicated to the aims of national freedom and progress under a capitalistic system dominated by the bourgeoisie. World War II brought no such social change. As part of the adjustment to the emerging new world, it left fewer gulfs and, except among some of the smaller countries, fewer permanent resentments. Moreover, it left Europe, if not all of Western civilization, weaker and with a deeper feeling of interdependence than had existed during the period following the Treaty of Versailles.

### Perspective

*Ten years after World War I and following the disruptions brought on by the Versailles Treaty, a worldwide depression set in. It led to fearful suffering for millions of people and forced adjustments upon the victors in regard to their economic demands. These adjustments came too late, however. The depression contributed to the expansion of Fascism from Italy to many parts of the continent, including Germany, where the National Socialists (Nazis) gained control. The Nazis immediately began rearming their country and eliminating all opponents. By so doing and by passing further social legislation, they succeeded in abolishing unemployment and thereby gained the support of businessmen and workers alike. Protective social legislation was also passed in the United States, and it too started on the road to recovery. The Communist world was less affected by the depression. Under a dictatorship that freely used police power, purges, and labor camps, the Soviets carried out the collectivization of agriculture and built up their industries. They too managed to strengthen their economy.*

*Depression and Fascism led, however, to war: first to civil war in Spain, then to a colonial war started by Italy, and finally—notwithstanding attempts at appeasing the dictators—to World War II. War brought early military victories to the Fascist powers. In the process, terrible new crimes were committed. The military position was reversed in 1941 when Germany attacked the Soviet Union, and the United States entered the war. The Fascist powers were defeated. After the United States exploded the first atomic bomb, Japan also fell. Italy, which had deserted its allies, was accepted as a "democracy" by the Western nations. Japan was stripped of both its early conquests and its military establishment. Germany was completely subdued, divided, occupied by the victors. It lost a quarter of its territory. A new international organization, the United Nations, was established by the victors.*

## Selected Readings

Arendt, Hannah. *The Origins of Totalitarianism* (New York: Harcourt, Brace & World 1966).
Carsten, F. L. *The Rise of Fascism* (Berkeley: University of California Press, 1980).
Clark, Martin. *Mussolini* (New York: Longman/Pearson, 2005).
Ellis, John. *Brute Force: Allied Strategy and Tactics in the Second World War* (New York: Viking, 1990).
Gilbert, Felix. *The End of the European Era, 1890 to the Present* (New York, Norton, 1991).
Joes, Anthony J. *The Rise of Fascism in the Contemporary World: Ideology, Evolution, Resurgence* (Boulder, Colo.: Westview Press, 1978).
Keegan, John. *The Second World War* (New York, Viking, 1990).
Kindleberger, Charles P. *The World in Depression, 1929–1939* (Berkeley: University of California Press, 1986).
Hitler, Adolf. *Mein Kampf* (Boston: Houghton Mifflin Company, 1971).
Marrus, Michael R. *The Holocaust in History* (Hanover, N.H.: Brandeis University Press, 1987).
Niewyk, Donald and Nicosia, Francis. *The Columbia Guide to the Holocaust* (New York: Columbia University Press, 2000).
Nolte, Enrest. *Three Faces of Fascism* (New York: The New American Library, Inc, 1969).
Rothwell, Victor. *The Origins of the Second World War* (New York: Palgrave, 2001).
Taylor, A. J. P. *The Origins of the Second World War* (London: Hamilton, 1961).
Thomas, Hugh. *The Spanish Civil War* (New York: Modern Library, 2001).
_____. *Armed Truce: The Beginnings of the Cold War, 1945–1946* (New York: Antheneum, 1987).
Thorne, Christopher. *Allies of a Kind: The United States, Britain and the War Against Japan, 1941-1945* (New York: Oxford University Press, 1978).
Ulam, Adam B. *A History of Soviet Russia* (New York: Praeger, 1976).

## Test Yourself

1. Included among the consequences of the Great Depression of 1929 was _____.
   A. The inability of farmers to find a market for their products
   B. Unemployment of millions of factory workers
   C. The crash of the New York Stock Exchange
   D. All of the above

2. The Italian Fascist regime in 1922 was led by _____.
   A. Mussolini
   B. Garibaldi
   C. Cavour
   D. Mazzini

3. In 1933, the Germans elected _____.
   A. Otto von Bismarck
   B. Adolph Hitler
   C. Oswald Spengler
   D. None of the above

4. The Spanish Civil War broke out in _____.
   A. 1931
   B. 1933
   C. 1936
   D. 1939

5. The American response to the Great Depression came in the form of a "New Deal" under the administration of _____.
   A. Calvin Coolidge
   B. Warren G. Harding
   C. Theodore Roosevelt
   D. Franklin D. Roosevelt

6. In 1936, a new constitution was adopted for the Soviet Union during which time the Union was composed of _____.
   A. Twenty Republics
   B. Thirteen Republics
   C. Fifteen Republics
   D. None of the above

7. The European powers appeased Germany in 1938 by surrendering the Sudetenland in Czechoslovakia in the treaty signed in the city of _____.
   A. Munich
   B. Berlin
   C. Moscow
   D. Frankfurt

8. World War II broke out in September 1939 with the German invasion of _____.
   A. Poland
   B. France
   C. Russia
   D. Belgium

## Answers and Explanations

1. **D.** By 1929, a depression had begun to develop in the Western economy. New industries were created, but older ones lost in importance. Ensuing unemployment brought a chain of reactions, inasmuch as even reduced production could no longer be absorbed, and further unemployment resulted. In October of 1929, the so-called crash on the New York Stock Exchange occurred, ruining many leading business enterprises. The close relationship between domestic business and foreign trade meant that a depression in any one country (especially the United States) inevitably affected all others—not excluding communist Russia, which was compelled to accept reduced prices for its exports. In 1931, the collapse of one of the great international banks, the Kreditanstalt in Vienna, intensified the downward turn of business in all countries. Most countries gave up the gold standard. Insecurity replaced complacency.

2. **A.** The Fascist leader Benito Mussolini established his regime in 1922.

3. **B.** In 1933, after repressive constitutional measures against the Nazis had proved to be useless, Adolph Hitler was entrusted with the formation of a government. He thus achieved power "legally." With the approval and assistance of some industrialists and the demoralized segments of the middle class and the proletariat who had suffered the consequences of Germany's defeat in 1918 and had been impoverished by inflation and depression, he substituted an authoritarian system for the national constitution.

4. **C.** Having failed to solve social as well as political problems, Rivera resigned in 1930. In the following year, the king, potentially an effective unifying influence for the country, was forced into exile. An election put into office a republican government (at first moderately liberal, later strongly socialistic), which aroused the bitter resistance of the conservatives by passing extensive anticlerical and anticapitalistic legislation. As a result, civil war broke out in 1936. In brutality, it was perhaps unequaled by any other modern war. Foreign interventionists soon participated—Communists, Fascists, and volunteers from democratic countries. For years, the triangular struggle raged among these three groups, until in 1939, Franco, leader of the. Falange, as the Spanish Fascists came to be known, emerged victorious. He achieved internal peace by rewarding his adherents and by crushing all opponents. His personal dictatorship solved few of Spain's domestic problems.

5. **D.** The influence of Fascist groups in the United States was kept at a negligible level, as social and economic changes similar to those in Europe were inaugurated during the New Deal administrations of Franklin D. Roosevelt. Social security laws were passed (such as those providing for old-age and unemployment insurance and minimum wages in industry); the gold standard was abandoned; debtors were granted a moratorium; huge government projects (e.g., the electrification of the Tennessee Valley) were undertaken; and some national planning was also attempted. Private enterprise and banking were brought under partial regulation by government, and thus a system of subsidies was used in order to influence the farmer's decisions regarding the types of crops and the acreage to be planted. Agriculture began to recover.

6. **B.** In 1936, a new constitution was adopted in the Soviet Union. By then, the nation consisted of 13 republics, each enjoying local autonomy, but subject to central political direction and central economic planning. The executive power remained in the hands of the Politburo, with Stalin at its head. Civil rights were formally extended to all Russians; thus after twenty years of discrimination, constitutional inequities directed against various "bourgeois" groups of the population were abolished.

7. A. Unprepared for war, even though the Spanish Civil War had served as a proving ground for weapons, the Western powers agreed to a series of conferences, and at Munich in 1938, they handed the Sudetenland over to Hitler. The Soviet Union, though affected by whatever position France and England would take, had not even been invited, and the French alliance system in the east thus collapsed.

8. A. The policy of appeasement was discarded, and no additional concessions were promised to Hitler, not even when, in August, the conclusion of a trade and nonaggression pact between Germany and the Soviet Union was suddenly announced, and the pro-Western diplomat, Maxim Litvinov, was replaced by the anti-Western, Vyacheslav Molotov, as Soviet foreign minister. The pact ended all hopes for collective security. In September, German armies marched into Poland. World War II had begun.

## CHAPTER 23
# The Postwar Era (1947-1967)

**1947** Marshall Plan for economic rehabilitation of Europe
India becomes independent from the British and is divided
**1948** Berlin blockade
State of Israel founded
Independence of Ireland
**1949** Triumph of communists in China
Establishment of a West German republic
**1950** Outbreak of Korean War
Schumann Plan for European steel and coal production
**1953** Death of Stalin
**1955** Germany enters NATO
**1956** Suez Canal nationalized by Egypt
Abortive invasion by England, France, Israel
**1957** First earth satellite *(Sputnik)* launched
**1961** Construction of Berlin Wall
**1962** Independence of Algeria
**1966** Vietnam War begins
**1967** Arab-Israeli War
Israel occupies Sinai Peninsula, Golan Heights, West Bank, Gaza, and East Jerusalem
**1975** Vietnam War ends

*In Western civilization, three trends, which had developed to some extent after World War I, rapidly gained headway after World War II. These trends included the use of mechanization in production and everyday living, the growing equalization of social classes, and the decline of Europe's power and prestige in international affairs. Human society—though still divided into classes, nations, and "two worlds" with opposing ideologies—was moving in the direction of one interrelated, interdependent world.*

## ■ INTELLECTUAL AND CULTURAL DEVELOPMENTS

Since the end of World War II, the West has devoted itself increasingly to science and technology and has achieved remarkable progress in these fields. There has been a growing realization that, contrary to the hopes of the ages of Enlightenment and Liberalism, "progress," though undeniable in material achievements, does not necessarily encompass the moral side of humanity. Preoccupation with personal "security" has acted as a check on original thought and has led to conservatism and the desire for conformity. This has been true for the Communist as well as the democratic nations of the world, both of which have sought to maintain the status quo, regardless of its manifold shortcomings.

## Science

Wars have always stimulated science and technology. Danger has always forced people to develop tools and processes that could save their lives and preserve their freedom. Insights into the mechanics of nature gained during war have furthered the progress of science in times of peace. World War II was no exception. Radar, rockets, and atomic fission were developed for military purposes in the period between 1939 and 1945. Afterward, they became important for peacetime use. Aviation in particular was greatly advanced during the war. Whereas, in 1927, Lindbergh made his lonely, first transatlantic flight to Paris, 25 years later, when the war was over, tens of millions of passengers were crossing continents and oceans by airplane each year. Countries of vast expanse and poor transportation systems, like Brazil, could now plan to skip the "railroad age" and immediately enter the "pair age."

In the fields of chemistry and nuclear physics, discoveries made under pressure of war by both victors and vanquished were exploited to serve new peaceful purposes. With the help of newly discovered vaccines and drugs, the effects of many diseases, including pneumonia, tuberculosis, and infantile paralysis, could be diminished. Nations increasingly put their faith in scientists to solve their problems. The Soviet Union trained scientists by the hundreds of thousands, and the United States showed an unaccustomed appreciation of pure science and mathematics, fields in which the country had long relied upon the work of Europeans. Wartime experiences had an effect on production methods. Automation—that is, the mechanization of industrial processes that had previously required supervision by human hands and minds—was introduced in large enterprises. Machines were used to replace technical, clerical, and even scientific personnel.

## Religion and Philosophy

After World War II, the memory of the horrors and uncertainties of war had the apparent effect of impelling humanity to intensify its search for security and comfort. Fearful of the dangers inherent in the growing mastery of natural forces—the development of atomic weapons, for instance—and disturbed by the use of such subtle physiological and psychological weapons as propaganda, indoctrination, and mental persuasion, many people turned anew to the consolations of religion. The consequent religious renaissance brought about a renewed emphasis on dogma, as seen in the spread of Neo-Orthodox beliefs. This led to the acceptance of long-submerged ecumenical ideas that promoted cooperation among the various faiths, and it caused a revival of religious experience in the Soviet Union, where the government eased its hostility toward church organizations and tolerated the extension of their activities. The revival embraced the older generation as well as younger people who had been brought up in a materialistic atmosphere.

In the face of invigorated religious trends and the growing realization of "puncertainty" in many of the conclusions to which the scientific ccommunity arrived, the positivist tradition lost some of its appeal. Logical positivism (or logical empiricism) continued to promote its faith in science as the only dependable source of knowledge and as an effective basis for solving social problems. It encountered growing competition from existentialism, however, which constituted a major new philosophical influence after World War II. Fearful of the dehumanizing effect of the Modern Age, existentialists affirmed the importance of the individual. They insisted that humans are not just "objects" to be described scientifically; they are "existing subjects." People gain authentic existence and knowledge of themselves through exercising their freedom. Existentialists emphasized the fact that each human being must realize and then resolutely face the inherent perils and predicaments of life.

### Education

In accordance with postwar political and scientific demands, new goals were established for education. A basic objective was to develop the character of children along the lines accepted by society. They were to become "well adjusted"—to a Communist, democratic, or Fascist society, the system within which they grew up. Society and its needs were stressed, as opposed to individualism and its demands. Therefore, the equalization of educational opportunity and aims was necessary.

Most governments, national and local, took a larger part than ever before in the conduct of education. They claimed more of the children's time, directed education toward natural and "social" (or politico-economic) sciences, and to an increasing extent, replaced the family and other educational agencies. National governments sponsored extensive programs of adult education and even assumed the task of "re-educating" entire nations. To promote their ideologies and policies, governments, particularly in the West, also carried on a large-scale exchange of students and scholars.

### Literature and Fine Arts

In literature and the fine arts, generalizations about the merits of what was created in the post–World War II period may well be premature. World War I marked the end of an age in Western civilization. Authors and artists in the 1920s had entered upon a new age and had used great artistic and social problems as their themes. New issues of similar dimensions did not appear in the 1940s or 1950s, nor did artists face a challenge like the preceding postwar periods had posed. Solid work was done by humanistic scholars, who were inclined to turn their attention more to historical and social aspects than to the aesthetic. Growing numbers of painters, musicians, and architects achieved much, but, to a large extent, Western people lived on their great cultural heritage, which they cultivated with care.

## ■ ECONOMIC, SOCIAL, AND POLITICAL DEVELOPMENTS

The dominating issue on the international stage was the rivalry between the United States and the Soviet Union. This rivalry was reflected first in the failure to reach a German settlement, then in a struggle over Communist penetration of other European nations, and eventually over influence in the Far East, the Middle East, and Africa. It embraced political, economic, cultural, and military issues. Its intensity shifted with temporary conditions and long-range developments over which the rivals themselves had no control. Thus, it depended upon factors such as the rapidly rising population figures in Europe and in other areas.

Unemployment along prewar lines did not reappear, despite the population surge and despite the fact that, within a decade, consumer goods were, at least in the Western countries, abundant again. Soon, production totals surpassed the highest prewar figures, even in the defeated nations, making possible improvements in their prewar living standards. Whether a better understanding of economic processes or more extensive state planning was the reason, a prolonged period of economic growth began.

### Postwar Economic Situation

The victors had planned to provide for the rebuilding of their own national economies and for the permanent economic subjugation of Germany. This plan was initiated by dismantling German industries; expropriating German ships, freight cars, locomotives, and other rolling stock; by seizing of its patents and production secrets; and by the forced recruitment of scientists, laborers, and prisoners into the service of the victors. For more than a year after the cessation of hostilities, this additional source of suffering impacted Germany without providing appropriate benefit to the victors. At this juncture, there was a drastic change in the relationship between the victorious and the defeated nations.

## Rebuilding the Western Economy

By 1947, it was clear that the intense struggle between the Communist East and the democratic West required a new approach to the task of rebuilding the Western economy. The United States took the initiative. During the war, it had outlined programs in various conferences at Dumbarton Oaks and Bretton Woods. Subsequently, the International Monetary Fund and International Bank for Reconstruction were founded, and preparations were made for the reduction of tariff barriers. The trend toward replacing national regulations with international rules grew stronger. Moreover, the nation had quickly "returned to normalcy" after the war. Rationing had been abolished, farm incomes had risen, a measure of controlled inflation had increased prices and wages, and a feeling of confidence and new incentives for greater production and broader employment were created. Successful restructuring of production facilities made it possible for the United States to propose, in 1947, the Marshall Plan, named after the American secretary of state. This made financial aid available to European countries. Ideological, humanitarian, and economic purposes were simultaneously served. England and France received most of the aid. To prevent impoverished peoples from falling prey to Communist doctrines, help was extended also to other Western nations, including former enemies. This program enabled almost all the European democracies to rebuild their production systems within a decade. By the mid-1950s, their economies flourished as never before. Germany, though deprived of the industries in its eastern zones, nevertheless regained its position as the leading industrial power of Europe through an effort that later became known as *Wirtschaftswunder* (economic miracle). Italy was also on the road toward economic recovery and stability.

## Rebuilding the Eastern Economy

In the East, Russia took the lead. New Five-Year Plans were drafted and coordinated with the industrial plans of regions controlled directly or indirectly by the Soviet Union. Important new centers of industry in Siberia, which had been built with the labor of Stalin's victims and which had benefited when factories were moved east during the war, proved now to be a major asset. Production in heavy industries increased rapidly. Within less than a decade, the Soviet Union attained the rank of second-largest industrial power in the world, surpassed only by the United States. It was thereby enabled to export surplus goods and to make investments abroad. However, since substantial amounts of labor were needed to create the production apparatus, little could be done to develop the industries manufacturing goods for civilian consumption. Consequently, standards of living remained at a low level. In agriculture, productivity did not increase adequately, and new experiments with collective farms, which were combined into larger units, did not bring the desired results.

## The Political Situation

Political readjustment came more slowly than economic recovery. No final war settlement was achieved, and no all-inclusive peace treaty negotiated.

## Eastern Europe

Russia enlarged its territories by incorporating parts of Finland, Poland, Germany, and Rumania. The formerly independent Baltic states, which Yalta and Potsdam kept in Soviet hands, were forced to remain within the jurisdiction of the USSR. Bolshevik governments were established in Poland and in occupied Balkan countries, and all were bound closely to Russia. Eastern Germany was assigned to Polish administration, and its inhabitants driven out, while Poles were settled there. In 1945, Czechoslovakia was reconstituted under a democratic government, with her borders approximately the same as those of 1937, and the Germans living there were brutally expelled. The democratic government was, however, overthrown in 1948 and replaced by a Communist regime closely allied to the Soviet Union. A special role in

*Figure 23–1 The United States and the Soviet Union and their Alliance systems during the Cold War*

world affairs was played by Yugoslavia under the leadership of Josip Broz Tito. During the war, Tito had directed the fight against the Nazis and insisted on independent policies. "Titoism" revealed tensions and dissensions among the Communist powers. Tito rejected the right of the Soviet Union to dictate policies to other Communist nations—notwithstanding the fact that Marxism had preached the identity of the interests of the workers in all countries, and the Soviet Union had previously been considered the leader and spokesman of true Marxism.

### Central and Western Europe

In the center of Europe, Germany—except for Polish-occupied territories—was divided: first into four zones, later into two. The latter zones became separate German states, a Western and an Eastern republic, both of which within a decade achieved virtual sovereignty, though each remained politically affiliated with its original occupying powers. This enforced duality reflected a continued shrinkage of the area of Western civilization and tradition, and it symbolized the division of the world into Eastern Communist and Western democratic areas. Austria was reestablished as a small, and eventually independent, nation—a neutral buffer between East and West. Italy regained most of its former European territories, but had to accord a measure of autonomy to the German population under its control, as well as to Sicily.

The other Western countries underwent no drastic territorial changes. Belgium, the Netherlands, and Luxembourg combined in a common customs area (Benelux) to obtain mutually beneficial trade advantages. Western Germany, France, and Benelux, with the blessing of the United States, formed a "coal and steel community," which provided for predetermined production quotas, a common market, and the elimination of tariff barriers for these products. Plans for a broader customs union, possibly including Great Britain, were formulated.

A "Council of Europe," constituting a consultative assembly of the Western European nations, was established in Strasbourg, at the very border between Germany and France. A bank to ease mutual convertibility of European funds and currencies was founded. Plans were made by the member states for cooperative atomic research and exploitation of atomic energy. Even though a unified military force was not organized, a military alliance joining the United States and England to the Continent was concluded in 1949. This alliance (the North Atlantic Treaty Organization, or NATO) had a central headquarters and an American supreme commander. As a whole, the idea of European unity made considerable progress. Cultural contacts and exchanges were augmented by political cooperation.

### United States

In the United States, the political impact of World War II was felt much more than that of World War I. A spirit of isolationism did not arise in the United States, as it did after 1918. Instead, the country took a leading role in almost all international decisions. Not only European countries, but former European colonies also came to be of concern.

The members of the British Empire, especially Canada and Australia, oriented themselves increasingly toward the United States. Economically weakened countries appealed to the United States and received aid designed to prevent them from turning to Communist Russia. Military bases were installed in France, England, Germany, Spain, Turkey, and other European countries, as well as in Asia and the Arctic and Antarctic. New treaties were made with Latin American nations, which were granted financial aid for economic development. Extensive programs for the exchange of teachers and students were inaugurated, and the unprecedented scale of travel of Americans abroad helped to establish numerous relationships with the Western nations.

### Colonial Areas

World War II accelerated the decline of colonialism. After Japan's defeat, China gained control over most of its former territories, including Western-held Shanghai and Russian-dominated Manchuria. Indochina rebelled against and eventually defeated France, which lost more than half of its former colony. A complete end to French rule came in 1954. Rebellious Indonesia separated from Holland and became an independent state. The United States granted independence to the Philippines. England granted statehood to the Gold Coast in Africa. India finally succeeded in bringing Gandhi's fight for freedom to a successful conclusion and abolished British rule. Though staying formally within the Commonwealth, it built a republic that envisioned neutrality in the East-West struggle.

Iran quarreled with the European powers over the possession and management of its oil industries and forced substantial concessions upon the Western owners. Arab states likewise asserted their independence in the conduct of their foreign policies and obtained a greater share of the profits from their oil. The people of Cyprus rose against England, as did native tribes in Africa. Egypt forced the British to withdraw military forces from the Suez Canal and nationalized the Canal Company in 1956 in order to use its revenue to build the Aswan High Dam. This led to an Anglo-Franco invasion, which, due to American and Russian opposition, failed to achieve its objectives, which included the toppling of the Egyptian regime of President Nasser. Within a few months, the invading forces had to be withdrawn, and Egypt's Nasser emerged with major political victory. A particularly bloody struggle occurred in France's North African possessions when the Arabs in Tunisia and Algeria rebelled. Tunisia gained especially far-reaching concessions and its independence in 1956. Shortly after, Algeria gained its independence in 1962.

The struggle was sharpened by the fact that, in 1948, a Jewish state, Israel, had been established in Palestine. As early as 1917, the Jews had been promised a homeland in Palestine by the British. After Hitler's persecutions and World War II had demonstrated the urgency of finding a refuge for Jews, the United Nations proposed the partition of Palestine into two states in 1947. This led to Israel's emergence.

*Figure 23–2  U.N. Partition of Palestine in Arab and Jewish States, 1947*

The establishment of Israel roused bitter resentment among all Arabs. Intermittent border clashes threatened the peace of the entire West.

    On the whole, the revolt of Asia and the culturally advanced areas of Africa was the result of the successful Westernization of former colonial regions. European ideologies of democracy and communism, European sciences, medicine, and technology, European habits, dress, and living modes, and European-born nationalism had penetrated to all parts of the world. The time was approaching when they were no longer needed. The division of the Western world into democratic and Communist segments gave the former colonies the opportunity to assert their independence. Eventually, there were more than 150 member states of the United Nations instead of the original fifty.

## Governmental Institutions and Ideologies

No new political ideology was developed as a result of World War II. Fascism in its extreme form was abolished, though not entirely eradicated.

Fascist regimes continued to function in countries such as Spain. Fascism was even introduced in a few other countries, such as Argentina, where Juan Perlin held power until 1955. Fascist principles also found their way into some of the democratic countries. In France and even in the United States, there was some fear that certain fascist tendencies might gain headway.

Communism continued in most of Eastern Europe. In Russia, where the enforcement of Communist doctrines had to be relaxed during the war so they would not interfere with the war effort, the government resumed the drastic application of its socialistic policies. Devaluation of the currency deprived people who had accumulated profits of their gains. Land that the peasants had taken from collective farms and used for private gardens had to be returned. Writers and scientists were compelled to follow strictly the party line.

Outside of the Soviet Union, Communism did not win the allegiance of Europe after the end of World War II, despite the widespread impoverishment and Russia's prestige as one of the principal victors. Except for Czechoslovakia, European countries did not establish a Communist government unless they were occupied by Russian military forces. Only in Asia, notably in China, did Communism spread under native leadership.

Democracy continued to be the predominant form of government in the Western countries. Democratic types of government were reintroduced in West Germany and Italy. Most democratic institutions, however, were affected by socialist ideas. In the United States, social reforms that had been assailed as "creeping socialism" in the 1930s were now accepted as a matter of course in the postwar period. Labor unions grew in influence, and employers had to make ever-increasing concessions to their workers.

In England, the Labor party, which came to power immediately after the war, socialized the steel and coal industries, nationalized the railways, and introduced a most comprehensive public health program. Subsequent conservative governments could not abandon all the new programs of socialization and reform, although they did prevent the nationalization of the steel industry. In West Germany, where a strong democratic government took office, socialists constituted the largest opposition group in the diet. Workers in the great coal and steel industries gained the right to share with owners in the functions of management.

In France and Italy, democratic governments remained in control, but they faced grave difficulties, owing to the opposition of socialists who followed a communist line on many issues. The French and Italian communists, instead of functioning as a loyal opposition within a democratic system, attempted to disrupt the governments and to swing their countries into the Soviet orbit. In the smaller Western nations—Scandinavia, the Netherlands, and Austria—moderate socialist trends prevailed. Here government seemed to be working toward the eventual consummation of many socialist ideals within a capitalist society.

## The United Nations

Persistent nationalism and the ideological conflict between East and West prevented any significant progress toward a world government. As the League of Nations had done after World War I, the United Nations provided an international forum for world opinion, and its sub-agencies accomplished a great deal in certain fields, such as economic affairs and education. In the political sphere, however, it fell far short of its goals. The veto power of a few large nations forestalled decisions on various important issues. Two of the five great nations—Russia and France—at one time or another resorted to boycotts. A third one, China, found itself represented by men who belonged to a regime ousted from China proper and holding no more than Formosa (Taiwan) and a few smaller islands. Neither West nor East Germany, despite their economic importance, became a member of the world organization. Small countries such as Holland and Israel refused to obey certain decisions of the United Nations. Disarmament issues, especially those involving atomic weapons, could not be agreed upon in the United Nations forum. As before, diplomatic action outside the United Nations was necessary to handle all important questions. Thus, traditional patterns for international negotiations were perpetuated.

## Postwar Crises

Under such circumstances, numerous international crises developed. The first major difficulty arose in 1948 when the Russians cut off the city of Berlin from land contact with the West. Supplies and personnel were transported to and from the city by air until the Soviet blockade ended.

In 1950, another major crisis arose when Communists in North Korea invaded South Korea, which had been under American control. This time war resulted. Various members of the United Nations, including the United States, participated on the South Korean side, while North Korea had the material and economic support of Russia and active military help from Communist China. This conflict, entailing heavy casualties on both sides, led to an uneasy truce, whereby the country was divided into two sections: a Communist state and a Western-supported one. Hardly had hostilities ended than a similar war developed in French Indochina, which led to a parallel result. The North became Communist and separate, while the South gained considerable independence from France, but remained in the Western camp.

In the meantime, crises developed in other regions: in Iran, over its decision to nationalize the foreign oil companies there; in the Middle East, over the Suez Canal and the conflict between Syria and Israel; and in North Africa over the question of freedom from French dominion. Behind all these issues loomed the greater struggle: the "cold" war between the Western democracies under American leadership and the Eastern communist nations under Russian leadership. Both sides built up their military potential and acquired vast stocks of atomic bombs and weapons. While they avoided an open break, they waged a bitter struggle over the allegiance of the "neutral" areas, such as India, Iran, and the Arab states, and of the colonies, where Russia had become a factor by aiding indigenous national movements.

## Coexistence and New Conflict

Stalin died in 1953. During his administration, he had concentrated upon the reconstruction of the Soviet Union so that it became the second greatest industrial power of the world, and he had preserved the Communist institutions of the nation. He had imposed his will on scholars, scientists, artists, and the masses of the Russian people. Under his regime, Soviet scientists made enormous advances, including discoveries in the fields of atomic energy and guided missiles, but because of his arbitrary and dictatorial ways, he had alienated even close collaborators. Owing to his ruthlessness and guile, he had forfeited the confidence of his European allies and aroused misgivings among even the Communists of other nations.

Stalin's death, therefore, marked a turning point—especially since dissension among his political heirs introduced a further element of weakness into the position of the Soviet Union. Promptly, the Russian policy of the Cold War was modified. Friendly words were addressed to the West. Amnesties were proclaimed in Russia, and travel restrictions were eased. A meeting between Eastern and Western statesmen at Geneva in 1955 seemed to herald an era of "peaceful coexistence." The Cold War proved not to have ended, but to have entered a new stage, however, when Stalin's successors consolidated their position after their sudden denunciation of Stalin's personal dictatorship. Practical concessions were few. Although the Soviet Union agreed to a peace with Austria and established diplomatic relations with West Germany, no progress was made in regard to the crucial problem of German reunification. Soviet disagreements with Tito's Yugoslavia were temporarily settled, but Soviet control of its satellites was not yielded, despite revolts in East Germany, Poland, and Hungary.

Western nations were invited to establish closer ties with the Communist world, especially in the economic field. Nevertheless, opposition to their policies was invariably encouraged.

On the positive side, open hostilities were avoided. In 1956, the cause of world peace was imperiled by events such as Anglo-French aggression in Egypt and the brutal Russian suppression of a revolt in Hungary. Other crises occurred in the following years. In 1958, the overthrow of the monarchy in the Arab state of Iraq threatened the political and economic position of the Western powers in the Middle East and the safety of their oil interests there. Uprisings in the African Congo followed upon the withdrawal of the Belgians in 1960 and the establishment of an independent nation there. Communists attacked Laos in 1961. Indian aggression took place in Portuguese Goa. In particular, the Soviet Union persistently refused to agree to supervised reduction of atomic armaments and attempted to force the Western powers to give up their position in Berlin. In 1961, the Communists built a wall through the center of Berlin with the purpose of further hindering East-West contacts and preventing Germans living in the eastern parts of the country from fleeing to the West, depriving their economy of competent workers.

The United Nations, challenged in its undertakings by its own members, lost more and more of its prestige and usefulness. Atomic testing was resumed in 1962, and new dissensions arose from continued Soviet demands with regard to Berlin, from simmering warfare in Laos and Vietnam, and ultimately from Soviet arms deliveries to Cuba. Only Western firmness in the face of this last challenge and the subsequent Soviet withdrawal, quickened perhaps by fears of a growing rift within the Communist world between China and the Soviet Union, led to a certain easing of the international tension. In 1963, there was a tentative agreement on suspension of testing of atomic weapons and to an increase in East-West trade.

## ■ NEW CHALLENGES

By the mid-1960s, many of the hopes held by the generation that had fought the two world wars were not realized, although in some ways, progress in that direction had been made. As always in the course of human affairs, the changes that had been brought about had created a new situation in which old solutions no longer served. New problems, too, had arisen, which demanded a new response and a fresh start.

### A Young Generation

By the mid 1960s, a generation had grown up that had lived through neither depression nor World War II. The old issue of Capitalist-Communist ideological rivalry had lost much of its meaning for this generation. Russian Communism had become more liberal, capitalistic, and ultra-nationalistic, Western capitalism more socialistic and authoritarian. The Soviet hold on its satellite countries had weakened, while United States leadership was challenged by France under President de Gaulle, as well as subsequently by Germany, England, and, despite the economic and military aid given to them, by Asian and African nations.

These political issues faced by the young generation were enhanced by economic and cultural changes. By 1967, the "economic miracles" of the postwar period had apparently come to an end. Rivalries over markets, problems of inflation and stability of currencies, especially the dollar and the pound, and struggles over tariffs reappeared. Subtly, power had begun to slip from the hands of leaders and their bureaucracies into those of small groups of scientifically trained experts—the technologists and economists who advised governments. A barrage of propaganda and advertising, seeking to hammer in ideas or sell goods, sought in vain to convince a new generation of the desirability of the status quo. Witnessing persisting social, national, and racial inequalities, continuing war preparations, and the depersonalization of society through technological advances, this young generation began to challenge prevailing morality, reject hypocrisy, and attack materialism and pragmatism.

### Demography

The outstanding event of the post–World War II period was the enormous population increase, not only in countries where, until then, lack of medical knowledge and care had checked population growth, but also among the highly developed countries. Once more the question posed by Malthus at the end of the 18th century—whether population increases would outstrip the available food supply—was raised. To meet the issue, a twofold attack was begun. To serve immediate needs, new scientific methods for improving agriculture were developed. Food grown in advanced countries was distributed to hungry populations, and technical knowledge was disseminated so that disadvantaged countries would be able to increase their own production. To provide a long-term solution, steps were taken to control birth rates, which were especially high in Latin America. Even governments and churches, traditionally opposed to such measures, began to support controls, reflecting a change in fundamental Western attitudes. A decrease in the birth rate, at least in the advanced countries, was noted by 1966.

## Science

Scientific progress made enormous advances. Physics, biology, chemistry, medicine, and astronomy, while revealing many complexities, also brought discoveries that involved increasingly difficult scientific and ethical problems. The discovery of the genetic code (DNA) by Crick and Watson in 1960 had revolutionary consequences in many areas outside of medicine and biogenetics because it created problems that could threaten human survival. New and hazardous chemical products were developed for use in agriculture.

Traditional products were replaced in the textile and building industries. Space travel opened possibilities for studies that could not be done successfully on earth, for weather forecasting, and for a better understanding of origin, shape, and conditions in the universe. Most of the discoveries could also be put to use for the perfection of destructive weaponry. Boundaries between these fields were difficult to draw. Scientific thinking also permeated social fields such as economics, psychology, history, and philosophy. A fundamental approach to quantification, often relying on mathematical studies and the help of statistical methods and computer sciences, was applied to these subjects. New machinery speeded up the process of obtaining solutions to problems and made obsolete the work of even skilled personnel. Computers became part of daily life, and computer science part of school curricula.

## Economy

The effect of technological evolution was felt when dealing with daily practical problems, as well as when considering long-term cultural trends. Production methods were as much affected as general social conditions.

### Industry

A steady growth of industrial productivity occurred. In competition with each other, the Soviet Union and the West helped spread industrialization—with all its consequences—to the underdeveloped countries. In continental Europe, owing to mutual assistance and cooperation, the Treaty of Rome in 1957 had created a Common Market of seven leading industrial nations, and these Common Market countries showed high rates of economic growth, at least for a decade. This stimulated ideas of a Common Market organization in Latin America as well. The unemployment of prewar years was replaced by an employment shortage in many trades, especially in areas of technological services. Significantly, this occurred despite the progress of automation in industry. Apparently, it was made possible by state economic planning, which did not reject deficit financing and which did provide for constant and coordinated economic growth in the sectors of production, wages, and prices.

Social security was steadily extended. While this policy heightened the dangers of monetary inflation, currency regulations diminished and tariffs were lowered. These developments were accompanied by general prosperity and a rapid rise in living standards in Western Europe and the United States. In the Soviet Union, challenged not only by Western skills but also by Communist China, which by 1965 had succeeded in producing its own atomic weapons, special attention was paid to the rapid refinement of industrial processes. Marked advances in space technology enabled the Soviet Union to launch the first space satellite *(Sputnik)* in 1957, and in 1961, they were the first to put a human being into orbit around the earth. In 1966, they achieved a "soft" missile landing on the moon. Yet, notwithstanding all achievements, living standards were not correspondingly improved because of the inefficiency of the entire system. Other countries, notably the United States, were also making great strides in space exploration.

### *Agriculture*
Outwardly less spectacular, but equally fundamental, were the changes in agriculture. Agricultural organization, whether of the nature of collective farms in Communist-ruled areas or individually owned farms in the West, moved toward consolidation of landholdings and the abolition of small farms. The peasantry as a class began to merge with the middle class. Production was influenced, if not directed, by government policies, price supports, setting of standards, international agreements, and mechanization in all sectors. In the West, these measures brought overproduction, despite a rapid population increase, and only the distribution of surplus products to underdeveloped parts of the world remained a serious challenge.

### Education
Modified and sophisticated production methods and the resulting social transformation required radical adjustments in education. The demand for unskilled laborers, who had made up the proletariat, declined, and their children swelled the ranks of the middle class because office workers were needed to operate the vast bureaucracies, as were technicians. For all these positions, training was required. Compulsory education was therefore extended. Universities, often teaching specialized knowledge, had to adjust to the influx of overwhelming numbers of students. For the few creative thinkers, the establishment of additional institutes became ever more urgent. The results were rewarding. Medical advances lengthened life expectancies, and many diseases were successfully treated. Studies of genetics and astronomy, of the weather, and of human behavior patterns, were promoted, and economic and historical scholarship profited thereby. An intellectual approach, often using mathematical methods, helped solve formerly unsolvable problems. Engineering benefited especially. An expanded media—a superabundance of paperback books and pictorial magazines, films, radio, and television—spread knowledge and entertainment, and scientific journals proliferated.

### Individualism
In a world so dependent on intricate scientific methods and technology and so subject to mass production and mass domination, the individual encountered ever greater difficulties in maintaining individuality and escaping the pressures of society with its set of values and tastes. Workers in factories, on the land, in the universities, and in research were dependent on others and had to pool their knowledge or skills, and much individual effort was absorbed by collective projects. Even the creative arts—architecture, literature, music—were affected. Tastes tended toward equalization. Mass-communication media—newspapers, films, and television—set the tone. Sociological aspects rather than problems of the individual fascinated the writer and the historian. Theater and musical concerts, as well as other artistic or scientific programs, usually funded by public and private support, envisaged "educational" effects upon the masses. Urban living and urbanization, whether in cities or suburbs, or in settlements erected uniformly by builders, contributed to the equalization trends, as did government policies in both capitalist and Communist countries. Perhaps as a reaction, abstract tendencies in painting and music, early medieval and Byzantine studies in history, Zen and other Oriental religions, gained the interest of those who tried to remain outside the collective pattern. Although, in the mid-60s, a certain rejection of abstract art was noticeable, the protest continued by a younger generation parallel to the *jeunesse doree* of Revolutionary France, which insisted on defying tradition in sexual behavior, dress, and taste.

## Nationalism

Not only the individual man or woman, but also the individual nation found itself exposed to the impact of new attitudes and economic forces.

### *Trends Toward International Organization*

While nationalism (in the sense in which it had developed in the Western world) was still increasing in areas where earlier colonial domination had hindered its growth, it began to wane among Western nations. The emphasis on national boundaries and on closed national economic units disappeared, as seen in the coordination of foreign policies, the pooling of armed forces (witness NATO and the Warsaw Pact), the partial disappearance of economic borders and customs barriers, mutual currency policies, the institution of common scientific projects, the easing of passport regulations, and increased tourism and exchange of labor forces. The division of Germany, the disintegration of the British Empire (in 1961 a dominion, South Africa, and in 1965 a colony, Rhodesia, left the Commonwealth), and the separation of Algeria from France in 1962 did not disturb the core of these leading nations, as would have happened only a few decades earlier. The European Common Market, under French-German leadership, became, despite attacks, a working reality. Communist Eastern Europe, through an emphasis on interdependence among its members, likewise contributed its share to the progressive decline of an older type of nationalism. Even such an institution as the Catholic Church felt the impact of the more cosmopolitan trends. In an ecumenical council convened by Pope John XXIII in 1961, and held in the Vatican (Vatican II) and lasting until 1965, rules were passed to "update" Church life, adjust to modern patterns, and ease long-existing antagonisms between Catholics and other Christian churches, as well as Eastern religions, Jews, and Arabs.

### *Trends Toward a Revival of Nationalism*

As the two world wars receded further into history, an opposite movement reappeared. In France, where a fifth republic with vast powers for its president, de Gaulle, was instituted in 1958, nationalism resurged. Appealing to the old concepts of "national sovereignty," de Gaulle insisted on completely independent rights for his country and did not hesitate to weaken such cooperative institutions as the Common Market or NATO, which the Western world had created in response to the bitter lesson of the world wars. Struggling England tried to keep alive ideas of its "special" position and was hesitant to enter a European community in which it could play no privileged role. Italy, ignoring its Fascist past, applauded nationalist aims.

In the Communist orbit, Yugoslavia under Tito pursued policies of national self-interest. By 1966, Rumania, Bulgaria, Poland, and Hungary also began to assert their national interests and to struggle for emancipation from Soviet domination. In defeated Germany, surrounded by increasingly nationalistic sentiments, national consciousness was ever more strongly reaffirmed despite the resolute support of all forms of European and transatlantic cooperation. The United States was no less concerned with the national question. Its bitter war in Vietnam, fought against native socialist forces supported by Communist China, involved to some extent national prestige and honor. By 1966, the Vietnam War constituted, indeed, the foremost international problem. Nationalism contributed also to the rift between the socialist worlds of Russia and China, and it threatened the peace in India, Pakistan, Indonesia, Malaysia, the Arab states, and in various parts of Africa.

## Democracy

The meaning of the term "democracy" changed. Communist countries used the word in a sense entirely opposed to that in Western countries. The latter, while holding on to the theories of the Age of Enlightenment, gave democracy in practice an entirely new content. Democratic forms taken over from

Anglo-Saxon countries—with free elections and powerful popular representative assemblies, with systems of checks and balances protecting the "rights of man," including the right of private property—were maintained in the West and the countries adhering to Western ideas. Democratic forms belittling these concepts and stressing a classless society, subordination of the individual to the common good, economic equality, and the conduct of affairs by a government and single party organization representative of the interests of all the workers in society were continued in the East and its dependencies.

Everywhere, "leadership," if not in the extreme form of Nazi patterns, was extolled. In Russia, the leadership principle predominated at least until 1964, during Nikita Khrushchev's premiership, which followed a two-year struggle for power after Stalin's death. In Germany, Chancellor Konrad Adenauer, who worked within a democratic framework, provided vigorous and capable leadership from 1954 to 1964. Between 1958 and 1969, France was led by Charles de Gaulle under a constitution that gave extensive powers to the president. The United States, where racial unrest threatened the traditional democratic fabric, looked to steadily enhanced authority, influence, and direction by its presidents. In Cuba, a Communist-supported leader, Fidel Castro, made himself the spokesman of democratic and national forces. Leadership rather than liberal democratic patterns was accepted also by new African nations, while army dictatorships either survived, or were reintroduced, in Brazil and some Central American nations. Threatened by totalitarian patterns, a changed democracy struggled to preserve for the individual those fundamental freedoms for which Western civilization had striven for centuries.

## Perspective

*The aftermath of World War II brought great advances in the natural sciences. The discovery of the genetic code (DNA) and discoveries in medicine, space exploration, cosmology, chemistry, and biology opened possibilities for fundamental developments. The world thus had the potential for vastly improving the quality of life, as well as destroying it utterly. Special attention was paid to education. Emphasis was placed less on the development of outstanding individuals than on an awareness of the individual's responsibilities as a member of society.*

*The economies of all countries improved rapidly, due to American generosity and cooperation and the determination of the European nations to strengthen their common interests through a Common Market. Governmental influence and interference increased everywhere. Recognizing that the interdependence of nations and people was steadily developing, various international organizations were founded to promote trade and cooperation in international questions.*

*Nevertheless, nationalism remained strong. Ethnic conflicts brought warfare and persecution. Uprisings occurred in former colonies and dominions until these gained full independence. In America, as well, nationalism lost little ground, even though it subsided somewhat in Europe. It showed itself in the struggle between the communist East and the largely democratic, capitalistic West. The "cold war" that resulted did not lead to open military action, even though outside of Europe numerous local wars occurred in which Western and Eastern countries interfered.*

*Attempts to reach a state of peaceful coexistence between East and West failed. Both sides continued to stockpile nuclear and conventional weapons. A new crisis occurred when the Communists built a wall dividing Berlin and a fortified border stretching from the Baltic Sea to the Adriatic, which made East-West personal contacts almost impossible.*

## Selected Readings

Grosser, Alfred. *The Western Alliance: European-American Relations Since 1945* (New York: Continuum Pub. Co., 1980).

Brower, Daniel R. *The World in the Twentieth Century: From Empires to Nations* (New York: Pearson Prentice Hall, 2006).

Jordan, Robert S. and Feld, Warner J. *Europe in the Balance* (Boston: Faber & Faber, 1986).

Kennedy, Paul. *The Rise and Fall of the Great Powers: Economic Change and Military Conflict From 1500-2000* (New York: Random House, 1987).

Moss, Walter. *A History of Russia* (London: Anthem, 2005).

Mafeber, W. *America, Russia, and the Cold War*: 1945-1996 (New York: McGraw-Hill, 1997).

## Test Yourself

1. When World War II came to an end, a new world order emerged with two leading super powers_____.
   A. Germany and France
   B. France and Britain
   C. The U.S. and Soviet Union
   D. China and the U.S.

2. NATO stands for_____.
   A. North Atlantic Treaty Organization
   B. North American Trade Organization
   C. North African Treaty Organization
   D. None of the above

3. In 1956, Egypt nationalized the Suez Canal Company prompting _____.
   A. An Anglo-Franco Invasion
   B. A German Invasion
   C. An American Invasion
   D. None of the above

4. The United Nations partitioned Palestine into two states in ____.
   A. 1945
   B. 1946
   C. 1947
   D. 1948

5. The discovery of the Genetic code (DNA) in 1960 was attributed to the work of_____.
   A. Crick and Watson
   B. Mendel and Newton
   C. James and Malthus
   D. None of the above

6. The Soviet Union was the first nation in 1961 to_____.
   A. Launch the first space satellite, *Sputnik*
   B. Put a human being into orbit around the earth
   C. Land a man on the moon
   D. None of the above

7. Between 1958 and 1969 France was led by_____.
   A. Francois Mitterrand
   B. Jacques Chirac
   C. Charles De Gaulle
   D. None of the above

8. The Federation of Yugoslavia was led by the communist _____.
   A. Milosevic
   B. Stalin
   C. Franco
   D. Tito

## Answers and Explanations

1. **C.** Since the war destroyed most of Europe, the two leading super powers after the war were the U.S. and the Soviet Union.

2. **A.** Even though a unified military force was not organized, a military alliance joining the United States and England to the Continent was concluded in 1949. This alliance (the North Atlantic Treaty Organization, or NATO) had a central headquarters and an American supreme commander. As a whole, the idea of European unity made considerable progress. Cultural contacts and exchanges were augmented by political cooperation.

3. **D.** Egypt forced the British to withdraw their military forces from the Suez Canal and nationalized the Canal Company in 1956 in order to use its revenue to build the Aswan High Dam. This led to an Anglo-Franco invasion, which, owing to American and Russian opposition, failed to achieve its objectives, including the toppling of the Egyptian regime of President Nasser.

4. **C.** Israel came about as a result of the partition of Palestine by the United Nations in 1947.

5. **A.** Scientific progress made enormous advances. Physics, biology, chemistry, medicine, and astronomy, while revealing many complexities, also brought discoveries that involve increasingly difficult scientific and ethical problems. The discovery of the genetic code (DNA) by Crick and Watson in 1960 had revolutionary consequences in many areas in addition to medicine and biogenetics, for it created problems that could threaten human survival. New and hazardous chemical products were developed for use in agriculture.

6. **B.** Marked advances in space technology enabled the Soviet Union to launch the first space satellite *(Sputnik)* in 1957; in 1961 they were the first to put a human being into orbit around the earth; and in 1966 they achieved a "soft" missile landing on the moon.

7. **C.** Between 1958 and 1969, France was led by Charles de Gaulle, under a constitution that gave extensive powers to the president.

8. **D.** A special role in world affairs was played by Yugoslavia under the Communist leader, Tito, who, during the war, had directed the fight against the Nazis and insisted on independent policies. "Titoism" revealed tensions and dissensions among the Communist powers. Tito rejected the right of the Soviet Union to dictate policies to other Communist nations—notwithstanding the fact that Marxism had preached the identity of the interests of the workers in all countries and the Soviet Union had previously been considered the leader and spokesman of true Marxism.

**CHAPTER 24**

# A World in Transition (1968-1984)

**1968** Students' and civil rights disorders
Soviet invasion and occupation of Czechoslovakia
**1969** Nuclear Nonproliferation Treaty
First manned landing on the moon
**1973** Arab-Israeli War
Oil crisis
Abortion legalized in the United States
**1974** Withdrawal of Portugal from its African colonies
**1975** Referendum in Britain confirms Britain's entry into Common Market
Franco, last Fascist dictator, dies
Helsinki Conference; rejection of force in order to achieve territorial changes
Communists win Vietnam War, country united; U.S. troops withdrawn
**1978** European Parliament created in Strasbourg
Camp David Accords
Israel agrees to return the Sinai Peninsula to Egypt for full diplomatic relations
**1979** Labor unrest in Poland (Lech Walesa)
The Signing of Egyptian-Israeli Peace Treaty
Afghanistan-Soviet Friendship Pact
Soviet troops dispatched to Afghanistan
**1981** Socialist party gains presidency in France
**1982** Falkland War
**1983** American invasion of Grenada
**1984** Recession in West ends; inflation lightened

*Shortly after World War I, Oswald Spengler stated in his famous work "The Decline of the West" that Western civilization had outlived its allotted time and was now facing dissolution to be succeeded by a new, fresh civilization.*

*Twenty years later, in his "Study of History," Arnold Toynbee agreed with some of Spengler's views, but suggested that a religious resurgence revitalizing the latent strength of its culture could prolong the life of Western civilization so that its early end was not inevitable. Another twenty years later, Karl Jaspers, dealing with the same question in his "Origin and Goal of History," concluded that even though a dangerous transition period must be anticipated, a new order, not necessarily a "Western" but a "world" civilization—would evolve. World unity was necessary and, Jaspers argued, was coming, as wars and revolutions became less and less feasible under the impact of scientific and technological developments. In a united world, humankind's soul and spirit, its aspirations and institutions, would be changed. A world civilization such as Jaspers envisioned still seems far off. Yet some general trends in that direction, distinctly Western in origin, seem to be evolving.*

## ■ INTERNATIONAL POLITICS

From the mid-1960s, the outstanding feature of the international scene was the increasing restraint that Communist and other nations of the Western world, wary of nuclear war, exercised whenever an occasion for confrontation arose. The danger spots had by then shifted from Europe to Asia and Africa, but no issue brought a military clash between the two strongest military powers, the USSR and the United States. The two superpowers confined themselves to a war of words and propaganda in the national news media of both countries and during meetings of the United Nations. Thus the racial question in South Africa and Rhodesia, where the white population sought to maintain dominance, remained a localized issue. Struggles between ethnic and political groups or tribes in central Africa—Ethiopia, where, in 1974, the emperor was deposed and supplanted by a military dictatorship, for example, or Bangladesh—did not bring military interference by the great powers. Neither did decolonization by the Netherlands in the West Indies (1973) and Portugal in Africa (1974), nor the further retreat of England from its naval bases abroad. Indeed, since 1969, some slight progress has been made in negotiations in regard to restraining the arms race, improving the exchange of information, and expanding East-West travel, trade, and scientific collaboration. Only two areas constituted a real threat to peace: Southeast Asia and the Middle East.

### Southeast Asia

Beginning in the late 1950s, after the French withdrawal from Southeast Asia, the United States allowed itself to be drawn into intervention in Vietnam to prevent a Communist takeover. By the mid-

*Figure 24–1 European colonial losses after 1945*

1960s, full-fledged military support was given to the non-Communist South. The tenacity of the Vietcong, combined with bitter disagreements among the American people regarding the country's war aims and policies, led to a military stalemate. After years of suffering by the Vietnamese people and the involvement of neighboring Cambodia and Laos, peace negotiations, concluded early in 1973, led only to a ceasefire agreement and the existence of two separate states, North and South Vietnam. Since neither side respected the peace terms, war broke out anew in 1975.

Despite continued United States support, the South Vietnamese resistance collapsed, and by May of 1975, the South had been conquered by the North. In the meantime, a coalition government that included Communists had already been established in Laos, and Cambodia too fell to the Communists.

### The Middle East

The situation in the Middle East constituted a still graver threat to world peace, but diplomacy and restraint once again prevented a direct confrontation of the superpowers. In June 1967, Egyptian provocations led to the outbreak of the Six-Day War, the third such conflict waged by Israel against its Arab neighbors. The extent of their military success surprised even the Israelis themselves. Aside from the capture of old Jerusalem, the Israelis were able to establish important buffer zones on the Golan Heights, the West Bank, and the Gaza Strip. A prolonged period of tension, broken by sporadic outbursts of fighting, followed. A full-scale Arab attack on Israel led to some initial successes before the Israelis stabilized the front and began to prepare for retaliation. Fearing an expansion of the war, the Soviet Union and the United States interceded, and buffer zones under United Nations supervision were established.

In the meantime, an entirely new situation had arisen, owing to a change in the economic scene. In order to gain consideration from the West, the Arabs began to use their economic strength, which rested on their oil resources. They tripled their price for oil, and the economies of the industrial nations seemed threatened.

## ■ INTERNATIONAL ECONOMY

In the course of the 1960s and the 1970s, socioeconomic patterns underwent a worldwide change that involved the most disparate economic systems. National and ideological boundaries began to lose their economic significance. Other issues came to assume greater importance. These crucial issues included population growth and starvation in Asia and Africa, pollution and exhaustion of natural resources, migrations of workers from underdeveloped countries into the foremost industrial states, and the rise and influence of multinational firms whose enterprises were carried on beyond national boundaries and beyond the reach of national legislation. This development demanded additional types of international regulations concerning not only the old political issues and the new technical ones, such as pollution and the waste of natural resources, but also problems of lawlessness, hijacking, kidnapping, and drug abuse on a global scale.

### The Monetary System

Under the impact of economic change, the monetary system in place since the end of World War II broke down. Unable to maintain its convertibility into gold, the United States devalued the dollar, and a substitute currency standard had to be sought. All exchange rates were repeatedly revised, and interest rates climbed. By 1974, inflation and rising unemployment beset most Western economies and endangered the security of the Western peoples. Economic growth slackened.

### East-West Economic Relations

Despite monetary problems, international trade increased. Trade between Communist and Western democratic countries especially accelerated in an atmosphere of political *"detente."* From 1969 on—and more especially after 1973—the Soviet Union and the nations allied to it in a common-market arrangement called Comecon showed more flexibility in their economic policies. They increased imports and exports, asked for credit, accorded industrial concessions, agreed to a measure of scientific cooperation, and hired the services of Western experts. With the help of the West and Japan, plans were made for huge developments to exploit natural gas and oil resources in Siberia and to lay pipelines from there to the seas. Although the West continued to rely on individual, capitalist initiative, and the less market-oriented East relied on socialist planning, a new economic mechanism was at work everywhere. A measure of economic "convergence" developed.

### Energy Crisis

It was in the face of such economic developments that the Arab oil-producing countries created a crisis. They drastically raised the price for their oil (other countries did likewise for other commodities, including wheat, soybeans, bauxite, sugar, and gold), placing a temporary embargo on oil deliveries to countries supporting Israel. The economy of the great industrial nations was thereby threatened. Simultaneously, Iran, Libya, and Morocco speeded up their nationalization of oil resources. However, through restraint and careful negotiations, as well as by exploiting the East-West rivalry, the oil-producing countries succeeded in avoiding a military response from the West. In an attempt to adjust to the situation, the industrial nations adopted the course of moderation advocated by the European consumer nations. They began to change their wasteful habits and to concentrate on developing their own sources of energy, including solar and nuclear, natural gas under the seas, coal, and so on. Better distribution, which could eventually benefit the underdeveloped countries, was initiated. These countries began to gain a better share in the wealth of nations. They could use it to industrialize, build schools, introduce social reforms, and enter an age of modernization.

## ■ NATIONAL POLICIES

Despite the increasing interdependence of all parts of the globe, national interests remained prevalent. Independence and power remained the goals of each nation. The political union of the European Economic Community (the Common Market) thus made hardly any progress. Indeed, local autonomy movements—such as in Britain's Scotland, France's Brittany, Italy's Sicily, Yugoslavia's Croatia, the Soviet Union's Ukraine, and Spain's Basque country—gained in significance.

### Germany

Somewhat contrary to the general trend was the policy of Germany. In 1969, the rule of the Christian Democratic Party under Konrad Adenauer and his heirs in West Germany (the Federal Republic) was replaced by a coalition led by the Social Democrats under Willy Brandt. In August 1970, the Federal Republic signed a treaty with the Soviet Union recognizing the territorial changes imposed by the Allies after World War II. West Germany subsequently regulated its relationship with other East European countries, recognized East Germany as a separate state—the German Democratic Republic—and agreed to the status of Berlin as arranged by the victors. Moreover, the country joined the United Nations simultaneously with East Germany. Internally, the Federal Republic continued to rebuild its economy, which was largely based on exports. Under pressure of vigorous radical movements, it introduced further social reforms and expanded its educational facilities. Brandt resigned in 1974 after the disclosure of a spy scandal involving a member of his staff. He was succeeded by Helmut Schmidt.

### England

Beset by determined labor-union demands and numerous strikes, England found itself in a deteriorating economic situation. The Labor party under Harold Wilson returned to power in 1974. Living conditions in Britain on the whole improved, and scientific work maintained high standards. Two other problems, however, disturbed English developments. First, England's entry into the European Common Market aroused widespread internal opposition because it implied increased involvement, both politically and economically, with European partners. Second, a new round of civil strife and unrest began in Ireland in 1969. At stake was the unification of the entire island under the leadership of the independent Catholic South, an outcome feared by the Protestant North, which formed part of Britain. No solution was found.

## Cyprus

As in Ireland, violent nationalism was a driving force at the other end of Europe, on Cyprus, where Greeks and Turks lived together in an uneasy relationship. Provoked by a Greek military *putsch*, Turkey sent troops and demanded the division of the island into two autonomous parts. The struggle not only endangered peace between Greece and Turkey, but also led to the collapse of the military dictatorship in Greece, its replacement by a more democratic regime, government crises in Turkey, and the possibility of a split in the NATO forces. A measure of order was precariously restored in 1974.

## Other European Countries

The year 1974 witnessed government changes in many Western countries, in addition to Germany and England. In France, General de Gaulle's regime had come to an end in 1969, and "Gaullism," with its nationalistic accent, was somewhat modified under his successors. Governments changed hands in Luxembourg, Belgium, Italy, and Portugal, where the long-time dictator Salazar had died in 1970, with the socialists generally gaining ground.

Economic difficulties and other problems beset most countries. For example, student unrest in France often led to violent riots in 1969, the issue of divorce laws disturbed Catholic Italy in the 1970s, and activists finally achieved voting rights for women in Switzerland. As the younger generation began to organize and assert its power, the voting age was lowered in many countries. The unrest and dissatisfaction with social and economic shortcomings indicated less a breakdown in Western ways and institutions than a change in attitudes that was to bring reform rather than revolution. In spite of difficulties, living standards almost everywhere improved. An egalitarian trend was noticeable in education and daily life, and social services, directed by an ever-increasing state bureaucracy, were extended.

## United States

More than any other Western nation, the United States was affected by the attitudes of the generation born since World War II. The country was internally beset by grave problems, including racial strife, which resolute legislation envisaging racial equality tried to mitigate. Other issues included women's rights, moral and sexual standards, prison reform, antiwar legislation, and demands for improved social welfare benefits. Economic uncertainties aggravated the situation. During 1974, inflation reached a level unequaled since the war, as did unemployment by 1975. Respect for the Constitution, law and order, and traditional values of American society diminished. Corruption penetrated many layers of society, and confidence in government was shaken as never before as a result of the Watergate scandal. This scandal involved an investigation into the break-in at Democratic campaign headquarters during the 1972 election in which it was revealed that President Richard Nixon had lied to the American people. To avoid impeachment proceedings, he resigned in 1974, the first president to do so. He was succeeded by his Vice-President Gerald Ford.

While *detente* with the Soviet Union relieved external pressures, diplomatic ties with China brought only meager results. The failure in Vietnam, the costs of that war in lives and money, and its moral implications upset traditional complacency and convictions. United States diplomatic efforts to settle the Middle East question failed, and cooperation with European allies and Latin America proved insufficient.

As in Europe, however, a readiness to introduce reforms prevented serious rifts. Except for the effects of lawlessness, living standards improved until the inflation of the 1970s, and by 1975, the economic climate had changed for the better. As a whole, the standing of the country was not seriously affected, and its power remained unchallenged.

### Latin America

The Latin American nations also faced inflation and other economic disruptions, especially with population pressures, but in some respects, their progress was remarkable. In many regions, modern factories were created, trade flourished, and social progress was observed. Politically, a measure of stability was gained under military dictatorships. In 1973, Argentina called back Juan Peron, who had been in exile since 1955. A socialist government in Chile under Salvador Allende (1970-1973), intent on social reform, came to a premature end with a rightist revolt. Only in Cuba did a Communist regime continue to flourish.

### The Soviet Union

While many of the problems besetting other Western countries left undisturbed those Eastern European nations under a Communist rule that could preserve strict order, other equally grave issues emerged. Progress in meeting shortages of capital, consumer goods, and housing was slow, and labor productivity was insufficient. Oppression of dissenting groups persisted, and freedom of movement remained limited. Public criticism of the system, while occasionally possible through private publications, remained risky. Under the impact of new technology, however, the relationship between state and society changed. Dissatisfaction increased, as was seen in growing conflicts between the political bureaucracy and the industrial managers. A new Soviet Five-Year Plan, announced in April 1971, provided for maintenance of previous goals rather than adaptation to new conditions. Still, increased collaboration and trade with the capitalist West could not be avoided. This meant not merely the exchange of goods, but also joint ventures and other business arrangements. Capitalist and Communist came into close and prolonged contact, which brought about the introduction and infiltration of unwanted ideas. This situation created dissension between the Soviet leadership under Leonid Brezhnev and other members of the Politburo. Yet, in view of the advantages gained by *detente*, the Communist successes in Southeast Asia (and to an extent, Portugal), and the misgivings about China's growing world role, the Soviets continued on the path of coexistence that had been decided upon for their external relations.

### East-Central Europe

In the smaller, Communist-dominated Eastern European states, progress toward modernization was rapid. East Germany, harshly controlled, could do nothing to challenge Soviet might, but in 1970, the Poles rioted and succeeded in replacing the old leadership with a somewhat more flexible one. Romanians and Hungarians emancipated themselves somewhat from close Russian supervision, adopted strongly nationalistic policies, liberalized their internal systems, and increasingly cooperated with the West. A serious clash occurred in Czechoslovakia in 1968, however, when the Czechs installed a more liberal government under Alexander Dubcek. Soviet troops were called in, "for the sake of socialism and the protection of socialist countries." They removed Dubcek and once more imposed strict Soviet control.

## ■ CULTURAL TRENDS

Student unrest, self-assertion of a new generation, and challenges to traditional standards opened new directions in creative thought. A good deal of intellectual effort was directed toward science and technology, as great strides continued to be made in these fields. Aside from improved industrial processes based on enormous research efforts, achievements were made in outer-space exploration and medical technology. Space walks by astronauts became almost commonplace, and a landing on the moon, watched by millions or people on live television, was achieved in 1969. The first transplant of a human heart was performed in South Africa in 1967, and other vital organs such as kidneys were also successfully transplanted. The laser beam became an important tool in surgery. Numerous studies going beyond those of Freud were undertaken to probe the human psyche. Cosmology, aided by radar instruments and far-reaching satellites, brought significant new working theories concerning the extent and nature of the universe. Most important was the discovery of a new nuclear particle that held the promise of making possible the formulation of a long-searched-for general field theory.

Writers like the French Albert Camus, the Swiss Friedrich Dürrenmatt, and the Russian Aleksandr Solzhenitsyn found a wide audience. Existentialism, as proposed by Jean-Paul Sartre and Martin Heidegger, lost some of its appeal. In music, Benjamin Britten held a foremost place, but in line with the mechanization of the age, the most conspicuous innovation came with the advent of electronic music, i.e., music composed by new, often mathematical techniques of composition for electronic sound equipment.

A reforming liberal movement asserted itself within the Christian churches, and some Eastern mysticism inspired Westerners struggling for a firm faith. However, as in other areas of life, conservative institutionalism proved stronger. The Second Vatican Council, which had started with high hopes under Pope John XXIII, did not achieve much under his successor. Many questions of the Modern Age received no creative answer, and arrangements for coexistence between the Catholic Church and the Communist countries were achieved more on the basis of expediency than conviction.

## ■ CRISIS OF CONFIDENCE

In November 1975, Francisco Franco died in Spain. With his death, the last Fascist dictatorship disappeared from Europe—about half a century after Fascism had started in Italy. With the death of China's revolutionary hero, Mao Zedong in September 1976, the greatest challenger to the Soviet Union's leadership of the Communist world passed from the scene. He left an unhealed breach in the Communist front, emphasized by the vigor of various socialistic, Communistic, and anarchistic movements separately pursuing, often within a narrow nationalist framework, the path to socialism.

### Political Scene

The new age following World War II was an age characterized by increasing uneasiness. No lasting solutions were found for the great political issues: for European unity (although England finally joined the Common Market in 1975); for East-West cooperation (which, if anything, declined somewhat); for tensions between developed and developing nations; for the Arab-Israeli conflict (despite the peace efforts of the Egyptian president Anwar Sadat in 1977-1979 and the signing of an Egyptian-Israeli peace treaty); for the Greek-Turkish strife over Cyprus; or the internal racial divisions in South Africa, which increasingly involved the policies of the West. The two great powers, the Soviet Union and the United States, had, in the meantime, lost some of their preeminence. Despite their military strength, they could no longer impose their will as they had before, not even in their own spheres of influence. International terrorism, aimed at the negative objectives of discrediting and undermining existing political patterns rather than constructive social objectives, became a major problem. Perhaps the most positive aspect of the late 1970s was the continued general realization that, under the atomic weapons threat, another world war could offer no solution to international problems. War, therefore, contrary to Clausewitz's dictum, could no longer be considered a means to promote national aims and to decide conflicts. Still, arms control made limited progress. Only isolated problems could be adjusted. For example, in 1978, the United States announced that it would relinquish control of the Panama Canal by the year 2000.

## Economic Scene

In both capitalistic and socialistic nations, material living standards continued to improve despite economic difficulties. Working hours were reduced and, thanks to computer techniques, work was lightened. Social services were broadened. A barrage of propaganda and advertisements through all public media sought to create, especially in the United States, ever new "needs" for ever new products, whereby the economy was to keep expanding and profiting.

In the process, most Western nations accumulated excessive public debts, quickened inflation, and steadily enlarged their political apparatus and their bureaucracies, which often failed to maintain standards of integrity. New currency troubles arose, and the dollar, in particular, faced a major decline in international value. In the eastern parts of Europe, unrest increased as the Soviet Union insisted upon economic integration among the member states of the Council for Mutual Economic Assistance (Comecon). Restrictions on the freedom of movement of the inhabitants of these countries were maintained. In many parts, doubt was voiced about the advantages of continuous industrial growth in the face of slowing birth rates, environmental consequences, potential shortages in safe energy supplies, and of the costs of social services.

## Cultural Scene

In the late 1970s, the Western world's attention continued to center on the natural sciences and technology. Research in astronomy, engineering, chemistry, and nuclear physics brought about new practical advances. Especially impressive were the achievements in bioengineering, genetic research, recombinant DNA (which also offered threatening perspectives), and medicine, in the diagnosis and prevention of some major diseases.

# ■ NEW CHALLENGES

By 1978, the effects of the Western way of life had spread so far in the economic, technological, and political arenas that it became almost impossible to restrict the term "Western civilization" to the West. Japan exemplified many aspects of that civilization. China, India (both of which had independently manufactured their own atomic bombs), the Arab states, and even newly formed African states reluctantly adopted some aspects of the West. Whether desired or not, a convergence occurred regarding tastes, building styles, dress, habits, and even forms of music and literature, as well as economic conditions, political systems, and thought patterns. Differences faded, and democratic institutions were reshaped under both capitalist and Communist systems. General issues of population growth, space, environment, technology, bureaucracy, interdependence, and humanitarianism gradually began to overshadow in importance the narrower perspectives of national policies and political ideologies. These issues became a common matter of survival, and a growing awareness of their importance constituted the promise of the future.

## Social Scene

With new production methods, computers, and robots, a fundamental shift occurred in social relationships and class structure. The traditional "proletariat" diminished in size and influence. Increasingly, it merged with the middle class and adopted middle-class standards. On the other hand, the modern state, which—conservative objections notwithstanding—had to assume ever more tasks and provide so many social and economic regulations, had to extend its bureaucracy. In conjunction with technicians working for the state, these groups constituted an ever more influential element in the social structure.

Moreover, the migration of poor people from less developed countries and of refugees from the East to highly industrialized nations altered the social composition of the populations. France, Switzerland, Germany, the United States, England, Holland, and others were affected and faced problems involving human rights, social services, and political prerogatives of the newcomers. In other words, the critical issue for those countries centered on how to utilize the skills and resources of the newcomers while attempting to positively integrate them in the larger fabric of society.

## Feminism and Civil Rights in the United States

For over two centuries, feminists in Western Europe and the United States have insisted that the principles of liberty and equality embodied in the French Declaration of the Rights of Man and of the Citizen and the American Declaration of Independence be applied to women. The feminist movements of the 20th century were able to substantiate women's gains. For example, in the United States, the Equal Pay Act, which established equal pay for men and women for the same kind of job and prohibited discrimination practices against women, was enacted in 1963. This act was further strengthened by the Civil Rights Act of 1964, which expressly prohibited all discriminations on the bases of race, religion, and sex. These laws were enforced by institutions like the Equal Opportunity Employment Commission, particularly in the case of the Civil Rights Act of 1964. The key component of the act deals with public accommodations, so that African Americans could no longer be excluded from restaurants, hotels and other public facilities. In other words, the act brought an end to legal segregation.

In education, women continued to fight for equality. In 1966, women created the National Organization for Women (NOW), along with the Women's Bipartisan Caucus in 1971, both dedicated to promote information and mobilize voters to demand equal education opportunities for women. These efforts did not fall on deaf ears. In 1972, the Education Act was created. This law prohibited sex discrimination. Finally, the courts, initially the chief enemy of feminist demands, let down their guard and became increasingly sympathetic to women's issues. They began to strike down discriminatory legislation and practices. Further, with the sexual liberation of women, there was talk about birth control and abortion for the first time. For the first time, women would have a choice in what happened with their bodies. An example of this is the case *Roe v. Wade* (1973), where a state's anti-abortion law was declared unconstitutional.

Moreover, women became somewhat more active in the political arena. For example, in the United States's state legislatures, the number of women increased. In the 1984 election, a woman, Geraldine Ferraro, was nominated for the position of vice-president.

## Perspective

*For centuries, philosophers had been predicting the decline of the West. Terrible wars ravaged Europe. Still, the West remained strong. In the 1980s, conservatism in politics was once more in the ascendancy. Yet the radical changes in attitudes and human and national values, which had been advocated in the late 1960s and 1970s and had attacked many of the traditional moral concepts, could not entirely destroy the basic themes of Western civilization.*

*The last of the Fascist dictators died and, injustices and ills in the capitalist world notwithstanding, democratic institutions continued to dominate in the West. Despite persistent nationalism, international cooperation as begun after World War II continued to make progress. Communism was in retreat. It had failed to achieve social justice and improve living standards. The conservative forces in the Soviet Union avoided the risk of abandoning the traditional patterns.*

*A number of wars occurred not in Europe, but in non-Western regions. When Western nations became involved, they often did not prevail. The excellence of their weaponry was of little avail, since its full weight could not be used. The power of the so-called "superpowers" diminished.*

*In the cultural field, every year brought new advances in the natural sciences. Philosophers, writers, and artists followed many new and interesting courses. Some of them were, however, passing fashions, which appealed mainly to a restricted intellectual audience, but were quickly replaced by others.*

## Selected Readings

Barnet, Richard J. *The Alliance* (New York: Simon and Schuster, 1983).

Briggs, Asa and Clavin, Patricia. *Modern Europe: 1789-Present* (London: Pearson Longman, 2003).

Foner, Eric. *Give Me Liberty: American History, vol. II* (New York: W. W. Norton & Company, 2004).

Lowenthal, Richard. *Social Change and Cultural Crisis* (New York: Columbia University Press, 1984).

Luxenburg, Norman. *Europe Since World War II* (Carbondale: Southern Illinois University Press, 1979).

Keylor, William. *The Twentieth-Century World: An International History* (Oxford: Oxford University Press, 2001).

Martiniello, Marco, ed., *Multicultural Policies and the State: A Comparison of Two European Societies* (Utrecht: The Netherlands: Utrecht University, 1998).

Postan, Michael M. *An Economic History of Western Europe, 1945–1964* (London: Methuen, 1967).

Urwin, Derek W. *A Political History of Western Europe Since 1945* (New York: Longman, 1997).

## Test Yourself

1. Egyptian provocations in 1967 led to the outbreak of war with_____.
   A. The United States
   B. England
   C. Israel
   D. France

2. The conflict in Cyprus was characterized by uneasy tensions between_____.
   A. Jews and Turks
   B. Greeks and Jews
   C. Jews and Christians
   D. Greeks and Turks

3. When it was clear that President Richard Nixon had lied to the American people in the context of the Watergate scandal he decided to avoid impeachment and resigned in the year_____.
   A. 1971
   B. 1972
   C. 1973
   D. 1974

4. The philosophy of existentialism was substantially contributed to by the work of _____.
   A. Jean Paul Sartre
   B. Martin Heidegger
   C. Sigmund Freud
   D. Both A and B

5. The Chinese Communist leader Mao Zedong died in September_____.
   A. 1972
   B. 1974
   C. 1976
   D. 1978

6. The American Civil Rights Act of 1964 called for_____
   A. An end to segregation
   B. An end to abortion
   C. An end to the war in Vietnam
   D. None of the above

## Answers and Explanations

1. **C.** In June 1967, Egyptian provocations led to the outbreak of the Six-Day War, the third such conflict waged by Israel against its Arab neighbors. The extent of their military success surprised even the Israelis themselves: Aside from the capture of old Jerusalem, the Israelis were able to establish important buffer zones on the Golan Heights, the West Bank, and the Gaza Strip. A prolonged period of tension, broken by sporadic outbursts of fighting, followed. A full-scale Arab attack on Israel led to some initial successes, before the Israelis stabilized the front and began to prepare for retaliation. Fearing an expansion of the war, the Soviet Union and the United States interceded, and buffer zones under United Nations supervision were established.

2. **D.** On the island of Cyprus, where Greeks and Turks lived together in an uneasy relationship. Provoked by a Greek military putsch, Turkey sent troops and demanded the division of the island into two autonomous parts. The struggle not only endangered peace between Greece and Turkey but also led to the collapse of the military dictatorship in Greece, its replacement by a more democratic regime, government crises in Turkey, and the possibility of a split in the NATO forces. A measure of order was precariously restored in 1974.

3. **D.** Corruption penetrated many layers of society, and confidence in government was shaken as never before as a result of the Watergate scandal. In the course of an investigation into the break-in at Democratic campaign headquarters during the 1972 election, it was revealed that President Richard Nixon had lied to the American people. To avoid impeachment proceedings, he resigned in 1974, the first president to do so. He was succeeded by his Vice-President Gerald Ford.

4. **D.** Existentialism was proposed by Jean-Paul Sartre and Martin Heidegger, but it later lost some of its appeal.

5. **C.** With the death of China's revolutionary hero Mao Zedong in September 1976, the greatest challenger to the Soviet Union's leadership of the Communist world passed from the scene. He left an unhealed breach in the Communist front, emphasized by the vigor of various socialistic, Communistic, and anarchistic movements separately pursuing, often within a narrow nationalist framework, the path to socialism.

6. **A.** The key issue of the Civil Rights Act deals with public accommodations, so that African Americans could no longer be excluded from restaurants, hotels and other public facilities. In other words, the act brought an end to legal segregation.

**CHAPTER 25**

# The End of the Cold War and the New Challenges (1985-Present)

**1985** Gorbachev becomes secretary general of the Soviet Union
**1986** Chernobyl atomic disaster
**1987** Soviets offer disarmament proposals
First Palestinian uprising (*Intifada*)
**1988** European Nations Conference: Single European Market irreversible
**1989** Conference of Nations on Human Rights
Hungary introduces "multiparty" government
Berlin Wall dismantled
United States invades Panama
**1990** Iraq annexes Kuwait
Soviets complete withdrawal from Afghanistan
German Federal Republic and German Democratic Republic become one nation
Communist governments in Czechoslovakia, Poland, Rumania, Hungary, and Bulgaria resign
**1991** War against Iraq
Gorbachev resigns presidency of the USSR
Civil War in Yugoslavia
Dissolution of USSR
**1992** Bill Clinton elected president of the United States
Czechoslovakia splits into Czech Republic and Slovakia
Maastricht Agreement
Israel and the PLO sign the Oslo Accords
**1994** War breaks out between Russia and Chechnya
**1995** Dayton Agreement ends civil war in Bosnia
**1996** Boris Yeltsin reelected president of Russia
Bill Clinton elected president of the United States for a second term
**1998** Serbian assaults on Albanians in Kosovo
**2001** Al-Qaida terrorist attacks in New York and Washington
U.S. Invasion of Afghanistan
**2002** European Union introduces the Euro

**2003** U.S.-led invasion of Iraq
**2004** European Union adds nine new states
NATO adds seven new members
Madrid train bombings
**2005** London public transport system suicide bombings

*Political stagnation came to an end in 1985. Fresh initiatives came from the USSR, where Mikhail Gorbachev, a younger member of the communist hierarchy, was elected to the post of secretary general of the Party. His program of glasnost (openness) introduced the disintegration of the Yalta agreements and a change in the traditional East-West confrontational posture. His program of perestroika (restructuring) envisioned the transformation of the Soviet economy. The West was unprepared, but it had to follow the Soviet lead, notwithstanding the fact that it was not strength but economic and political weakness that had prompted the reversal of Soviet policy.*

*The collapse of the Soviet Union and the end of the Cold War ushers in a new world order. Europe became more economically and politically unified as a result of the newly expanded European Union and its inauguration in 2002 of a unified currency, the Euro. Violence and civil wars in the Yugoslavia led to its breakup but also contributed to more international involvement in decisively stopping ethnic cleansing and atrocities in Bosnia and Serbia.*

*The terrorist attacks against the United States on September 11, 2001, galvanized international effort to combat terrorism at its root. American-led invasion of Afghanistan and Iraq in 2001 and 2003 may contribute to defeating terrorists and regimes sponsoring them but may also stir an important debate about the pre-emptive use of military force as a means to eradicate terror around the globe.*

## ■ THE INTERNATIONAL SCENE

The system of international relations was greatly affected by revolutionary changes in Eastern Europe. Meanwhile, global interdependence encouraged peaceful coexistence and cooperation, but also caused tension that contributed to violence and war.

### Glasnost and Western Policies

The opening of barriers to the outside world began in Hungary, with the consent of the Soviet government. The eagerness with which citizens took advantage of travel opportunities to the West and access to Western information speeded up the process of *glasnost*. A grave nuclear disaster in the Ukraine at Chernobyl (1986), only seven years after a nuclear accident in the United States at Three Mile Island (1979), demonstrated to what extent dangers in one country could engulf others.

### *Germany*

The decisive breakthrough on the road to reunification came in 1989 when, taking advantage of *glasnost*, East German citizens, demonstrating peaceably, breached the Berlin Wall (after being allowed to be opened by the East German government), which for almost three decades had separated them from their relatives in the western parts of Germany. Thus, they challenged their communist rulers, who were forced to back down. One barrier after another fell. Free movement back and forth between East and West was reintroduced. These events in Germany stunned the Western world, especially when it became clear that the Soviets were willing to stand aside and let Germany remain a member of NATO and the EEC.

The events in Germany paralleled liberation movements in Czechoslovakia, Hungary, Bulgaria, and Rumania. Everywhere the communist rulers were being removed. The reunification of Germany was completed by a national referendum in October of 1990.

This fundamental change which Gorbachev's *glasnost* had achieved in the existing balance of power had worldwide repercussions. In particular, it led to significant reductions in armaments and occu-

*Figure 25–1 German Reunification in 1990*

pation troops, not only in Central Europe but also in non-European countries, such as Angola. Self-determination and autonomy movements everywhere were given new hope.

### United States and Global Affairs

*Glasnost* necessitated a reversal of American foreign policy and a shift from confrontation to peaceful cooperation far beyond the European arena. The perception of Third World struggles as "an extension of the cold war" had to be discarded. Still, Washington continued to hold as its leading principle the policy of "keeping governments in power that would not challenge U.S. policies." The United States supported the government of President Ferdinand Marcos in the Philippines until he was ousted in 1986. It indirectly involved itself in the internal struggles in Nicaragua and El Salvador. In 1989 it invaded Panama and helped overthrow the formerly friendly government of Manuel Noriega. It thus sought to reassert its power and leadership.

In 1990, a graver test came in the Middle East, when Iraq invaded neighboring Kuwait and seized this oil-rich country. An embargo on all shipments to and from Iraq was declared, and a large American military force, which included some troops from allied nations, was dispatched to the Persian Gulf. With the economic sanctions not bringing quick results, the United States sought permission from the United Nations to use military force. The brief war for the liberation of Kuwait began in early 1991 and ended successfully after causing terrible human losses. From 1991 to 2001, The Iraqi regime was subjected to economic sanctions that crippled the economy and caused the death of so many ordinary Iraqis.

Israelis and Palestinians continued their violence against each other. A Palestinian uprising in 1987 against Israel's occupation of Gaza and the West Bank eventually led both Palestinians and Israelis to negotiate an end to the conflict. With Norway's mediation, they met in Oslo and negotiated the 1993 Oslo Accords that called for Palestinian autonomy in Gaza and the West Bank and ultimately the creation of a Palestinian state to peacefully co-exist with Israel. American efforts to broker peace between the two parties led to a number of bilateral negotiations but without a final settlement.

### The Soviet Union

*Glasnost* obviously had its greatest impact on the USSR itself. Access to information from abroad was no longer forbidden to its citizens; travel abroad became easier. In foreign affairs, aside from changing its German policies, the Soviet Union tolerated the abolition of the dominating communist governments in its satellite states and the virtual dissolution of the Warsaw Pact. The Soviets completed the evacuation of Afghanistan, thereby eliminating a point of dissension, especially with the United States. Gradually they reduced their troops stationed in Central Europe; they engaged in negotiations with the European powers and the United States concerning common action in other areas of the globe where local struggles threatened peaceful developments. When the war in Iraq broke out in 1991, they refrained from military intervention but participated in the efforts to persuade Iraq to leave Kuwait.

### Perestroika and the Western Economy

Just as *glasnost* had consequences not only for the Soviet Union but elsewhere, so did *perestroika*.

During the years between 1985 and 1990, notwithstanding pockets of poverty and ignorance in Western Europe and the United States, living standards in these areas were high. But those in the Soviet Union deteriorated. Severe drought conditions had contributed to the economic problems in the years 1979 to 1981, but the organization of the Soviet economy remained largely at fault. Gorbachev attacked the problem by seeking to bring about what his predecessors since Khrushchev had envisioned but not achieved. He reduced the number of central agencies directing the economy and put more responsibility as well as greater authority into the hands of industrial and agricultural units. Where discipline and obedience were formerly demanded, a measure of pluralism would now be allowed.

### Economic Aims

In 1988, steps were taken to enlarge the private sector of the economy. Peasants could use more of the available land for growing crops for private consumption and for sale. Small businesses could be founded, as long as they did not employ external help. Newspapers and books could give expression to dissenting opinions. Also the government permitted the Orthodox Church wider activities; Gorbachev even visited the pope in Rome.

But the ownership of land as well as industries remained in the hands of the state; central planning was maintained. No unifying ideology was devised that could inspire and also satisfy people trained along old Soviet lines, who preferred security to Western-type freedoms. Within the confines of socialist ownership and control, no method was found to create the open-market arrangements and free competition that the West had found useful in raising its living standards.

In 1990, Gorbachev was elected president; additional executive authority was given him. A popularly elected legislature was instituted, and the monopoly of the Communist Party was dissolved. A 500-day plan was worked out to integrate the Soviet Union into the world economy by permitting joint ventures with foreign enterprise. In the future, a measure of private ownership of land and various types of ownership in industry were to be allowed. The convertibility of the Russian currency was envisioned. For this purpose, an exchange of the existing currency into new bills took place in 1991 under harsh conditions, which created much discontent; the more so as all changes needed time to bring about the desired results. In the meantime, the economy deteriorated further. Food in the cities became still scarcer. Price increases followed. Large parts of the population had to rely on the black market, which flourished.

### *Opposition*

Dissatisfaction on the side of devoted communists as well as opponents of the system and a feeling of insecurity followed. It brought a widening gap between reformers and conservatives and a tightening of the reins by Gorbachev. Fears prevailed that with the replacement of some of the reformers in the government by old-line communists, as had happened late in 1990 and early 1991, private ownership could eventually encounter renewed persecutions.

Independence movements in several of the Soviet Union's constituent republics added to Gorbachev's problems. In the Baltic countries as well as in the Caucasus, in Asian regions and the Ukraine, and even in the republic of Russia itself, autonomy and independence were demanded. Where action in this direction was undertaken, the government did not permit it. In a few instances it used force. The 500-day plan did not, however, exclude the possibility of reforming the Union in an orderly way into a federation of sovereign states and allowing some republics to withdraw from the Union.

### *Reaction*

At the beginning of 1991, the policy of *perestroika*, as opposed to that of *glasnost*, had brought insufficient results. The conservative forces in the country sought to reassert themselves. But when they attempted to regain power through a coup in the middle of 1991, they failed and the opposition under the president of the Russian republic, Boris Yeltsin, triumphed. The reform work was now speeded up and in December 1991 Gorbachev resigned from his office. This signified the dissolution of the Soviet Union. Practically all member republics of the Union declared their independence. A "Commonwealth" was proposed by Boris Yeltsin and others to take its place, and in the economic sphere communism was to be replaced by a freer, market-oriented economy—largely in private hands.

The execution of this plan met, however, with grave obstacles. The problems of borders, of new ethnic disagreements, of the possession of military weapons, of finance and debts (notwithstanding the help extended by European countries), and of foreign relations were overwhelming and results remained in doubt.

## The United States

*Perestroika* and German unification opened up opportunities to United States industries and service enterprises. But by 1990, the dollar had fallen to an all-time low. With military expenditures rising dramatically, national indebtedness had risen to an all-time high. Third World countries could not repay their debts. Foreign industrial competition, especially by Japan and, to a lesser degree, other Asian nations, threatened American industries, which failed to keep up with technical advances. Once a creditor nation, the United States had become a debtor nation. Industrial productivity lagged.

Yet, after a brief recession (1982-1984), inflation and unemployment were kept in check; credits could be extended wherever new markets opened. General living standards, notwithstanding pockets of poverty and rapidly increasing homelessness and crime in some urban centers, remained high. Achievements in the natural sciences, and especially in medicine, were outstanding. Gains were made in the struggle for integration of its black population; for the full achievement of women's equal rights; for an end to hatred toward, and discrimination against homosexual men and women; for prison reform; and for civil rights at home and abroad.

## Europe

Events in the USSR and the United States reinforced the role played by Europeans in world affairs. The opening of Eastern Europe did not interfere with the maintenance of close ties with the United States, nor did the determination of the Continental powers to strengthen European unity.

England, too, adjusted to the emerging pattern and its need to cooperate with the Continental powers. Somewhat reluctantly, it yielded in 1990 with regard to the establishment of a common monetary unit.

Economic conditions in Europe were satisfactory, allowing for higher standards of living, even in less industrially advanced nations, such as Spain and Portugal. However, unemployment was high. A fair system of social security helped to mitigate its consequences in most countries. Special problems were caused by the integration of formerly communist countries into the Western economy, by the stream of immigrants from Eastern Europe and also from Asia and Africa, and by the breakup of Yugoslavia, where bitter internal warfare raged. The usual inefficiency of communist industry necessitated huge foreign investments in production centers and factories and for the improvement of environmental conditions.

## Ethnic Conflict in East-Central Europe Since 1989

An energetic Eastern Europe began to follow a western model of society. Poland achieved a quick transition to free-market economy; Hungary took steps to gradually follow Poland's lead. Czechoslovakia followed a similar course and by January 1993 the country split into two separate states: the more industrialized Czech Republic and the more agriculturally oriented Slovakia. Economic development in most Eastern European countries were, however, held down by inflation, unemployment, and outdated industrial enterprises.

After 1995, the economic conditions began to change for the better and by 1999 Poland, Hungary and the Czech Republic were admitted to the North Atlantic Treaty Organization (NATO). They also, along with Bulgaria, Estonia, Latvia, Lithuania, Slovakia and Slovenia, joined the European Union in 2004, thus enhancing European socio-economic and political stability.

Conditions were not as good in Yugoslavia. The post World War I Yugoslav Federation was undermined by the separation of Slovenia and Croatia in 1991. Bosnia with its three ethnic groups: Catholic Croats, Muslims, and Orthodox Serbs seceded in 1992. This action promoted Serbia to react. The three ethnic groups brutally fought each other and a process of Serbian ethnic cleansing of Muslims provoked moral outrage. It took United Nations and NATO intervention in 1995 to stop Serbian atrocities. The United States hosted a conference in Dayton, Ohio, that led to the Dayton Agreement in November 1995. The agreement proposed was equally represented by Muslims, Serbs, and Croats. But this agreement was a bit late for the thousands who had lost their lives.

Ethnic tension continued in Serbia as another civil war erupted between ethnic Serbs and ethnic Muslim Albanians in the Kosovo region of Serbia. This time NATO reacted swiftly to punish Serbia with

*Figure 25–2 The Balkans in 2000, after the breakup of the Yugoslav Federation*

air strikes in March 1999 that eventually ended the brutal rule of Serbia's dictator Milosevic. Further, Milosevic was put on trial for his policies of ethnic cleansing.

## Post-Communist Russia

Formerly the dominant republic of the Soviet Union, Russia became an independent Republic after the dissolution of the union in December 1991. Under Yeltsin leadership, Russia was committed to promoting democracy and a free-market economy. However, the old Communist hard liners dominated the first Duma election in December 1993 and forced Yeltsin to slow down his economic liberalization policies. Yeltsin was re-elected for a second tern in 1995 but his poor health coupled with his inability to steadily improve the Russian economy and inability to control the ethnic claims to independence by Chechnya, a small Muslim enclave in the Caucasus at war for centuries with conquering Russians. Yeltsin resigned in 1999 but not before naming a successor, a former member of the KGB, Vladimir Putin. Putin was elected President of the Russian Federation twice, in 2000 and 2004. Under his leadership, Russia's economic and political conditions drastically improved. However, the war in Chechnya continued and Putin vowed not to relinquish Russia's military campaign; Chechnya's rebels are defeated.

## Contemporary Western Europe

Developments in Western Europe continued throughout the 1990s. France, German, and England continued to play the most significant roles individually and with the newly established European Union.

### European Union

The end of the cold war added urgency to the process of European integration. From the start, its supporters had hoped that the Common Market could accomplish wider uniformity in areas like tax policy and business law, in which national difference created obstacles to economic activity across national borders.

Meeting at Maastricht, in the Netherlands, in 1992, the members of the European Community (EC) committed to fiscal austerity to prepare for the unification of their economies. They also agreed to a common policy of workers' rights, and to a common currency and central banking structure by 1999. But the agreement, in order to be affective, required the approval of all members. Although some provisions of the Maastricht agreement were controversial, in November1993 the European Union (EU) was formally established and by 1999 a unified currency, the euro, was introduced.

### England

In England, Prime Minister Margaret Thatcher resigned in 1991 after losing support from her conservative party. She was succeeded by John Major who led the country until the 1997 election. The Labor Party, revitalized under the leadership of Tony Blair, won the election. Under Blair's leadership, the Labor Party moved more to the political center and gained popular support as it enacted pro-business, pro-enterprise policies. Blair helped to end the conflict in Northern Ireland between Catholics and Protestants. Blair continued to lead the country after his reelection in 2001 and 2005.

### France

In France, President Francois Mitterrand was reelected in 1988 for a second 7-year term. In 1995 Mitterrand was succeeded by his Prime Minister, Jacques Chirac. Chirac promised vigorous attack on unemployment and deficit reduction. However, in order to balance France's budget, Chirac advocated cuts in health benefits and transportation services that led to nationwide protests. Yet, despite his policies of austerity, Chirac was re-elected for a second term in 2002.

### Germany

The re-unification of East and West Germany in 1990 into the German Federal Republic created enormous economic problems for most Germans. Restructuring the East German economy and integrating with its West German counterpart caused increased unemployment and budget deficits. Unemployment reached 12.8 percent in late 1997 and it soared to 20 percent in the eastern region. Germany's substantial social welfare benefits eased some of the economic difficulties, but for many Germans their economic well-being was in jeopardy. Chancellor Kohl, of the Christian Democratic Union, became the first Chancellor of reunified Germany in 1990, but was defeated in 1998 as the German economy continued to suffer. Gerhard Schroeder, of the Socialist Democratic Party won the chancellorship post in the 1998 election and retained it in the 2002 election.

## The United States and the War on Terrorism

The United States-led war to liberate Kuwait from Iraq promoted both hatred and admiration for future American policies. In the 2000 election, an energetic George W. Bush won the American presidency with a slim margin. Shortly after, on September 2001, an orchestrated attack by members of the Islamic terrorist group "al-Qaida" destroyed the World Trade Center in New York and caused extensive

*Figure 25–3 European Union membership extended to Eastern Europe in 2004* damage to the Pentagon building in Washington, D.C. Bush vowed to punish the perpetrators and in October 2001 the United Stated invaded Afghanistan, where al-Qaida leader Osama bin Laden was believed to hide, and destroyed the Afghan pro al-Qaida regime of Taliban. The American war on terrorism continued with the invasion of Iraq in 2003 to remove the brutal regime of Saddam Hussein. The invasion was based on the grounds that the Iraqi regime possessed weapons of mass destruction and financially supported terrorists to attack the United States and its allies. While the vast majority of peoples around the world believe that terrorism must be defeated, they equally believe that war, on the scale of the one in Iraq, may not be the answer.

## The Twenty-First Century and Global Prospects

With the end of the Cold War, the world's regions are no longer divided into pro-United States, pro-Soviet, and "non-aligned" states; rather, new configurations of allegiance based on economics, ideology, and strategic interest are still emerging. The emergence of the United States as the only remaining superpower; the end of the nuclear arms race between the U.S. and Soviet/post Soviet Russia; the expansion of NATO with the addition of former Soviet republics; and the resurgence of virulent nationalism and several bloody conflicts in Eastern Europe and elsewhere around the world have shaped the early history of the 21st century.

In the Muslim world, conflicts over the right for self-determination and the degree to which Islam will have an integral role in national identity, law, and government have taken center stage as the Israeli-Palestinian struggle devolves into civil war and as Islamist movements (through peaceful and violent means) move to more directly challenge the legitimacy of secular government. The recent confrontation between the West and the Islamic world was mounted not by secular regimes in Muslim countries, whose rulers were economically linked to and militarily dependent on the West, but rather by varied militant groups that operated both openly and underground. Since these groups do not possess the conventional armed forces of a sovereign state, they recruited fighters among alienated, underemployed young men from the Middle East and South Asia, whose societies had failed to capitalize on a globally driven economy that enabled peoples of other developing regions to prosper and flourish. The rise of religious extremism, suicide bombing, and martyrdom in the name of religion pushed these young men to become a dangerous force that resorted to the acts of terrorism to achieve its goals.

The September 11, 2001, attacks on the United States, the March 11, 2004, Madrid train bombing, and the July 5, 2005, London public transport system suicide bombing represent a fundamental turning point in Western history because they directly allude to an emerging global war of ideas: democracy vs. theocracy and authoritarianism; tolerance vs. intolerance; modernism vs. traditionalism; peace and co-existence vs. war and violence; and poverty vs. prosperity. The fear and anxiety caused by the new threat of international terrorism at the beginning of the 21st century makes it essential for the West to win this war of ideas, if it hopes to continue and prevail as the World's leading civilization.

## Perspective

*The great events and significant trends from 1985-2004 included (1) the reunification of Germany and, to an extent, Western Europe itself; (2) the reduction of national ambitions among the technically developed nations and the decline of the superpowers; (3) the continued increase of world population and the steady Westernization of all nations under the impact of technology; (4) further realization of the need for determined environmental improvement and the accelerated progress of the natural sciences, especially medicine; (5) the international effort to combat terrorism and the pre-emptive use of military force as a means to do so. All this is perhaps evidence that a new period in Western civilization, sometimes labeled "postmodern," has indeed dawned. In this new world, neither war nor money holds out the promise of solving major problems. Even from a geographical point of view, a new age had begun. If the Mediterranean area circumscribed what historians call "ancient" history, Europe the "medieval" world, and the entire planet "modern" times, then it may be that expansion into air and space justifies the view that a new age is beginning. Only future historians will be able to tell whether Western civilization has retained its place in this new world.*

## Selected Readings

Gorbachev, Mikhail S. *Memoirs* (New York: Doubleday, 1996).

Keylor, William. *The Twentieth-Century World and Beyond: An International History* (Oxford: Oxford University Press, 2006).

Lepor, Keith Philip, ed. *After the Cold War: Essays on the Emerging World Order* (Austin: University of Texas Press, 1997).

Pond, Elizabeth. *Beyond the Wall: Germany's Road to Unification* (Washington, D.C.: Brookings Institution, 1993).

Reminck, David. Resurrection: *The Struggle for a new Russia* (New York: Random House, 1997).

Reynolds, David. *One World Divisible: A Global History since 1945* (New York: Penguin Books, 2001).

Brower, Daniel R. *The World in the Twentieth Century: From Empires to Nations* (New York: Pearson Prentice Hall, 2006).

## Test Yourself

1. The reunification of Germany was completed by a national referendum in_____
   A. October 1990
   B. December 1989
   C. October 1989
   D. December 1990

2. The two words *glasnost* and *perestroika* are translated as:_____
   A. Freedom and Democracy
   B. Socialism and Equality
   C. Openness and Restructuring
   D. None of the above

3. In 1993, Palestinians and Israelis signed the_____
   A. The Geneva Accords
   B. The Jerusalem Compromise
   C. The Cairo Agreement
   D. The Oslo Accords

4. The following East European countries were admitted to membership in NATO, except_____
   A. Hungary
   B. Romania
   C. Czech Republic
   D. Poland

5. The first Chancellor of reunified Germany in 1990 was _____
   A. Willy Brandt
   B. Helmut Kohl
   C. Gerhard Schroeder
   D. None of the above

6. The 1995 Dayton Agreement brought and end to the civil war in _____
   A. Bosnia
   B. Romania
   C. Croatia
   D. Montenegro

7. In 1997 election in England led to Labor Party victory, headed by____
   A. John Major
   B. Margaret Thatcher
   C. Anthony Eden
   D. Tony Blair

## Answers and Explanations

1. **A.** After the collapse of the Berlin Wall in 1989, East and West Germany were reunited once a national referendum was endorsed in October of 1990.

2. **C.** Mikhail Gorbachev, a younger member of the Soviet communist hierarchy, was elected to the post of secretary general of the Party in 1985. His program of *glasnost* (openness) and *perestroika* (restructuring) envisioned the transformation of the Soviet economy.

3. **D.** With Norway's mediation, Palestinians and Israelis met in Oslo and negotiated the 1993 Oslo Accords that called for Palestinian autonomy in Gaza and the West Bank and ultimately the creation of a Palestinian state to peacefully co-exist with Israel.

4. **B.** After 1995, the economic conditions began to change for the better in Eastern Europe and by 1999 Poland, Hungary and the Czech Republic were admitted to the North Atlantic Treaty Organization (NATO).

5. **B.** Chancellor Kohl, of the Christian Democratic Union, became the first chancellor of reunified Germany in 1990.

6. **A.** Bosnia with its three ethnic groups: Catholic Croats, Muslims, and Orthodox Serbs seceded in 1992. This action promoted Serbia to react. The three ethnic groups brutally fought each other and a process of Serbian ethnic cleansing of Muslims provoked moral outrage. It took United Nations and NATO intervention in 1995 to stop Serbian atrocities. The United States hosted a conference in Dayton, Ohio, that led to the Dayton Agreement in November 1995. The agreement proposed was equally represented by Muslims, Serbs, and Croats.

7. **D.** In the 1997 election, the Labor Party, revitalized under the leadership of Tony Blair, won a major victory.

# Index

**A**

Aachen (Aix-la-Chapelle), Congress of, 156, 166
Abelard, Peter, 14
Adenauer, Konrad, 331, 339
Aeschylus, 4
Afghanistan, 199, 202, 222, 250, 288, 336, 348, 349, 351, 357
   Soviet invasion of, 348
   US invasion of, 348, 349, 357
"Age of Reason", 75, 83, 110
Aix-la-Chapelle, Peace of (1668), 95
Aix-la-Chapelle, Peace of (1748), 109, 116, 118
Albania, 259, 298, 308, 348, 353
Al-Qaida, 348
Alsace and Lorraine, 50, 59, 79, 89, 197, 218, 258, 270
America, 23, 27, 30, 36, 37, 42, 60, 64, 68, 75–77, 84, 89, 92, 98, 102, 105, 110, 115–120, 122, 124, 129–133, 137, 146–148, 151, 157, 171, 173, 184, 185, 199, 202, 203, 207, 227, 232, 240, 241, 243, 248, 252, 255–257, 288, 292, 305, 323, 328, 331, 341
   Balboa, 23, 25, 27
   Canada, 76, 82, 118, 119, 129, 199, 253, 323
   Caribbean, 99, 101, 118, 120, 129
      Cuba, 255, 327, 331, 341
         Castro, Fidel, 331
         Cuban crisis, 327
      Jamaica, 102
   Central America, 146, 221, 233, 247, 255, 256, 288, 327, 331, 341, 342, 348, 351
      El Salvador, 351
      Nicaragua, 351
      Panama, 221, 233, 247, 255, 256, 342, 348, 351
         Panama Canal, 247, 256, 342
         US invasion, 348, 351
      Puerto Rico, 255
   colony, 37, 42, 60, 64, 75–77, 89, 92, 98, 102, 105, 110, 115–120, 129–133, 137, 146, 151, 199, 203, 207, 232, 248
      Dutch, 76, 98, 102
      English, 76, 98, 102, 105, 110, 115, 117–119, 120, 129–131, 146, 199
         Cornwallis, 131
         Ghent, Treaty of, 39, 146
         North American Act (1867), 199
         Stamp Act, 110, 120
      French, 76, 102, 117–119, 129, 131
      Jesuits, 60
      Portugal, 102, 105, 132, 146
      revolutions, 137
      slaves and slave trade, 105, 203, 207
      Spanish, 37, 42, 60, 75, 76, 89, 105, 118, 131, 132, 146, 232, 248
      Swedish, 76
   discovery by Columbus, 23, 27, 36
   Gomara's history of, 30
   Latin America, 157, 227, 240, 241, 252, 255, 256, 292, 305, 323, 328, 340, 341
      First Pan-American Congress (1889), 227
      "Monroe Doctrine", 157
      see also South America
      see also Central America
      see also North America, Mexico
      see also Caribbean,
   Native Americans, 76, 184, 226
      extermination of, 184
   North America, 27, 76, 84, 92, 102, 115, 118–120, 129, 146, 151, 185, 202, 292
      Mexico, 25, 27, 35, 43, 76, 89, 146, 179, 192, 194, 227, 279, 292, 306
   Pan-American Union, 257, 305
   settlements and colonists, 75, 118
   South America, 84, 132, 146, 151, 202, 255, 341
      Argentina, 146, 325, 341
      Bolivar, 146, 155
      Bolivia, 43
         Potosi silver mines, 43
      Brazil, 37, 42, 76, 89, 102, 113, 146, 155, 238, 319, 331
         independence of, 155
      Chile, 146, 155, 341
         Allende, Salvadore, 341
      Columbia, 76, 89, 255
      Miranda, 146
      Morelos, 146
      Paraguay, 76, 89, 146
      Peru, 27, 43, 76, 89, 146, 252
      Republic of Gran Columbia, 155
      San Martin, 146
      Uruguay, 146
      Venezuela, 146, 255
      Vespucci, Amerigo, 27
Amundsen, 243, 247
   North Pole, discovery of, 243
   South Pole, discovery of, 243, 247
Anarchism and Anarchists, 171, 172, 200, 212, 213, 223, 224, 236, 251, 253, 342, 347
   Bakunin, see Russia, Bakunin
   Kropotkin, see Russia, Kropotkin
   see also Nihilism and Nihilists
Andersen, Hans Christian, 252
Anti-Semitism, 251, 252, 263
Aquinas, St. Thomas, 14, 17
Arabs, 1, 15, 140, 142, 147, 154, 155, 172, 194, 202, 207, 217, 221–223, 231, 241, 249, 251, 257, 258, 288, 296, 308, 311, 318, 323, 324, 326, 327, 330, 335, 336, 338, 339, 342, 343, 347–349, 351, 355, 357
   Arab-Israeli war (1967), 318
   Arab-Israeli war (1973), 336, 338, 342, 347
   energy crisis, and 339
   states, 140, 142, 147, 154, 155, 172, 194, 202, 207, 217, 221–223. 231, 241, 249, 251, 257, 258, 288, 296, 308, 311, 318, 323, 324, 326, 327, 335, 336, 338, 339, 342, 347–349, 351, 355, 357
   Algeria, 155, 318, 323, 330, French occupation, 155
      independence, 318
   Egypt, 1, 140, 142, 147, 154, 172, 194, 202, 207, 217, 222, 223, 231, 288, 308, 311, 318, 323, 326, 327, 335, 336, 338, 342, 347
      ancient Egyptian hieroglyphic language, 147
      British occupation, 217, 223, 231, 288
      revolutionary movement against, 223, 231
      Egypt-Israeli peace treaty, 336, 342
      Napoleon's campaign, 140, 142, 147, 154
      Nasser, 323, 335
      "Rosetta stone", 154
      Sadat, Anwar, 342
      Suez Canal, 194, 202, 207, 217, 222, 308, 318, 323, 326, 335
         construction of, 202
         invasion by England-France-Israel, 318, 323, 335
         nationalization of (1956), 318, 323
         opening (1869), 207
   Iraq, 288, 296, 327, 348, 349, 351, 355, 357
      economic sanctions against, 351
      Hussein, Saddam, 357
      US invasion of, 349, 357
   Kuwait, 348, 351, 355
   Libya, 339
   Morocco, 194, 249, 251, 257, 258, 339
   Palestine, 288, 296, 318, 323, 324, 335, 348
      Intifada, 348
      partition of, 323, 324, 335
      PLO, 348
   Sudan, 249, 257
   Syria, 194, 326
   Tran Jordan, 288, 296
   Tunisia, 217, 221, 223, 323
      French protectorate, 217, 221, 223, 323
      rebellion against French rule, 323
Architecture, 2, 3, 4, 7, 11, 60, 84, 85, 90, 95, 99, 104, 108, 149, 174, 209, 238, 239, 279, 280, 284, 293, 329
   17th Century, 84
   Baroque style, 84, 85, 90
   Greek, 2, 3, 4
   Roman, 7
   Spanish, 60
Aristocracy, 16, 21, 97–99, 101, 111, 125, 156
   see also Nobility
Aristophanes, 4
Aristotle, 1, 3, 11, 14, 21
Arkwright, 110, 120
Art, 3, 5, 15, 17, 23, 24, 26, 29, 30, 32, 35, 44, 47, 56, 65, 66, 84, 85, 90, 92, 99, 104, 122, 123, 125, 147, 149, 168, 174, 207, 209, 214, 236, 238–240, 242, 243, 246, 247, 279, 283–285, 303, 310, 329
   Abstract, 329
   Baroque style, 84, 85, 90
   Expressionism, 236, 239, 240, 243, 247, 283–285
   Greek, 5, 15
   Impressionism, 207, 209, 214, 236, 239, 240
   Mannerism, 65
   Medieval, 15
   Neoclassic, 149, 174, 209
   neo-Gothic, 174, 209
   pre-Raphaelite, 209
   Rococo, 125, 149
   Roman, 47, 56
      destruction of, 47, 56
   Romantic, see Romanticism
   Surrealist, 239, 246
   see also Architecture
   see also Literature
   see also Music
   see also Painting
   see also Sculpture
Augustus, Cesar, 1, 8
Aurelius, Marcus, 1, 8
Australia, 132, 181, 253, 304, 323
Austria, 38, 60, 68, 77, 96, 99, 100, 104, 108, 110, 111, 113, 115, 116, 117, 135, 136, 139, 141–145, 156–158, 182–184, 186, 187, 191, 192, 194, 195–197, 203, 207, 217, 220–223, 225, 237, 238, 240, 243, 246, 248–251, 258, 259, 263–268, 270, 271, 275, 290, 298, 301, 307, 322, 325, 326
Aztecs, 27, 35, 172

**B**

Bach, Johann Sebastian, 109, 125, 149
   *Art of Fugue*, 109, 125
   *St. John Passion*, 125
   *St. Matthew Passion*, 109, 125

## 362  Index

Bacon, Francis, 58, 67, 74
   Novum Organum, 74
Bacon, Roger, 14
Bagehot, 247
Balkans, 39, 42, 99, 108, 179, 186, 225, 227, 247, 250, 252, 258, 259, 260, 263, 271, 292, 308, 321, 354
   Balkan Wars, 247, 259
      First Balkan War (1912), 247
      Second Balkan War (1913), 247
   Pan-Slav Congress, 179, 186, 225
   see also Bosnia
   see also Croatia
   see also Serbia
   see also Slovenia
   see also Yugoslavia
Balzac, 173, 179, 239
   Comedie Humaine (The Human Comedy), 173, 179
Basle, Peace of (1795), 130
Batavian republic, 142
Becquerel, 237
   radioactivity, discovery of, 237
Beethoven, 141, 149, 155
   Fidelio, 149
   Ninth Symphony, 155
Belgium, 132, 145, 161, 163, 179, 187, 227, 252, 263, 266, 267, 272, 273, 278, 299, 308, 322, 340
Bell, Graham, 217
   Telephone, invention of, 217
Bergson, Henri, 238
Berlioz, 167, 174, 178, 209
   Symphonie Fantastique, 167, 174, 178
Bernardin de Saint-Pierre, 124
   Paul et Virginie, 124
Bernini, Giovanni, 85, 90
Bernstein, Eduard, see Germany, Social-Democratic Party, Bernstein, Eduard
Berlin Wall, see Germany, Berlin Wall
Biology and Biological Science, 85, 104, 125, 147, 156, 207, 210, 237, 282, 296, 328, 331, 335, 343
   biogenetics, 328, 335
   DNA, 328, 331, 335, 343
   see also Medicine and Medical Science
Bismarck, Otto von, see Germany, Bismarck, Otto von
Bizet, 209
   Carmen, 209
Boccaccio, 16
Bologna, University of, 12
Bolshevik Revolution, see Russia, Revolutions, October, 1917
Bonaparte, Napoleon, see France, Bonaparte, Napoleon
Bohr, Niels, 247, 280
   atomic structure, description of, 247
Bosnia, 258, 259, 263, 270, 348, 349, 353, 360
   Dayton Agreement, 360
   see also Balkans,
   see also Croatia
   see also Serbia

   see also Slovenia
   see also Yugoslavia
Bossuet, 102
Bourbon dynasty, 62, 83, 116, 145, 158, 163, 181, 183, 187, 198
Boyle, 103
   Properties of Gases, 103
Brahe, Tycho, 67
Brandt, Willy, see Germany, Brandt, Willy
Britain, 12, 16, 17, 21, 25, 26, 28, 29, 36, 37, 38, 40, 42–44, 47–51, 56, 58, 59, 63, 64, 67, 68, 74–78, 80–82, 85, 89, 91, 92, 95–99, 102, 104, 105, 108–110, 112–122, 124, 125, 129–132, 136, 137, 139, 140, 142–148, 151, 154, 155, 157–161, 163, 166–168, 170–175, 178–182, 184, 185, 188, 191, 192, 194, 197, 199, 200, 202, 203, 206–208, 211, 212, 217, 219, 220–223, 225, 227, 231, 233–236, 238, 242, 246–259, 263, 265–268, 270–272, 278, 286–290, 293, 296, 298, 300, 304, 307–312, 317, 318, 321–323, 325, 327, 330, 335–337, 339, 340, 342, 343, 353, 355, 360
   Anglican Church, see Church,
   Anti-Communist policy, 286
   Art and Literature, 173, 174, 208
   Asquith, 236, 246, 252
   balance of power in Europe, 116, 118, 146, 157, 194, 248, 249
   loss of Calais, 63
   Balfour, 252
   "Bill of Rights", 92, 98
   Blair, Tony, 355, 360
   Boleyn, Anne, 49
   Boleyn, Thomas, 49
   Burke, Edmund, 158
   Chamberlain, Joseph, 247, 252
   Charles I, 74, 81, 82, 89, 91, 96, 97
      execution of, 91
   Chartist rising, 179, 180, 181, 191
   Chevalier-Cobden Treaty, 192, 194
   Civil War, 75, 81, 82, 85, 96
   colonies, 76, 89, 105, 118–121, 131, 137, 142, 146, 151, 154, 181, 191, 199, 202, 203, 217, 222, 223, 225, 231, 247, 249, 250, 252–255, 257, 258, 270, 288, 293, 296, 311, 323, 330, 335
      Africa and Near East, 217, 222, 223, 231, 257, 270, 288, 323, 335
      Boer War, 257
      Suez Canal, 202, 217, 222, 318, 323, 335
         Suez crisis, 318, 323, 335
      America, 76, 89, 105, 118, 120, 121, 131, 137, 142, 146, 151, 154, 199, 255
         slave trade, 105, 121
      Clive, Robert, 118
      Colonists, 118

      disintegration of, 330
      East India, 118, 181, 199, 202, 222, 288, 298, 318
         Gandhi, Mahatma, 288, 298, 323
      Far East and Pacific, 179, 181, 191, 202, 222, 247, 254, 257, 288, 311
      French and Indian War, 118
      Ireland, 67, 68, 119, 222, 293
      King George's War, 118
      Middle East, 258, 270
      Statute of Westminster, 288
      War of Jenkins's Ear, 118
   Commonwealth, 132, 288, 304, 323, 330
   Corn Law, 159, 179, 180, 181, 191
      Anti-Corn Law League, 180, 181, 191
   Cranmer, Archbishop, 49
   Cromwell, Oliver, 82, 89, 91, 96–98, 102
   Cromwell, Thomas, 49
   Disraeli, 199, 206, 222
   emigration, 242
   Entente Cordiale, 247–249, 258
   Fabian Society, 222, 231, 236
   Fisher, John, 49
   George, Lloyd, 236, 246, 252, 265, 270, 288
   Gladstone, 253
   "Glorious Revolution", 92, 97, 98, 105, 108
   Great Fire in London (1665), 91
   Henry VIII, 38, 43, 49, 50, 56, 63
   industry and industrial revolution, 148, 167, 168, 170, 172, 174, 178, 194, 199, 219, 233, 234, 289
      reforms, 167, 172, 178
   Labor Party, 289, 300, 325, 339, 355, 360
   Levelers, 82
   Major, John, 355
   More, Thomas, 23, 30, 31, 49, 59, 172
   Navigation Act, 91, 96
   Nelson, Admiral, 143, 154
   parliament, 38, 49, 64, 81, 82, 89, 92, 96–98, 105, 110, 114, 115, 125, 159, 161, 163, 166, 167, 180, 248, 253, 263
      electoral system, 163
      "Long Parliament", 81
      "Rump" Parliament, 82, 89
   Petition of Rights, 74
   population, 171, 233
   Reform Bill, 161, 179, 180, 199, 206, 207, 222
   Romantic Movement, see Romanticism, England
   Salisbury, 252
   Scotland, 49, 51, 63, 64, 66, 82, 89, 92, 98, 119, 336, 339
   Seven Years' War, 116, 117, 119
   Socialism and Socialists, 236, 246
   "South Sea Bubble", 109
   Stuarts, 81, 114
   Thatcher, Margaret, 355
   Thirty Years' War, 85, 99

   Tory party, 97, 114, 159, 161, 166, 180
   Triple Entente, 247, 248–250, 263, 266
   Tudor dynasty, 36, 38, 44, 63, 81
   "Victorian" era and style, 199, 238–240
      Queen Victoria, 180, 222, 238, 248
   War of the Roses, 36
   Whigs, 97, 114, 161, 180, 188
   Wolsey, Cardinal, 49
   Women, 168
Britten, Benjamin, 342
Browning, Elizabeth, 208
Browning, Robert, 208
Bulgaria, 225, 231, 252, 258, 259, 266, 268, 270, 330, 348, 349, 353
Bunyan, 91, 104
   Pilgrim's Progress, 91, 104
Burghers, 26, 28, 29, 30, 32, 35–37, 42, 65, 80, 81, 134, 142
Burke, Edmund, see Britain, Burke, Edmund
Byron, 140, 150, 173
   Childe Harold's Pilgrimage, 140, 173
Byzantine Empire, 15, 29, 329

## C

Caesar, 8, 52
Calderon, 84
Calvin, John, see Church, Reformation, Calvin, John
Cambodia, 338
Camus, Albert, 342
Canaletto, Antonio, 125
Carlyle, 167, 179, 208, 247
   Heroes and Hero-Worship, 179
Carnegie, 233
Carnegie Peace Endowment, 256
Castro, Fidel, see America, Caribbean, Cuba, Castro, Fidel
Catholic, see Church, Roman Catholic
Cavour, 192, 197, 198, 207
Cellini, Benvenuto, 29, 30
Celsius, 109
   Thermometer, invention of, 109
Cervantes, 67, 72, 74
   Don Quixote, 67, 72, 74
Cezanne, 239
Chaplin, Charles, 284
Charlemagne, 12, 16, 21, 59
Charles de Gaulle, see France, Charles de Gaulle
Chateaubriand, 150
Chekhov, Anton, 239
Chemistry, 103, 123, 147, 174, 210, 214, 237, 238, 281, 282, 319, 328, 331, 335, 343
Chernobyl atomic disaster (1986), 348, 349
China, 28, 77, 101, 122, 181, 191, 192, 199, 200, 202, 222, 241, 247, 254, 256, 257, 288, 311, 312, 318, 323, 325–328, 330, 340–343, 347
   Mao Zedong, 342, 347
   "Opium War", 181, 191
Chirac, Jacques, see France, Chirac, Jacques
Chopin, 174

# Index

Church, 12, 14, 16, 21, 24, 28, 30, 35, 37, 38, 44–46, 48–52, 56, 58, 60, 63–66, 72, 76, 78, 80–84, 89, 94, 95, 97, 100, 133, 134, 137, 142, 145, 149, 156, 158, 161, 174, 181, 182, 194, 197, 209, 211, 214, 218, 220, 222, 231, 235, 240, 241, 243, 252, 291, 296, 301–303, 330, 342, 351
   abuses, 44
   clergy, 24, 35, 44, 45, 51, 52, 60, 84, 133, 134, 156, 194, 240, 241, 303
   Dominicans, 76, 89, 197
   English (Anglican), 49, 58, 63, 64, 81, 82, 97, 161
      "Thirty-nine Articles", 58, 63
   Fascism, and, 301
   France, and, 134, 137, 142, 145, 181, 194, 211, 241
      French Revolution, and, 134, 137
      Napoleon, and, 142, 145
   Franciscans, 76, 89, 197
   Germany, in, 45, 46, 49, 51, 220, 222, 231
   Jesuits, 43, 52, 60, 64, 76, 77, 84, 89, 94, 111, 113, 240
   Orthodox, 12, 14, 100, 113, 209, 211, 235, 240, 241, 274, 285, 291, 293, 296, 319, 351, 353, 360
      Greek, 240
      Neo-Orthodox, 285, 293, 319
   Pope and Papacy, 14, 23, 27, 36, 37, 44, 45, 47, 49, 51, 52, 56, 59, 100, 124, 134, 142, 143, 179, 183, 187, 194, 197–199, 206, 207, 211, 214, 216, 220, 223, 231, 235, 240, 279, 302, 330, 342
      Alexander V (Borgia), 23
      Gregory XIII, 52
         "Gregorian Calendar", 52
         replacement of Julian Calendar, 52
      John XXIII, 330, 342
      Leo XIII, 235
      Papal infallibility, dogma of, 207, 211, 216, 220, 231
      Papal states, 143, 183, 187, 197, 198, 206, 207, 279
      Pious IX, 211, 214, 235
   Protestant, 43, 44, 47, 49, 50, 52, 56, 57, 62, 63, 66, 68, 76, 78, 82–85, 98, 105, 111, 113, 211, 216, 217, 220, 231, 235, 240, 241, 283, 285, 296, 340, 355
   Reformation, 23, 43–53, 56, 58, 59, 62, 65, 83, 101, 137, 209, 264, 283, 296
      Calvin, John, 43, 50, 51, 59, 61, 62, 64, 79, 82, 83, 85, 89, 94, 95, 97
         Servetus, burning at stake, 31, 44, 51
      Catholic Reformation, 51
      Counter Reformation, 51, 52, 56, 78, 84
         Council of Trent (1563), 52, 58, 66

Luther, Martin, 23, 29–31, 43, 45–51, 56, 59, 61, 64, 72, 78, 79, 89, 100
   *95 Theses*, 23
   Puritans, 63, 76, 81, 82, 85, 89
   Savonarola, 23, 45
   Ulrich Zwingli, 48, 49, 56
   Roman Catholic, 12, 14, 16, 21, 30, 44–47, 49–51, 52, 56, 57, 59–66, 68, 76–79, 81–85, 89, 94, 98, 100, 105, 108, 113, 142, 144, 145, 148, 150, 155, 159, 161, 181, 183, 184, 209, 211, 214, 216–218, 220, 221, 231, 235, 240, 241, 243, 251, 285, 302, 303, 330, 340, 342, 353, 355, 360
   Russia, in, 65, 72, 100, 235, 241, 291, 296, 351, 211
   Schmalkaldic war, 50
   St. Peter's Church in Rome, 85, 90, 211, 216
   state and, 240
   Vatican, 199, 223, 240, 251, 279, 302, 330, 342
Churchill, Winston, 308
Cicero, 1, 8
Clausewitz, 342
Clive, Robert, *see* Britain, colonies, Clive, Robert
Clouet, Jean, 29
Colbert, 91, 95, 102, 108, 139
Cold War, 318, 322, 326, 327, 331, 339, 348–350, 355, 357, 360
   Berlin Blockade (1948), 318, 326
   Berlin Wall, 318, 327, 348, 349, 360
      demolition of (1989), 348, 349, 360
Coleridge, 140, 150
Columbus, Christopher, 23, 25, 27, 36
   America, discovery of, 23, 25, 27, 36
Common Market, *see* EEC (European Economic Community)
Communist Manifesto, *see* Marx, Karl, Marxism, Communist Manifesto
Comte, Auguste, 179, 209, 216, 251, 282
   *Cours de philosophie positive*, 179
   *see also* Positivism and Positivists
Congress of Vienna (1815), 140, 145, 155, 167, 252, 269
Conrad, 239
Constable, 174
Constantinople, 225, 231, 257, 259
Cook, 110, 147
   Trip around the World, 147
Cooper, James Fenimore, 173
   *Leatherstocking tales*, 173
Copernicus, Nicholas, 31, 43, 59, 67, 72
   *De Revolutionibus Orbium Coelestium (On the Revolutions of the Heavenly Spheres)*, 43
Corelli, 125
Corneille, 74, 104
   *Le Cid*, 74, 104

Cortes, Hernan, 27, 35
Cranach, 29
Crick and Watson, 328, 335
   biogenetics, 328, 335
   genetic code (DNA), 328, 331, 335, 343
Croatia, 339, 353, 360
   Croats, 353, 360
   *see also* Balkans,
   *see also* Bosnia,
   *see also* Serbia
   *see also* Slovenia,
   *see also* Yugoslavia
Crusades, 12
   First, 12
   Second, 12
   Third, 12
Curie, Mary and Pierre, 232, 237
   Radium, discovery of, 232, 237
Cyprus, 225, 323, 340, 342, 347
Czech Republic, 348, 353, 360
Czechoslovakia, 270, 271, 286, 292, 298, 307, 321, 325, 336, 341, 348, 349, 353
   Communist regime, 321
   end of, 348
   Dubcek, Alexander, 341
   German invasion, 298, 307
   Soviet invasion, 336, 341
   *see also* Bohemia
   *see also* Czech Republic
   *see also* Slovakia

## D

Dante, 150
   *Divina Commedia*, 150
Danton, *see* France, French Revolution, Danton
Darwin, Charles, 207, 210, 211, 214, 216, 237
   Theory of Evolution, 207, 210, 211, 216
Darwin, Erasmus, 210
Debussy, 240
Defoe, Daniel, 109, 124
   *Robinson Crusoe*, 109, 124
Delacroix, 174
Denmark, 47, 49, 64, 72, 75, 78, 101, 110, 122, 145, 174, 186, 192, 195, 222, 227, 270, 285, 299, 308
Derby, 199
Descartes, 74, 83, 84, 101, 209
   *Discours de la Methode*, 74
De Vries, 237
Dewes, Charles G., 300
Dewey, John, 282
Dickens, Charles, 173, 179
   *Oliver Twist*, 179
Diets, 16, 21, 36, 38, 43, 46, 47, 59, 65, 100, 113, 186, 236, 246, 325
   *see also* Russia, Duma
   *see also* Parliament
Dürrenmatt, Friedrich, 342
Donizetti, 174
Don Quixote, *see* Cervantes, Don Quixote
Dostoevsky, Feodore, 207, 208, 239
   *Brothers Karamazovs*, 208
   *Crime and Punishment*, 207, 208
Drake, 63
Dreiser, Theodore, 283
Droste-Hülshoff, 208

Dubcek, Alexander, *see* Czechoslovakia, Dubcek, Alexander
Dumas, 173, 179, 239
   *Count of Monte Cristo*, 179
   *The Three Musketeers*, 173
Dupleix, *see* France, colonies, Dupleix
Durer, 29, 43
   *Four Apostles*, 43
Dvorak, 240, 285

## E

East India Company, 59, 118
   Dutch, 59
   English, 59, 118
Edict of Nantes, 58, 62, 83, 91, 95
Edison, Thomas Alva, 217, 255
   Electric Light Bulb, invention of, 217
   Phonograph, invention of, 217
EEC (European Economic Community), 339, 349
Eichendorff, 150
Einstein, Albert, 236, 237, 246, 247, 280
   Theory of Relativity, 236, 237, 246, 247, 280
El Greco, 66, 72
Eliot, George, 208
Eliot, T.S., 284
Emerson, 208
Emily, 173
   *Wuthering Heights*, 173
Engels, Friedrich, 212, 224
   *Communist Manifesto*, 212
England, *see* Britain
Enlightenment, Age of, 109, 110, 112, 123–125, 129, 130, 131, 137, 148, 156, 167, 173, 208, 209, 211, 256, 264, 301, 318, 330
Epstein, Jacob, 284
Erasmus of Rotterdam, 30, 31, 43, 59
Estonia, 64, 65, 271, 299, 302, 353
European Common Market, *see* EEC (European Economic Community)
European Union (EU), 348, 349, 353, 355, 356
Euro, 348, 349, 355
European Parliament, 336
Existentialism and Existentialists, 319, 342, 347
Expressionism and Expressionists, 240, 247, 283, 284

## F

Falkland war, 336
Faraday, Michel, 174, 179
Fascism, 279, 284, 298, 299, 301–308, 311–313, 316, 320, 325, 330, 336, 342, 344
   Characteristics, 301
   Communism versus, 305
   defeat of, 311, 312
   Democracy versus, 304
   Fascism in action, 302
   World War II, in, 306–308, 311, 312
   "quislings", 308
   spread of, 302

Fascism *(Continued)*
  see also Germany, Nazism and Nazi (National Socialist) Party
  see also Italy, Fascist rule
  see also Mussolini, Benito
Fashoda, crisis, 249, 257, 258
Fichte, 148, 158, 173, 209
Finland, 100, 144, 145, 224, 254, 271, 273, 278, 284, 298, 308, 321
Fitzgerald, F. Scott, 283
Flaubert, 173
  *Madame Bovary*, 173
Fleming, Alexander, 282
  Penicillin, discovery of, 282
Fourier, Charles, 172, 178
France, 12, 16, 17, 21, 23, 29, 30, 36, 38, 39, 40, 42, 43, 47, 49–51, 56, 58, 59, 61–64, 67, 68, 74–79, 82, 83, 91–93, 95–100, 102–105, 108–120, 122–125, 129, 130–137, 139–146, 149, 150, 151, 154–160, 163, 166–168, 170–175, 179, 181–183, 185, 187, 188, 191, 192, 194–199, 200, 202, 203, 206–209, 211, 213, 217, 218, 220–223, 227, 232, 234–237–240, 247–251, 253, 254, 257–259, 263, 266–268, 270–272, 278, 279, 283, 284, 286–290, 297, 299, 300, 304, 307, 308, 311, 312, 317, 318, 321–323, 325–327, 329–331, 335–337, 339, 340, 342, 343, 344, 355
  absolutism, 82, 83, 92
  Alsace and Loraine, dispute with Germany, *see* Alsace and Loraine
  Blanc, Louis, 172, 185
  Bonaparte, Napoleon, 140–147, 149, 151, 154–156, 158, 159, 161, 162, 166, 167, 173, 181, 208, 221, 256, 270
    Austerlitz, battle of, 140
    *Code Napoleon*, 142, 144, 147, 154, 158
    Constitution, 142
    Consulate, the (1799–1804), 142
    decline, 143
    Directorate, 145
    Egypt, conquest of, 142, 147, 154
    as Emperor, 140
    European conquests, 142
    exile of, 145
    exile to St. Helena, 140, 145, 151, 154
    Italian campaign, 142
    Leipzig, battle of, 145
    Napoleonic Code, 158
    Napoleonic wars, 142–146, 159, 161, 166, 173
    Parliament, 133
    Russian campaign, 140, 144, 154
    Trafalgar, battle of, 140, 143
    Waterloo, battle of, 140, 145, 154
  Catherine de Medici, 62
  Charles de Gaulle, 312, 327, 330, 331, 335, 340
  Chevalier-Cobden Treaty, 192, 194
  Chirac, Jacques, 355
  Civil War, 58, 62, 82
  Clemenceau, 251, 263, 270
  Colbert, 91, 95, 102, 108, 139
  colonies, 76, 118, 119, 155, 217, 218, 257, 258, 288, 311, 312, 323, 330
    Africa, 217, 218, 257, 258, 330
    Algeria, seizure of, 155
    Dupleix, 109, 118
    East India, 118
    Far East, 257, 311, 312
    French America, 76, 118, 119
    French and Indian war, 117, 118
    Tollendal, Lally, 118
  The Consulate (1799–1804), 142
  Dreyfus affair, 232, 251, 263
  Dubois, 114, 116
  Entente Cordiale (1904), 247–249, 258
  February Revolution (1848), 179, 181, 183, 185
  Fleury, 114, 116
  French Revolution (1789), 130, 132–137, 139, 140, 144, 146, 151, 156, 163, 167, 185, 191, 208, 288, 344
    Committee of Public Safety, 136, 137
    Cordeliers, 134
    Danton, 134, 136, 139
    Declaration of the Rights of Man, 134, 139, 344
    Estates-General, 38, 82, 83, 94, 134
    Fall of Bastille, 130, 134, 139
    Feuillants, 134
    Girondins, 136
    Jacobins, 134, 136, 213
    Marat, 134, 136
    "Reign of Terror", 136, 139
    Robespierre, 130, 134, 136, 137, 139, 141
  House of Valois, 38, 42
  Huguenots, 58, 62, 99, 105
  July Revolution (1830), 155, 159, 161, 163, 166
  Lorraine, France's claim of, 79, 89
  Louis IX, reign of, 36
  Louis XI, reign of, 42
  Louis XIV, reign of, 93, 98, 100, 104, 110, 116
  Louis XV, 113
  Louis XVI, 134, 135, 136
  Louis XVIII, 145, 158, 166
  Louis Napoleon Bonaparte (Napoleon III), 186, 191, 192, 194–199, 203, 206, 207
  Maginot Line, *see* World War II, Maginot Line
  Mazarin, 91, 93
  Michelet, 208
  Mirabeau, 134
  Mitterrand, Francois, 355
  Montaigne, 58, 67
  Napoleon III, *see* Louis Napoleon Bonaparte
  Paris Commune, rising of, 207, 213
  Peace of Paris (1763), 110, 118, 119, 129
  Peace of Paris (1783), 130, 145
  Peace of Paris (1857), 192, 225
  Peace of the Pyrenees (1659), 79, 91
  Peace of Westphalia, 93, 108
  Petain, Marshal Henri, 308
  religious wars, 58, 62, 68
    Night of St. Bartholomew (1572), 62
    War of the three Henrys, 62
  Richelieu, 74, 83
  Rollin, Ledru, 185
  slave trade, 145
  Suez Canal, 194, 202, 318, 323
  Suez crisis, 318, 323
  Thiers, 181, 182, 208, 213
  "Vichy" government, 308
  "War of Devolution", 95
France, Anatole, 239
Franck, Cesar, 240
Francke, 124
Franklin, Benjamin, 109, 119, 123, 131
  experiments with lightning and electricity, 109
Freud, Sigmund, 237, 246, 247, 282, 342
Fugger Family, 26, 28, 43
  Fugger, Jacob, 43

**G**
Galicia, 270
Galileo, 67, 72, 74, 83
  Law of Falling Bodies, 74
Galsworthy, John, 283
Galvani, 147
  Animal electricity, discovery of, 147
Garbo, Greta, 284
Garibaldi, 183, 187, 191, 198
Gauguin, Paul, 239
Gauss, 174
George, Lloyd, 236, 246, 252, 265, 270, 288
George, Stefan, 284
Germany, 7, 12, 13, 16, 17, 21, 24, 26, 29–31, 36, 38–40, 42, 43, 45–48, 50, 52, 56, 59–62, 64, 66, 68, 72, 73, 75, 77–80, 82, 83, 85, 89, 92, 95, 96, 99, 100, 103–105, 109–117, 119, 122, 124, 125, 129, 136, 139–145, 143–145, 149, 150, 154, 156, 158, 159, 161, 163, 168, 170, 171, 173, 174, 178, 179, 182–184, 186, 187, 191–199, 203, 206–208, 210, 212, 217, 218, 220–223, 225, 227, 231, 233–240, 242, 243, 246–252, 256–259, 263–275, 278, 279, 283–290, 293, 296–303, 306–313, 316–318, 320–323, 325–327, 330, 331, 339, 340, 341, 343, 348–352, 355, 357
  Alsace and Loraine, dispute with France, *see* Alsace and Loraine
  Austro-Prussian dualism, solution of, 196
  Berlin Wall, 318, 327, 348, 360
  Bismarck, Otto von, 192, 195–197, 206, 207, 217–222, 225, 227, 231, 235, 236, 246, 247, 248, 250, 258, 259, 263, 266, 269
  Brandt, Willy, 339
  Brest-Litovsk Treaty, 264, 268, 274, 278
  *Bundesrat*, 218
  *Burschenschaften* (fraternities), 158
  Christian Democratic Party, 339, 355, 360
  Congress of Carlsbad (1819), 155, 156, 159
  Diet of Worms (1521), 43, 46
  Division of Germany, 318, 321, 322, 330
  East Germany (German Democratic Republic), 321, 322, 325, 339, 341, 348–350, 355
  emigrants, 101, 242
  Frankfurt Parliament, 186, 195
  Franco-Prussian War (1870–71), 197, 206, 225, 248
    Sedan, 206
  German Confederation (1848–1858), 193, 195
  German-Danish war (1864), 192
  German Empire, 38–40, 42, 43, 46, 47, 50, 68, 77, 79, 89, 115, 196, 197, 206, 207, 218, 231
  German-Russian Reinsurance Treaty (1887), 217, 221, 225, 248, 263
  German States and Territories, 38, 45, 60, 64, 78, 79, 89, 92, 96, 99, 100, 104, 105, 109, 110, 111, 113, 115–117, 122, 124, 129, 136, 139–145, 154, 158, 161, 182–184, 186, 191, 192, 194–198, 203, 206–208, 218, 240, 248, 266, 268, 270, 271, 290, 298, 300, 307
    Austria, *see* Austria
    Bavaria, 38, 60, 290
    Bohemia, 78, 186, 240, 270
    Brandenburg, 38, 60, 79, 89, 92, 99, 100, 105, 113, 115
    Moravia, 124, 270
    Prussia, 64, 96, 100, 104, 105, 110, 111, 113, 115–117, 122, 129, 136, 139–145, 154, 158, 161, 182–184, 186, 191, 192, 194–198, 203, 206–208, 218, 248, 266, 268, 270
    Rhineland, 186, 270, 298, 300, 307
    Saxony, 38, 45, 60, 78, 79, 89
    Silesia, 109, 111, 116, 117, 129, 271
    Silesian Wars, 109, 111, 129
      First Silesian War (1740), 109, 111
      Second Silesian War (1744), 109

## Index

German Unity, problems of, 161, 218, 219
   Unification movement, 161
Germanic ethnic groups and Germanic roots, 12, 13, 16
"Holy Roman Empire of the German Nation", 92, 140, 143
House of Hapsburg, 38, 39, 42, 50, 52, 56, 59–62, 72, 75, 77, 78, 80, 82, 83, 89, 95, 96, 99, 111, 115, 116, 143, 144, 182, 183, 186, 195–197
House of Hohenzollern, 99, 100, 196
industrial development, 170, 219, 225, 233
Kohl, Helmut, 355, 360
*Kulturkampf*, 217, 220, 231, 240
Locarno Conference (1925), 279, 287, 290, 293, 297
NATO, membership of, 318, 349
Nazism and Nazi (National Socialist) Party), 303, 307, 308, 310–313, 316, 322, 331, 335
   extermination campaign against Jews, 310
   Goebbels, Joseph, 308
   Holocaust, Jews, 311, 312
   *Kristallnacht*, 308
   seizure of power, 303
   see also Fascism
Partition of Poland, see Poland, Partition of Poland
Peace of Augsburg (1555), 44, 50, 78
Peace of Utrecht (1713), 92, 96
Peace of Westphalia (1648), 75, 78, 79, 83, 89, 92, 93, 99, 108, 264
Peasants' revolt in Germany (1524), 43, 46, 47, 66
population, 171, 233
Reformation in Germany, 45–48, 50, 56
*Reichstag*, 218, 220, 235
Reunification of Germany (1990), 348, 350, 352, 355, 357, 360
Revolution (1848), 179, 186
Schlieffen Plan, 266, 267, 278
Schroeder, Gerhard, 355
Schmidt, Helmut, 339
Schroeder, Gerhard, 355
Social-Democratic Party, 236, 246, 339
   Bernstein, Eduard, 236
   Kautsky, Karl, 236
Spartacists, 289
Soviet-Nazi Pact, 298
Sudetenland, incorporation of, 298, 307, 317
Thirty Years' War (1618–1648), 78, 85, 99
Three Emperors' League (1872), 217, 220, 221, 225
Treaty of Rapallo (1922), 279, 287, 290, 291, 296
Treaty of Versailles (1918), 264, 269–271, 275, 278, 286, 287, 288, 290, 293, 297, 303, 306–308, 312

reparations, 270, 272, 274, 275, 279, 285, 286, 287, 289, 290, 293, 297, 298, 300, 303
Weimar Republic, 283, 289, 296, 303
West Germany (Federal Republic of Germany), 318, 322, 325, 326, 339, 348, 350, 355, 360
Women, 168
*Zollverein*, 161, 179, 182
Gibbon, 124
Gide, Andre, 283
Gilbert of Colchester, 68, 72
Gioberti, 158
"Glorious Revolution", English, see Britain, "Glorious Revolution"
Gluck, 109, 149
   *Alceste*, 149
   *Iphigenie en Tauride*, 149
   *Orfeo*, 109
Goethe, 110, 140, 141, 150, 154, 158, 173, 179, 210
   *Faust*, 140, 179
   *Goetz*, 150
   *Sorrows of Young Werther*, 110
   *Wilhelm Meister*, 150
Gogol, 173
   *Dead Souls*, 173
Gorbachev, Mikhail, see Russia, USSR, Gorbachev, Mikhail
Gorky, Maxim, 283
Gounod, 209
Goya, 149
Great Britain, see Britain
Great Depression, 235, 279, 298, 299, 313, 316
   New York Stock Exchange, crash of, 279, 299, 316
Greco, El, 66
Greece, 1–8, 11, 12, 14, 15, 17, 22, 30, 124, 150, 155, 157, 161, 163, 166, 240, 258, 259, 271, 302, 308, 340, 342, 347
Greenback, 255
Grieg, 240, 252
Grotius, Hugo, 74, 84, 103
   *De Jure Belli et Pacis (Law of War and Peace)*, 74
Guardi, Francesco, 125
Guilds, 17, 21, 30, 35, 144, 170
Guizot, 182
Gutenberg, 48

## H

Hakluyt, 67
Hals, Frans, 91, 105
Handel, George Frideric, 109, 125, 149
   *The Messiah*, 109, 125
Hannibal, 8
Hardy, Thomas, 283
Hargreaves, 120
Haydn, 140, 149
   *Creation*, 149
   *Emperor Quartet*, 140
*Te Deum*, 149
Hertz, 237
Hauptmann, 239
Hawkins, 63
Hawthorne, 208
Hebbel, 173

Hegel, 148, 149, 155, 173, 209, 210
Heidegger, Martin, 342, 347
   see also Existentialism and Existentialists
Heine, Heinrich, 155, 173
Heisenberg, Werner, 280, 298
   indeterminacy theory, 298
Helmholtz, 174, 179
   on the Conservation of Energy, 179
Helsinki Conference (1975), 336
Hemingway, Ernest, 283
Herodotus, 1, 4, 8, 11
Hesse, Hermann, 283
Hitler, Adolf, 290, 298, 302, 303, 306–311, 316, 317, 323
   see also Germany, Nazism and Nazi (National Socialist) Party)
   see also World War II
Hobbes, 91, 102, 103
   *Leviathan*, 91
Hoffmann, E.T.A., 150, 173
Holbein, 29, 43
   *Anne of Cleves*, 29
   *Erasmus*, 29
Holland, 75, 79, 80, 83, 89, 95, 97–99, 112, 119, 136, 139, 142, 144, 145, 161, 187, 227, 233, 242, 250, 252, 257, 289, 299, 304, 308, 323, 326, 343
   see also Netherlands
"Holy Alliance", 140, 145, 148, 157, 168, 271. 278
Holy Roman Empire, 79, 92, 140, 143
Homer, 1, 4, 8, 11
Horace, 8
Hugo, Victor, 155, 167, 173, 178
   *The Hunchback of Notre Dame*, 167, 173, 178
Huguenots, see France, Huguenots
*The Human Comedy*, see Balzac, *Comedie Humaine (The Human Comedy)*
Hume, 109, 123
   *Treatise of Human Nature*, 109
Hundred Years War, 12
Hungary, 16, 28, 39, 42, 47, 49, 50, 56, 60, 66, 99, 108, 186, 187, 195, 196, 207, 220, 251, 252, 259, 266, 268, 270, 271, 292, 302, 312, 326, 327, 330, 348, 349, 353, 360
   Austria-Hungary, dual monarchy, 196, 207, 220, 251, 259, 266, 268, 270
   Magyar, 186, 270
Hutten, Ulrich von, 24, 30, 66

## I

Ibsen, 207, 217, 239, 252
   *The Doll's House*, 217
   *Peer Gynt*, 207
*Iliad*, 1, 4, 8, 11
IMF (International Monetary Fund), 321
Impressionism and Impressionists, 207, 214, 240
Inca, 27
India, 1, 23, 25, 27, 28, 35, 37, 39, 42, 59, 60, 74, 95, 109, 110, 117–120, 129, 132, 142, 148, 155, 160, 181, 191, 192, 199,

202, 222, 225, 253, 258, 271, 288, 298, 318, 323, 326, 327, 330, 343
   Gandhi, Mahatma, 288
   independence, 318, 323
   Indian Mutiny, 192, 199
Indonesia, 74, 202, 311, 323, 330
   Dutch colony, 74, 202, 311, 323
   rebellion against Holland, 323
   Japanese invasion, 311
International Bank for Reconstruction, 321
International Court of Justice, 271
Ireland, 64, 68, 82, 119, 181, 222, 293, 298, 318, 340, 355
   Church of, 222
   Eire, 298, 318
   Independence, 318
   Northern Ireland (Ulster), 82, 355
Israel, 318, 323, 324, 326, 335, 336, 338, 339, 342, 347, 348, 351, 357, 360
   Camp David Accords, 336
   Egyptian-Israeli Peace Treaty, 336, 342
   Jewish State Founded, 318, 323, 324
   Partition of Palestine, 335
   Oslo Accord with PLO, 348, 360
   Suez Canal crisis, 318
   War with Arabs (1967 – Six-Day War), 318, 338, 347
   War with Arabs (1973), 326
   see also Arabs, Palestine
Italy, 1, 12, 16, 17, 23, 26, 29–31, 36–39, 42, 47, 49, 50, 52, 56, 59, 61, 63, 64, 66–68, 78, 85, 95, 96, 100, 115, 125, 132, 140–142, 145, 150, 155, 157, 158, 161, 163, 170, 173–175, 179, 182, 183, 186, 187, 191, 192, 194–200, 203, 206, 207, 209, 211, 217, 220–223, 227, 240, 242, 247, 248, 250, 251, 258, 259, 263, 266, 270, 271, 279, 284, 287, 292, 298, 300–304, 307, 308, 311–313, 316, 321, 322, 325, 330, 339, 340, 342
   colonies, 247, 251, 257, 258, 259, 298, 307, 308, 311, 313
      Abyssinia, annexation of, 298
      Albania, invasion of, 298, 308
      Ethiopia, 251, 257, 258, 307
      North Africa, 311
      Turkish Tripoli, annexation of, 247, 259
   Communists, 325
   Emmanuel III, Victor, 302
   Fascist rule, 279, 284, 301, 302, 304, 307, 312, 313, 316, 325, 330
      Black Shirts, 302
      see also Mussolini, Benito
   Mazzini, 158, 179, 187
      "Young Italy" movement, 179, 183, 191
   Napoleon's campaign and rule, 140–142, 144
   revolution (1820), 155
   revolution (1848), 179, 187
   Roman Control, under, 1
   secret societies, 158
      Carbonari, 158

Italy *(Continued)*
  Sicily, 183, 187, 198, 322, 339
  States and Territories, 1, 6–8, 11, 12, 14–17, 21–23, 36, 37, 42, 43, 45, 47, 49, 52, 56, 60, 61, 66, 68, 72, 85, 90, 124, 142, 154, 174, 183, 186, 187, 191, 196, 198, 199, 207, 208, 211, 216, 220, 233, 240, 287, 293, 298, 302, 307, 328, 351
    Florence, 23, 45, 66, 72, 187, 198
    Genoa, 183, 191, 287, 293
    Milan, 186, 187
    Naples, 183, 187, 198
    Rome, 1, 6–8, 11, 12, 14–17, 21, 22, 36, 37, 43, 45, 47, 49, 52, 56, 60, 66, 68, 72, 85, 90, 124, 142, 154, 174, 187, 198, 199, 207, 208, 211, 216, 220, 233, 240, 298, 302, 307, 328, 351
    Roman Empire, 1, 6, 8, 14, 21, 124
    Venice, 37, 42, 61, 174, 187, 196, 198
  Triple Alliance (1882), 217, 220, 248, 263
  Unification, 197, 203, 206
  "Young Italy" movement, 179, 183, 191

**J**
Jamaica, 102
Jenkinson, 63
Jesuits, *see* Church, Jesuits
Jew, 15, 60, 77, 80, 100, 111, 136, 139, 142, 168, 222, 224, 251, 252, 263, 273, 302, 303, 308, 311, 312, 318, 323, 324, 326, 330, 335, 336, 338, 339, 342, 347, 348, 351, 357, 360
  anti-Jewish legislation, 222
  "Dreyfus Affair", 251, 263
  extermination campaign against, 310
  Holocaust, in Nazi rule, 311, 312
  Israel, Jewish state, 318, 323, 324, 326, 335, 336, 338, 339, 342, 347, 348, 351, 357, 360
    Egyptian-Israeli Peace Treaty, 336, 342
    Gaza Strip, 318, 338, 347, 351, 360
    Oslo Accord with PLO, 348, 351, 360
    war with Arabs, 335, 338, 342, 347
    West Bank, 318, 338, 347
    *see also* Arabs, Palestine
  Zionism, 251
Joyce, James, 279, 283
  *Ulysses*, 279
Juvenal, 8

**K**
Kafka, 239, 246
  *Metamorphosis*, 239, 246
Kandinsky, 239
Kant, Emmanuel, 123, 130, 141, 148, 154, 209

*Kritik der reinen Vernunft (Critique of Pure Reason)*, 130, 148, 154
Karlowitz, Peace of (1699), 92, 99, 108
Kautsky, Karl, *see* Germany, Social-Democratic Party, Kautsky, Karl
Kay, 109
  Flying Shuttle, invention of, 109
Keats, 150, 173
  *Ode to a Nightingale*, 173
Kemal, Mustafa (Ataturk), *see* Ottoman Turkey, Kemal, Mustafa (Ataturk)
Kepler, 74, 83
  "Kepler's Laws", 83
  Laws of Planetary Motion, 74
Keynes, John Maynard, 282
Kipling, 239
Klee, Paul, 239, 284
Kleist, 150
Knox, John, 51, 58
Koch, 210, 237
Kohl, *see* Germany, Kohl, Helmut
Kropotkin, *see* Russia, Kropotkin
Kutuzov, 144

**L**
labor, 17, 21, 26, 28, 32, 60, 76, 95, 120, 122, 133, 134, 148, 159, 168, 170–172, 178, 184, 185, 187, 191, 213, 216, 222, 226, 232, 235, 236, 243, 251, 253–255, 260, 265, 271, 280, 286, 289, 292, 293, 299–301, 303–305, 308, 310, 313, 316, 320, 321, 325, 328, 330, 336, , 338–341, 353, 355, 360
  cheap labor, 170
  communal labor of Middle Ages, 17, 21
  compulsory national labor service in Nazi Germany, 303
  division of labor, 17, 28, 32, 170, 171, 178, 265
  forced labor, 60, 120
  free labor, need for, 26
  industrial labor, 120, 168
  labor as a commodity, 213, 216
  labor camps of Soviet Union, 292, 305, 308, 313, 321
  labor legislation, 159
  labor market, 120
  labor movement, 213, 222, 226, 235, 236, 243, 251, 253, 254, 260, 293, 301, 305, 325, 336, 339
    labor revolts, 185, 191, 254
    labor strikes, 253, 293
    labor unions and organizations, 213, 222, 235, 236, 243, 251, 301, 305, 325, 336, 339
      American Federation of Labor, 226
      "First International", 213
      "Second International", 236
    Socialist movement, 236
  labor parties, 236, 260
  labor problems, 226

Labor Party of Britain, 289, 300, 325, 339, 355, 360
  Labor Cabinet, British, 289, 300, 339, 355, 360
labor shortage, 303
  manual labor, reduction of, 171
  productivity in Soviet Union, 341
  slave labor, 28
  skilled labor, 235
  unemployment, 26, 133, 134, 148, 159, 171, 172, 235, 253, 255, 286, 289, 299, 300, 303–305, 313, 316, 320, 328, 338, 340, 353, 355
  women's labor, 168
La Fontaine, 104
Lagerlof, 239, 252
*Laissez-faire*, 115, 122, 170, 171, 174, 175, 178, 180, 222, 300
Lamarck, 147, 210
Laos, 327, 338
Lasalle, 236
Latvia, 65, 271, 299, 302, 353
Lausanne Reparation conference (1932), 298
Lawrence, D.H., 283
League of Nations, 264, 270, 271, 275, 278, 285, 287, 297, 298, 300, 306, 307, 312, 325
Leibnitz, 91, 92, 103, 104, 209
  differential calculus, 91
  monadology, 92
Lenin, Vladimir Illych, 264, 272–274, 278, 279, 286, 290, 291, 296, 309
  *see also* Russia, Communism and Communists
  *see also* Russia, Revolutions
  *see also* Russia, Socialism and Socialists
  *see also* Russia, Soviet Russia
  *see also* Russia, USSR, Bolshevik government
Leonardo da Vinci, 23, 29, 31, 66
  *Last Supper*, 23, 29
  *Mona Lisa*, 29
Lessing, 124, 150, 154
Liberals and Liberalism, 95, 108, 114, 142, 144, 148, 154–161, 163, 166, 168, 170, 178, 180–183, 185–188, 191, 193–195, 197, 199, 201, 206, 209, 211–213, 218, 220–222, 226, 227, 232, 235, 236, 246, 250, 251, 254–256, 264, 265, 268, 269, 271–273, 275, 279, 281, 286, 288–290, 292, 299–302, 304, 305, 308, 312, 316, 318, 327, 331, 341, 342, 354
Lincoln, Abraham, 192, 201, 206, 207
  assassination of, 207
  *see also* United States of America
Lindberg, Charles, 280, 281, 296, 319
Linnaeus, 109, 122
  *Systema Natura*, 109
Lister, 237
Liszt, Franz, 174, 208
Literature, 4, 7, 8, 13, 15, 17, 22, 23, 26, 30, 31, 32, 35, 59, 60, 63–65, 67, 77, 84, 99, 104, 111, 122, 124, 149, 150, 151, 173–175, 207, 208, 238, 239, 243, 279, 280, 283, 292, 306, 320, 329, 343
  17th Century, of, 104
  18th Century, of, 124
  Classical, 31, 35
  Elizabethan age, 64
  Greek, 4
  Individualism, 329
  Medieval, 15, 22
  Renaissance, 8, 59, 63
  Roman, 7
Lithuania, 39, 42, 49, 56, 58, 64, 65, 100, 113, 271, 299, 302, 308, 353
Litvinov, Maxim, *see* Russia, USSR, Litvinov, Maxim
Livius, 7, 8
Livonia, 49, 56, 58, 59, 65, 66, 69, 78, 100, 113, 116, 268
Locke, John, 47, 92, 103, 108, 110, 123
  *Essay concerning Human Understanding*, 92, 103, 108
Lomonosov, 124
Longfellow, 208
Lorenzo de Medici, 23
Low Countries, 39, 42, 61
Lublin, Union of, 58
Luther, Martin, *see* Church, Reformation, Luther Martin
Lyell, Charles, 174

**M**
Maastricht Agreement, 348, 355
Mabillon, 104, 124
Macaulay, 192, 208
  *History of England*, 192
Machiavelli, 23, 31, 35, 59, 61
  *The Prince*, 23, 31, 35, 61
*Madame Bovary*, *see* Flaubert, *Madame Bovary*
Magellan, Ferdinand, 25, 27, 43
Magna Carta, The, 12
Magnus, Albertus, 14
Mahler, 240
Maillol, Aristide, 284
Malaysia, 330
Malraux, Andre, 283
Malta, 145, 199, 223
Malthus, 140, 170, 210, 328
  *Essay on the Principle of Population*, 140
Mann, Heinrich, 283
Mann, Thomas, 283
Manzoni, 158, 173
  *Promised Bride*, 173
Marat, *see* France, French Revolution, Marat
Marcator, 58, 68, 73
Marlowe, 67
Marx, Karl, 179, 185, 188, 191, 207, 208, 212, 213, 214, 224, 225, 236, 241, 251, 256, 282, 283, 285, 296, 306, 322, 335
Marxism, 179, 185, 188, 191, 207, 208, 212, 213, 214, 224, 225, 236, 241, 251, 256, 306, 322, 335
  *Communist Manifesto*, 179, 185, 188, 191, 212
  *Das Kapital*, 207, 212

Marxist movement, 251, 256, 283, 285
  Revisionism, 236
  see also Engels, Friedrich,
  see also Germany, Social-Democratic Party
  see also Germany, Spartacists
  see also labor, labor movement, labor unions and organizations, "First International
  see also labor, labor movement, labor unions and organizations, "Second International"
  see also Russia, Socialism and Socialists, Marxism and Marxists
Matisse, 239
Maupassant, 208, 239
Maximilian I, 39, 192, 194
Maxwell, 174, 207
  *Treatise on Electricity*, 207
Mayakovsky, Vladimir, 283
Mazarin, see France, Mazarin
Mazzini, see *Italy*, Mazzini
Medicine and Medical Science, 3, 15, 22, 66, 121, 123, 125, 147, 171, 210, 214, 233, 237, 242, 255, 282, 324, 327–329, 331, 335, 342, 343, 353, 357
  biogenetics, 328, 335
  DNA, 328, 331, 335, 343
  see also Biology and Biological Science
Melville, 208
Mendel, 237
  laws of heredity, 237
Mendeleev, 210
Mendelssohn, 174
Mercator, 58, 68, 73
Mestrovic, Ivan, 284
*Metamorphosis*, see Kafka, *Metamorphosis*
Metternich, 145, 156–159, 179, 182, 183, 186, 188, 193, 195, 218, 271, 278
Meyer, 210
Michelangelo, 23, 29, 59
  *Ceiling of Sistine Chapel*, 23, 29
  *Moses*, 29
Mickiewicz, 173
Mill, John Stuart, 171, 178, 179, 192, 209
  *Principles of Political Economy*, 179
Millikan, 237
Milton, 91, 104
  *Paradise Lost*, 91, 104
Moliere, 104
  *Bourgeois Gentilhomme*, 104
  *Tartuffe*, 104
Molotov, Vyacheslav, see Russia, USSR, Molotov, Vyacheslav
Mommsen, Theodore, 7, 208
Montaigne, 67
Montenegro, 258
  see also Balkans
  see also Serbia
  see also Yugoslavia
Montesquieu, 109, 123, 129
  *Lettres Parsanes (Persian Letters)*, 109, 123
  *L'Esprit des Lois (Spirit of Laws)*, 109, 123, 129

Moore, Henry, 284
Moors, 60, 77
More, Sir Thomas, 23, 30, 31, 49, 59, 172
Morike, 150
Morse, 179
  Telegraph, invention of, 179
Mozart, 130, 149
  *Don Giovanni*, 130, 149
  *Magic Flute*, 149
  *Marriage of Figaro*, 149
Mun, Thomas, 74
  Theory of Mercantilism, 74
Munich Conference (1938), see World War II, Munich Conference ("appeasement")
Murillo, 105
Music, 16, 30, 66, 85, 125, 149, 174, 175, 208, 238, 240, 284
  16th Century ("The Golden Age of Song"), 30
  Baroque style, 85
  Romanticism, 174
  "Victorian style", 238
Mussolini, Benito, 279, 302, 307, 308, 311, 316
Mussorgsky, 240
  *Boris Godunov*, 240
Mysticism, 2, 14, 124, 125, 148, 342

**N**
Nansen, discovery of North Pole, 243
Napoleonic wars, see France, Bonaparte, Napoleon, Napoleonic wars
NATO (North Atlantic Treaty Organization), 318, 323, 330, 335, 340, 347, 349, 353, 357, 360
Netherlands, 26, 35, 39, 49–52, 56, 58, 59, 61, 62, 64, 66, 68, 78, 80, 84, 95, 96, 98, 163, 170, 257, 264, 284, 322, 325, 337, 355
  War of Independence, 58, 68
Newton, Isaac, 91, 92, 103, 108, 110, 236, 237, 246, 280
  Law of Gravitation, 91, 110
  Optics, 92
  *Philosophiae Naturalis Principia Mathematica*, 91, 103, 108
Nietzsche, Friedrich, 217, 238
  *Thus Spake Zarathustra*, 217
Nihilism and Nihilists, 224, 236
Nobel, Alfred, 207, 233, 256
  Dynamite, invention of, 207, 233
  Nobel Prize, 256
  Nobel Peace Prize, 256
Nobility, 24, 26, 30, 31, 35–38, 40, 42, 60, 64, 65, 77, 80–83, 89, 93, 95, 100, 108, 114, 125, 133, 134, 139, 144, 160, 161, 166, 167, 180, 182, 200, 224, 233, 250, 259, 273, 274, 290
  see also Aristocracy
Nominalist scholastic effort, 14, 21, 92
Nordenskjold, discovery of North Pole, 243

Norman Conquest of England, 12
Norway, 49, 56, 64, 72, 145, 239, 240, 243, 247, 252, 299, 304, 308, 351, 360
Nuclear Nonproliferation Treaty (1969), 336

**O**
*Odyssey*, 1, 4, 8, 11
Orthodox Church, see Church, Orthodox
Ottoman Empire, see Ottoman Turkey
Ottoman Turkey, 38–40, 43, 47, 58, 60, 61, 91, 99, 100, 105, 108, 115, 117, 130, 144, 157, 161, 163, 166, 184, 187, 191, 199, 200, 202, 206, 217, 221, 225, 227, 231, 247, 252, 258, 259, 263, 264, 266, 268, 270, 271, 288, 302, 305, 311, 323, 340, 347
  Battle of Lepanto, 58
  Battle of Navarino, 166
  Kemal, Mustafa (Ataturk), 302
  Kuprili, Ahmed, 99, 108
  Russian-Turkish Peace of Jassy (1792), 130
  Russo-Turkish War (1768–1774), 117
  Russo-Turkish War (1877–1878), 217, 225, 231
  Suleiman the Magnificent, 43
  "Young Turk" Movement, 225, 247, 258, 263
Owen, Robert, 155, 171, 172, 178

**P**
Paganini, 174
  *Carnival of Venice*, 174
Paine, Thomas, 120
Painting, 29, 105, 149, 209, 239, 284
  Expressionists, 239
  "Fauvists", 239
  Impressionists, 239
  Neoclassic, 209
  neo-Gothic, 209
  neo-Impressionists, 239
  pre-Raphaelite, 209
  Surrealism, 284
Pakistan, 330
Palestrina, 58, 66
Palmerston, 180, 199
Papal States, see Church, Pope and Papacy, Papal states
Paracelsus, 31, 43
Pareto, Vilfredo, 301
Parliament, 16, 21, 36–38, 49, 64, 81, 82, 89, 92–94, 96–98, 100, 105, 108, 110, 114, 115, 120, 125, 133, 159, 161, 166, 167, 180, 182, 186, 194–196, 206, 213, 221, 223, 236, 248, 250–253, 256, 263, 272, 273, 289, 301, 302, 307, 336
  see also Diets
  see also Russia, Duma
Pascal, 91, 103
  Barometer, invention of, 103
  *Pensees*, 91
Theory of Probability, 103
Passos, John Dos, 283
Pasteur, Luis, 210, 237

Pavlov, 237, 246
  Conditioned Reflexes, 237, 246
Peary, discovery of North Pole, 243
Petrarch, 16
Physics, 3, 5, 68, 72, 83, 85, 103, 104, 108, 123, 148, 154, 174, 209, 210, 214, 216, 217, 237, 238, 246, 280, 282, 305, 310, 319, 328, 335, 343
Physiocrats, 109, 122
  Quesnay, 109, 122
  *Tableau economique*, 109
Picasso, Pablo, 284
Plague, 91, 97
Planck, Max, 237, 247
  Quantum Theory, 237, 247
Plato, 1, 3, 11, 14, 21, 172
Plautus, 8
Poe, Edgar Allen, 173, 179
Poland, 26, 39, 42, 51, 58, 59, 64, 65, 68, 69, 78, 79, 80, 99–101, 105, 108–110, 113, 116, 130, 132, 136, 145, 163, 173, 174, 192, 195, 239, 248, 266, 268, 270, 271, 279, 286, 292, 298, 302, 308, 312, 317, 321, 322, 326, 330, 336, 348, 353, 360
  Communist regime, 312, 321, 326, 336, 348
  Labor unrest (1979), 336
  Resignation of Communist governments, 348
  "Curzon Line", 271
  First Partition of Poland (1772), 110
  Fourth Partition of Poland between Germany and Russia (1939), 298, 308, 317
  Kosciusko, 136
  NATO, admission in, 360
  Pilsudski, Joseph, 302
  Polish Corridor, 270
  Polish-Russian War (1920), 279
  Revolt in Poland, 192
  Second Partition of Poland, 136
  Third Partition of Poland (1795), 130
  Walesa, Lech, 336
  War of Polish Succession (1733–1735), 109, 116
Populist, 225, 236, 246, 255
  American populists, 236, 246, 255
  see also Russia, Populists (Narodniki)
Portugal, 16, 25–27, 35, 37, 42, 61, 68, 74, 75, 77, 102, 105, 110, 113, 132, 143, 146, 157, 227, 302, 336, 337, 340, 341, 353
Salazar, 340
Positivism and Positivists, 209, 216, 251, 282, 319
  Logical Positivism, 282, 319
Prevost, Abbe, 124
  *Manon Lescaut*, 124
Proudhon, 172, 178, 212
Proust, Mercel, 239, 246, 283
Psychology, 3, 31, 35, 173, 208, 211, 224, 231, 237, 239, 243, 246, 280, 282–284, 328
  Abnormal, 243, 282
  Conditioned Reflexes, 237, 246
  Normal, 243, 282

Psychology *(Continued)*
 Psychoanalysis, 237, 246, 247
   First Congress of (1908), 247
   *see also* Freud, Sigmund,
Puccini, 240
 *La Boheme*, 240
 *Tosca*, 240
Purcell, 125
Pushkin, Alexander, 167, 173, 178
 *Eugene Onegin*, 167, 178
 *Queen of Spades*, 167, 178

**Q**
"Quislings", 308

**R**
Rabelais, 43, 67
 *Gargantua*, 43, 67
Racine, 104
 *Athalie*, 104
 *Britannicus*, 104
Raleigh, 63
Ranke, Leopold von, 174, 179, 208
 *History of the Popes*, 179
Rapallo, German-Russian Treaty of (1922), 279, 287, 290, 291, 296
Raphael, 23, 29, 209
 *Madonna of the Chair*, 29
 *Pre-Raphaelites* art movement, 209
 *Sistine Madonna*, 23, 29
Realism and Realists, 4, 14, 21, 29, 92, 283, 284
 inner reality, 284
 Realistic form of Art, 4, 29
 Realist scholastic effort, 14, 21
 *see also* Nominalist scholastic effort
Religious liberalism, 148
Rembrandt, 74, 91, 105
*Remembrance of Things Past*, 239, 246, 283
Renaissance, 8, 15, 24, 26, 28, 29, 32, 39, 42, 52, 53, 58, 59, 63, 65–67, 75, 84, 85, 101, 104, 108, 150
Reuchlin, Johann, 30, 59
Rhodes, Cecil, 257
Rhodesia, 330, 337
Ricardo, David, 170
Richelieu, *see* France, Richelieu
Rilke, Rainer Maria, 284
Rimsky-Korsakov, 240
Rivera, Diego, 284, 304, 316
Robespierre, *see* France, French Revolution, Robespierre
Rodin, 239
Roentgen, 232, 237
 X-rays, discovery of, 232, 237
Roman Catholics, *see* Church, Roman Catholic
Romanticism, 149, 150, 173, 174, 209, 239, 240
 Romantic Movement, 150, 173
  English, 150, 173, 174, 239, 240
  France, 150, 239, 240
  German, 150, 173, 240
  Polish, 239
  Swedish, 239
 "Romantic Age", 150
Rome, 1, 6–8, 11, 12, 14–17, 21, 22, 36, 37, 43, 45, 47, 49, 52, 56, 60, 66, 68, 72, 79, 85, 90, 92, 124, 140, 142, 143, 154, 174, 187, 198, 199, 207, 208, 211, 216, 233, 240, 258, 298, 302, 307, 328, 351
 History, 208
 "Holy Roman Empire", 36, 79, 92, 140, 143
 Roman Catholics, *see* Church, Roman Catholic
 Roman Catholic Church, *see* Roman Catholics
 Roman Empire, 1, 6–8, 12, 14, 16, 21, 124
 Roman heritage, 6–8, 11, 14–17, 22
 Roman Law, 7, 11, 16, 37, 142, 154, 174
 Rome-Berlin axis, 298, 307
 Treaty of 1957, 328
Rolland, Romain, 283
Roosevelt, Franklin, *see* United States of America, Roosevelt, Franklin
Roosevelt, Theodore, *see* United States of America, Roosevelt, Theodore
"Rosetta stone", 154
Rossini, 174
Rousseau, Jean Jacques, 109, 123, 124, 129, 136, 139
 *Contrat Social (Social Contract)*, 109
Rubens, Peter Paul, 85
Rumania, 252, 307, 312, 321, 330, 348, 349
Russell, Bertrand, 199, 282
Russia, 16, 17, 21, 23, 26, 28, 36, 38–40, 42, 58, 59, 63–65, 68, 69, 72, 80, 91, 92, 100, 101, 104, 105, 110–113, 115–117, 122, 124, 129, 136, 140, 142–145, 148, 150, 151, 154–161, 163, 166, 168, 171, 173, 175, 178, 183, 184, 187, 188, 191–195, 197, 199–203, 206–208, 210, 211, 212, 214, 217, 220–225, 227, 231–242, 246–251, 253–255, 257–260, 263–268, 270–275, 278, 279, 283–293, 296, 298, 299, 300, 301, 305–309, 311–313, 316–323, 325–331, 335, 337–344, 347, 348–352, 354, 355, 357
 Alaska, sale of, 202
 Alexander I, 145, 148, 157, 160, 159, 160, 166
 Alexander II, 192, 200, 217, 224, 225
  assassination of, 217, 225
 Alexander III, 225
 Anglo-Russian Treaty over Persia (1907), 247
 Asia, expansion in, 199, 200, 225, 22
 Bakunin, 212
 Catherine the Great, 110, 112, 129, 136
 Chechnya, war with, 348, 354
 Chernobyl atomic disaster (1986), 348, 349
 Colony, competition for, 254, 257
 Communism and Communists, 286, 287, 290, 291, 293
 *see also* Revolutions
 *see also* Socialism and Socialists
 *see also* USSR
 Cossacks, 65, 80, 100
 Crimean War, 192, 197, 199, 200, 206, 224
  Sebastopol, battle of, 206
 Dekabrist revolt (1825), 155, 160, 161, 166, 183
 Duma (Russian Parliament), 236, 247, 250, 254, 255, 272, 273, 354
 Emigration, 233
 Enlightenment, 112, 1297
 Franco-Russian alliance (1891), 232, 287
 Great Northern war (between Sweden and Russia)(1700–1721), 116
  Peace of Nystad (1721), 116
 Industry and industrialization, 168, 163, 224, 253, 257, 339
  Trans-Siberian Railway, 257
 Ivan IV (Ivan the Terrible), 58, 59, 65, 72
 Ivan the Great, 36, 65, 72
 KGB, 354
 Khrushchev, Nikita, 331, 351
 Kropotkin, 212
 Kulak, 224, 231, 292
 *mir*, 200, 224, 255
 Narodnik, *see* Russia, Populists (Narodniki)
 Napoleon's invasion (1812), 140, 144, 151, 154
 Navarino, naval battle of, 155, 161, 166
 Nicholas I, 160, 166, 184, 187, 200, 225
 Nicholas II, 258, 272
 Peace of Adrianople, 155, 161, 184, 191
 Peace of Brest-Litovsk (1918), 264, 268, 274, 278
 Peace of Jassy (1792), 130
 Peter I (Peter the Great), 92, 112, 117, 129
 Peter III, 116
 Polish-Russian war (1920), 279
 Population, 171
 Populists (Narodniki), 225
 Post-Communist, 354
 Pugachev revolt, 110, 113, 129
 Putin, Vladimir, 354
 Rasputin, 272
 Russian-German Reinsurance Treaty, 217, 221, 225, 248, 263
 Razin, Stenka, 101
 Religion, 210, 235, 241
  Orthodox, 210, 235
  Protestant, 235
 Revolutions, 250, 254, 264, 268, 272, 274, 275, 286, 290, 291, 293, 296
  1905, of, 250, 254, 272, , 274, 279, , 290, 291, 293, 305, 307
  Allied intervention in Russia, 264, 293
  Bolshevik reconstruction, 274, 326
  Comintern (Third International), 286
  Anti-Comintern pact between Germany and Japan, 307
  Counter-revolution, 264, 274, 286
  Civil war in Russia, 264, 274, 286, 293
   Denikin, Anton, 286
   Kolchak, Aleksandr, 286
   Wrangel, Pyotr, 286
  February, 1917, 264, 268, 272
  Five Years' Plan, 279, 291–293, 305, 321, 341
  Kerensky, 273, 278
  NEP (New Economic Policy) of Soviet Russia, 279, 291, 292, 296
  October, 1917, 264, 268, 273, 278
  War Communism, period of (1919–1921), 290
 Russo-Japanese war (1904–1905), 247, 249, 254
 Russo-Turkish war (1768–1774), 117
 Russo-Turkish war (1877–1878), 217, 221, 225, 231
 Serfs and Serfdom, 80, 101, 112, 129, 159, 183, 187, 192, 199, 200, 201, 203, 207
  emancipation of (1861), 192, 200, 201, 203, 207
 Seven Years' War (1756–1763), 116, 117
 Siberia, 58, 65, 69, 101, 112, 122, 199, 224, 247, 253, 257, 274, 286–288, 290, 291, 296, 305, 321, 339
  Russian expansion in, 58, 65, 69, 199
 Socialism and Socialists, 225, 236, 253, 254, 264, 268, 272–274, 286–288, 301, 305–307, 309, 321
  Bolshevik, 254, 264, 268, 272–274, 286, 290, 301, 305–307, 309, 321
  Marxism and Marxists, 225, 236, 254, 264, 268, 272–274, 286, 290, 301, 305–307, 309, 321
  Menshevik, 236, 254
  Plekhanov, Georgi, 225
 Soviet Russia, 279, 283, 287, 293, 307, 312, 357
 *see also* USSR
Soviet Union, *see* USSR
Sputnik (First earth satellite), 318, 329, 335
Stolypin reform, 272
Three Emperors' League (1872), 217, 220, 225
Treaty of Rapallo (1922), 279, 290
Treaty of Unkiar Skelessy, 191
"Triple Entente" of Russia-England-France, 248–250, 263, 266
Ukraine, 91, 100
 incorporation of, 91
 Peace of Andrusovo (1667), 100

# Index

USSR, 285, 286, 289, 291, 293, 296, 298, 305–309, 311–313, 316–323, 325–331, 335, 336, 337–344, 347, 348–352, 354, 355, 357
   Bolshevik government, 274, 286, 305, 321
   China, rift with, 330
   "Cold War", 322, 326, 331, 348–350, 355, 357
   Constitution of 1936, 316
   detente, 338, 340, 341
   dissolution of, 348, 352, 354
   East Europe, influence on, 321, 325–327, 341, 351
      dissolution of Warsaw Pact, 351
   Economic Depression of 1929–1933, effect of, 316
   Five-Year Plans, 279, 291–293, 305, 321, 341
   formation of, 291, 296
   German invasion and defeat, 299, 309, 311, 312
   Glasnost, 349–351
   Gorbachev, Mikhail, 348, 349, 351, 352, 360
   Korean War, 318, 326
   labor camps, 292, 305, 308, 313
   League of Nations, entry in, 298, 307
   Litvinov, Maxim, 308, 317
   Molotov, Vyacheslav, 308, 317
   Partition of Poland, 298
   Perestroika, 349, 351, 352, 360
   Purges in Russia, 298, 305, 306, 313
   Russian society, 306
   Soviet-Finland war, 298
   Soviet-Nazi pact, 298
   Suez Canal crisis, 318, 323, 326, 335
   Vietnam war, 318, 327, 330, 336–338, 340
   World War II, 298, 299, 307–309, 311–313, 317, 321
      Finland, attack on, 298, 308
      German invasion of, 299, 309, 311
      German defeat at Stalingrad, 311
      occupation and division of Germany, 312
      Soviet occupation troop, 312
      Japan, war against, 311
      Poland, partition between Germany and Russia, 298, 308
      Russian troops enter Germany, 311
      Soviet-Nazi Non-aggression Pact, 298, 308, 317
Rutherford, Ernest, 280

## S

Saint-Pierre, Bernardin de, 124
Saint-Simon, 172, 178
San Stefano, Peace Treaty of, 225, 231
Sartre, Jean-Paul, 342, 347
   see also Existentialism and Existentialists
Savonarola, see Church, Reformation, Savonarola
Scandinavia, 16, 17, 30, 43, 47–49, 64, 68, 168, 170, 187, 243, 250, 252, 325
   Scandinavian Union, 43
Scarlatti, Alessandro, 85, 125
Schiller, 140, 150, 154
   *The Robbers*, 150, 154
   *Wallenstein*, 150, 154
   *Wilhelm Tell*, 140, 154
Schmidt, Helmut, see Germany, Schmidt, Helmut,
Schelling, 148, 173
Schonberg, Arnold, 240, 284
Schopenhauer, 173
   *The World As Will and Idea*, 173
Schroddinger, Erwin, 280
Schroeder, Gerhard, see Germany, Schroeder, Gerhard
Schubert, Franz, 155, 174
   Trout Quintet, 155
Schumann, 174
Schumann Plan for European steel and coal production, 318
Schumpeter, Joseph, 282
Science and Technology, 3, 4, 14, 15, 23, 24, 26, 29, 31, 44, 59, 64, 66–69, 73, 83–85, 92, 95, 99, 103–105, 108, 110, 112, 122, 123, 141, 147, 148, 151, 154, 167, 168, 173, 174, 182, 183, 195, 207–212, 214, 216, 217, 232, 236–238, 240, 241, 243, 248, 255, 256, 264, 280–283, 285, 292, 293, 299, 303, 306, 311, 318–320, 324, 328, 329, 331, 335, 341–344, 353, 357
Scotland, see Britain, Scotland
Scott, Sir Walter, 155, 167, 173
   *Ivanhoe*, 155, 167, 173
Sculpture, 4, 7, 29, 30, 63, 84, 85, 90, 149, 174, 239, 284
Seneca, 8
Serbia, 225, 252, 258, 259, 263, 266, 270, 348, 349, 353, 360
   assassination of Archduke Francis Ferdinand in Sarajevo, 259, 263
   Dayton Agreement, 360
   Kosovo region, 348, 353
   Milosevic, 354
   NATO intervention, 353, 354
   see also Balkans,
   see also Bosnia,
   see also Croatia,
   see also Montenegro
   see also Slovenia
   see also Yugoslavia
Servetus, 31, 44, 51
   see also Church, Reformation, Calvin, John, Servetus, burning at stake
Seurat, 239
Seven Years' War (1756–1763), 109, 110, 116, 117, 119
Shakespeare, William, 59, 63, 67, 72, 84, 124
Shaw, Barnard, 239, 247, 284
   *Man and Superman*, 247
Shelley, 150, 173
   *Ode to the West Wind*, 173
Sicily, see Italy, Sicily
Sinclair, Lewis, 279, 283
   *Babbitt*, 279
Sinclair, Upton, 283
Slaves and Slavery, 5, 13, 28, 37, 42, 60, 76, 89, 96, 105, 113, 118, 121, 129, 131, 145, 156, 160, 166, 180, 184, 199, 201, 203, 206, 207, 208, 220, 271
   antislavery groups, 184
   slave trade, 28, 37, 42, 96, 105, 113, 118, 121, 145, 156, 166, 271
   see also United States of America, Civil War
   see also United States of America, slavery
Slovakia, 348, 353
Slovenia, 353
   see also Balkans,
   see also Bosnia,
   see also Croatia,
   see also Serbia,
   see also Yugoslavia,
Smetana, 285
Smith, Adam, 122, 130, 148, 170, 178
   *The Wealth of Nations*, 122, 130
see also laissez-faire
Socialism and Socialists, 137, 172, 182, 185, 188, 191, 193, 194, 211–213, 218, 220–222, 225, 227, 231–233, 235, 236, 243, 246, 250–256, 264, 268, 269, 271–275, 279, 287, 289–291, 296, 301–304, 313, 316, 325, 327, 330, 336, 339–343, 347, 352, 355
Society of Jesus, see Church, Jesuits
Sociology, 156, 200, 237, 238, 243, 265, 280, 282, 283, 296, 301, 329
Socrates, 1, 3, 11
Solzhenitsyn, Aleksandr, 342
Sophocles, 4
Spain, 12, 16, 17, 23, 25–30, 36–40, 42–44, 47, 49, 50, 56, 58–64, 66–68, 72, 75–81, 84, 85, 89, 90, 92, 95–99, 101, 102, 105, 108, 110, 113, 115–119, 125, 129, 131, 132, 136, 139, 141, 143–146, 149, 154, 155, 157, 158, 163, 166, 170, 171, 183, 187, 194, 196, 198, 202, 227, 232, 240, 242, 246, 248, 252, 255, 256, 284, 298, 302–304, 307, 313, 316, 317, 323, 325, 339, 342, 353
   Basque country, 339
   Bourbon, 196, 198
      see also Bourbon dynasty
   Catherine of Aragon, 49, 56
   Charles III, 110, 113, 129
   Charles V, 36, 39
   civil war, 298, 302, 304, 307, 313, 316, 317
   colony, 25, 27, 28, 36, 39, 40, 58, 60–62, 68, 75–78, 89, 96, 101, 102, 105, 113, 129, 132, 146, 155, 232, 246, 248
   encomienda system, 60, 75, 113, 129, 132
   settlers, 102
   slave trade, 96
      see also Slave Trade
   Spanish America, 60, 75–77, 113, 129, 132, 146, 155
   Spanish Netherlands, rising in, 58, 61, 62, 68, 78
   conservatism versus liberalism, 158
   Cortez, Hernando, 43
   decline of, 77, 105
   Empire, 39, 102
   Falange, 304, 316
   Fascism, in, 302–304, 313, 316, 325
   Ferdinand and Isabella, 36, 37, 42
   Franco, Francisco, 302, 304, 316, 342
   industry and industrialization, 170
   Low country's rising, see Spain, colony, Netherlands, rising in
   "Monroe Doctrine", effect of, 166
   Muslim rule, end of, 23
   Napoleon, and, 144–146, 154
   Peace of the Pyrenees (1659), 79
   Peace of Vervins, 58
   Phillip II, 59, 60, 63, 72, 75
   Pizarro, 25, 27, 43
   population, 171
   Rivera, Diego, 284, 304, 316
   Seven Years' War (1756–1763), 116, 117
   Spanish Armada, destruction of, 58, 59, 64
   Union of Aragon and Castile, 36, 37
   United States, war with, 232, 246, 248, 255
   War of Spanish succession, 92, 96, 116
   William of Orange, 58, 61, 98
Spengler, Oswald, 282, 296, 336
   *Decline of the West*, 282, 296, 336
Spenser, 67
Spinoza, 91, 103, 209
   *Ethics*, 91
Sputnik (First earth satellite), see Russia, Sputnik (First earth satellite),
Stalin, Josef, 274, 279, 291, 296, 298, 305, 306, 311, 316, 318, 321, 326, 331
   see also Russia, Revolutions
   see also Russia, Socialism and Socialists, Bolshevik
   see also Russia, USSR, Purges in Russia
Stendhal, 173, 239
   *The Red and the Black*, 173
Stephenson, George, 140, 147
   Steam Locomotive, building of, 140, 147
Stowe, Harriet Beecher, 192, 208
   *Uncle Tom's Cabin*, 192, 208
Strauss, David Friedrich, 179, 210, 211, 214, 216
   *Life of Jesus*, 179
Strauss, Johann, 209

Strauss, Richard, 240
  *Rosenkavalier*, 240
  *Salome*, 240
Strindberg, 239, 252
Suez Canal, 194, 202, 207, 217, 222, 308, 318, 323, 326, 335
Suvorov, 142
Sweden, 43, 49, 59, 64, 66, 69, 72, 75, 78, 79, 85, 89, 92, 95, 100, 101, 105, 110, 113, 116, 122, 144, 145, 233, 239, 252
  *see also* Scandinavia, Scandinavian Union
Swift, Jonathon, 124
  *Gulliver's Travels*, 124
Switzerland, 16, 38, 47–49, 51, 56, 59, 79, 89, 104, 119, 123, 144, 147, 161, 174, 187, 197, 227, 233, 250, 252, 284, 340, 342, 343

**T**

Tacitus, 7, 8
Tasso, 67
Tchaikovsky, 240
Tennyson, 208, 239
Terence, 8
Theresa, Empress Maria, 109, 111, 116
Thirty Years' War, *see* Germany, Thirty Years' War (1618–1648)
Thomson, 237
Thoreau, 208
Three Mile Island, Nuclear accident (1979), 349
Thucydides, 1, 4, 5, 8, 11
  History of the Peloponnesian War, 1
Tiepolo, Giovanni, 125
Tilly, 78
Titian, 29, 58, 59
Tito, Josip Broz, 322, 326, 330, 335
Tollendal, Lally, *see* France, colonies, Tollendal, Lally
Tolstoy, Alexei, 283
Tolstoy, Leo, 144, 154, 207, 208, 239, 241
  *Anna Karenina*, 208
  *War and Peace*, 144, 154, 207, 208
Transylvania, 270
Trotsky, Leon, 273, 274, 279, 291, 296, 305
  banishment from Soviet Union, 279, 305
Turgenev, 208
  *Fathers and Sons*, 208
Turgot, 110, 133
Turkey, *see* Ottoman Turkey
Turner, 174
Twain, Mark, 239

**U**

*Ulysses*, *see* Joyce, James, *Ulysses*
Ukraine, 80, 91, 100, 268, 286, 291, 296, 309, 339, 349, 352
*Uncle Tom's Cabin*, *see* Stowe, Harriet Beecher, *Uncle Tom's Cabin*
United Nations, 299, 312, 313, 323–327, 335, 337–339, 347, 351, 353, 360

United States of America, 120, 130, 131, 132, 139, 140, 145, 146, 151, 154, 157, 158, 160, 163, 166, 168, 173, 178, 184, 187, 192–194, 199, 201–203, 207, 208, 218, 223, 225, 226, 227, 232–236, 238, 239, 246–248, 252, 254–257, 259, 260, 263–266, 268, 270–273, 275, 278, 280, 283–289, 292, 296, 297, 299, 300, 301, 304, 305, 307, 309–313, 316, 319–323, 325–331, 335–338, 340, 342–344, 347, 349–353, 355, 357, 360
  abortion legalized, 336
  Adams, 131, 146
  Afghanistan, invasion of, 349
  African-Americans, 344, 347
  Agriculture, 234
  Alaska, purchase of, 202
  anti-Communism, 286
  "Articles of Confederation", 131
  Bancroft, 208
  "Bill of Rights", 146
  Bretton Woods, 321
  Briand-Kellogg Pact (1928), 287, 296
  Central America, and, 288, 348
    Panama, and, 247, 255, 256, 348
    invasion of, 348
  Civil Rights, 184, 344, 347
    Civil Rights Act, 344, 347
    Equal Pay Act, 344
  Civil War, 201, 207, 265
  Clayton (anti-trust) Act, 247
  Clinton, Bill, 348
  Cold War, 320, 321, 326, 337, 342
  Declaration of Independence, 120, 130, 131, 344
  Dumbarton Oaks, 321
  Far East, 257, 309
    Open-Door Policy, 257
  Fascist groups, 304, 305, 316, 325
  Feminism, 344
  Ford, Gerald, 340, 347
  Great Depression, 235, 299, 300, 316
  Grenada, invasion of, 336
  Hamilton, Alexander, 131
  immigrants and settlers, 160, 201, 223, 226
    fear of "Yellow Peril", 227
  industry and trade, 140, 168, 226, 233, 252, 255, 280, 281, 305, 353
    Ford, Henry, 255, 280, 281
    Fulton's steamship, 140
    Morgan, 255
    Rockefeller, 233, 255
  Jackson, Andrew, 160
  Jefferson, Thomas, 131, 146
  Kellogg, Frank, 287, 296
  Korean War, 326
  labor, 226, 236
    American Federation of Labor, 226
  Latin America, and, 256, 292
  Louisiana, purchase of, 140

  Marshall, 321
  Marshall Plan, 321
  Madison, James, 139
  Middle East, 338, 340, 347, 348, 351
    Iraq, invasion of, 348, 351
    Israel and Palestine, and, 351
  "Monroe Doctrine", 157, 166
  native Americans, 226
  NATO, 323, 335, 360
  New Deal, 304
  Nixon, Richard, 340, 347
  Nuclear accident at Three Mile Island, 349
  Pacific region, 227, 232, 309–311
    Hawaii, 227, 232, 255, 310
      Pearl Harbor, bombardment of, 310
    Japan, occupation of, 311
    Midway Islands, 227
    Philippines, 323
  Paine, Thomas, 120
  Parkman, 208
  Penn, William, 91
  population, 226
  Populists and Populism, 236, 246, 255
  Roosevelt, Franklin, 300, 305
  Roosevelt, Theodore, 254, 255, 263
  slavery, 160, 199, 201, 203, 207
    abolition of, 199, 203
    Missouri compromise, 160
  Social reforms, 325
  Socialists and Socialism, 227, 236, 246
  Society, 340
  Spanish-American war, 232, 246, 248, 255
  Suez Canal, involvement in, 194, 323, 335
    Suez Canal crisis, 323, 335
  Terrorism, war against, 349, 355, 357
  Three Mile Island, Nuclear accident (1979), 349
  United Nations, participation in, 312
    veto power, 312
  Vietnam War, 330, 337, 338
  War of Independence, 131
  Washington, George, 131, 146
  West-ward expansion, 160, 227
  Wilson, Woodrow, 255
  Women, 168, 178
  *see also* America

**V**

Van Dyke, 85
Valery, Paul, 284
Valois, House of, 38, 39, 42
Vasa, Gustavas, 30, 43, 47, 64
Vasco da Gama, 23, 27, 35
Vega, Lope de, 84
Velasquez, 85, 90, 91
Verdi, 207, 209, 214
  *Aida*, 207, 209
  *La Traviata*, 209
  *Rigoletto*, 209
Vermeer, 105
Verne, Jules, 207
  *Twenty Thousand Leagues under the Sea*, 207

Vesalius, 31, 43
  *De Humani Corporis Fabrica (The Structure of the Human Body)*, 43
Vespucci, Amerigo, *see* America, Vespucci, Amerigo
Vietnam, 318, 327, 330, 336, 337, 338, 340
  communist win, 336, 337
  North Vietnam, 338
  South Vietnam 338
  unification of, 336, 338
  US failure, 340
  war in, 318, 330, 336, 340
Viking invasion, 12
Vincent van Gogh, 217, 239
  *Sunflowers*, 217
Virgil, 8, 11
  *Aeneid*, 8, 11
Volta, 147
  Work on electrical current, 147
Voltaire, 109, 123, 124
  *Candide*, 109

**W**

Wagner, 209, 214, 248
  *Nibelungen Ring*, 209
  *Meistersinger*, 209
  *Parsifal*, 209
  *Tristan and Isolde*, 209
Wallenstein, 74, 78
Wandiwash, Battle of (1760), 109, 118
War of Devolution, 91, 95
Watt, James, 110, 123, 130
  Steam Engine, invention of, 110, 130
Weber, 155, 174
  *Der Freischutz*, 155
Weber, Max, 283, 296
Weismann, 237
Werfel, Franz, 283
Whistler, 239
Whitehead, Alfred North, 282
White Russia, 271
Whitman, 208
Whitney, 120
William of Orange, 58, 61, 98
  Low Countries, war of Independence against Spain, 61
Wilson, Harold, 339
Wilson, Woodrow, 255, 268, 270, 271, 278
Winckelmann, 124, 147, 154
Wittgenstein, Ludwig, 282
Wordsworth, 140, 150, 173
Workers' Movement, 192, 236
  First International, 192
  Second International, 236
World War I, 235, 236, 243, 247, 249–252, 256, 259, 260, 263–269, 272, 273, 280, 282, 283–288, 292, 296, 299, 301, 307, 308, 312, 318, 320, 323, 327, 330, 336, 353
  Armistice, 268
  Balkans, 259
  Britain, in, 259
  Ferdinand, Archduke Francis assassinated in Sarajevo, 259

Germany, in, 247, 263, 301
    Germany's arms build-up, 247
    invasion of Belgium, 263
Italy in, 251, 259, 301
Map of Europe, changed after, 269
Marne, first battle of, 264, 267
Russia, in, 259
    Treaty of Versailles (1918), 264, 269–271, 275, 278, 286, 287, 288, 290, 293, 297, 303, 306–308, 312
    reparations, 270, 272, 274, 275, 279, 285, 286, 287, 289, 290, 293, 297, 298, 300, 303
    Trench warfare, 267
    "Triple Alliance" of Germany-Austria-Italy, 263
    "Triple Entente" of France-England-Russia, 263
    plan, 266
Verdun, battle of, 264, 267
War Guilt, 266
World War II, 298, 299, 302, 306–313, 317–320, 323, 325, 327, 330, 331, 338–340, 342, 344
    Allies, 311
        attack Japan, 311
        invade Italy, 311
    Atomic bomb, 299, 313
    Axis powers, 298, 307, 311
    Rome-Berlin Axis, 298, 307
    Czechoslovakia, collapse of, 298
    Germany, in, 307, 308, 311
        anti-Comintern pact, 307
        invasion of Poland, 308, 317
        occupation of France, 308
        Stalingrad, defeat at, 311
        surrender of, 299
    Italy, in, 298, 307, 308, 311
        annexes Abyssinia, 298
        invades Albania, 298, 308
        invades Ethiopia, 307
    Japan in, 298, 299, 306, 307, 310, 311, 313, 323
        anti-Comintern pact, 307
        atomic bomb dropped by USA, 299, 313
        expansion in China, 298, 306, 311
        Japanese policy and strategy in, 309
        Manchuria, establishment as a separate state, 306
        Russian entry in war against Japan, 311
        surrender of, 299
    Maginot Line, 308
    Munich Conference ("appeasement"), 298, 307, 317
    Occupation of Germany and Japan, 311
    Pacific, in, 310, 311
        Hiroshima, atomic bombing on, 311
        Nagasaki, atomic bombing on, 311
        Pearl Harbor, attack on, 299, 310
    Potsdam Conference, 312, 321
    Soviet Union and, see Russia, USSR, World War II
    Teheran Conference, 312
    United States, entry into the war, 311
    Yalta Conference (1945), 299, 312, 321, 349
Wright brothers, 233, 247
    Airplane, invention of, 233, 247
Wright, Frank Lloyd, 284

**X**
Xavier, Francis, 77

**Y**
Yeats, William Butler, 284
Yeltsin, Boris, 348, 352, 354
Young, Owen D., 298, 300
    Young Plan, 298, 300
Yugoslavia, 270, 286, 302, 322, 326, 330, 335, 339, 348, 349, 353
    civil war and break-up of, 348, 349, 353
    King Alexander, 302
    NATO intervention, 353
    Tito, Josip Broz, 322, 326, 330, 335
    see also Balkans,
    see also Bosnia
    see also Croatia,
    see also Montenegro
    see also Serbia
    see also Slovenia

**Z**
Zola, Emil, 208, 239, 251, 263
Zwingli, Ulrich, see Church, Reformation, Ulrich Zwingli

# Collins College OUTLINES
*Fully Revised and Updated*

**INTRODUCTION TO BUSINESS**
H. James Williams
ISBN 978-0-06-088149-8 (paperback)

**WESTERN CIVILIZATION FROM 1500**
Ahmed Ibrahim and Walter Kirchner
ISBN: 978-0-06-088160-3 (paperback)

**COLLEGE CHEMISTRY***
Drew H. Wolfe and Steven Boone
ISBN: 978-0-06-088147-4 (paperback)

**COLLEGE BIOLOGY***
Marshall Sundberg
ISBN: 978-0-06-088161-0 (paperback)

**BASIC MATHEMATICS**
Lawrence A. Trivieri
ISBN 978-0-06-088146-7 (paperback)

**INTRODUCTION TO CALCULUS**
Joan Van Glabek
ISBN 978-0-06-088150-4 (paperback)

**INTRODUCTION TO AMERICAN GOVERNMENT***
Larry Elowitz
ISBN 978-0-06-088151-1 (paperback)

**INTRODUCTION TO PSYCHOLOGY***
Joseph Johnson and Ann L. Weber
ISBN 978-0-06-088152-8 (paperback)

**MODERN EUROPEAN HISTORY**
John R. Barber
ISBN 978-0-06-088153-5 (paperback)

**ORGANIC CHEMISTRY**
Michael Smith
ISBN 978-0-06-088154-2 (paperback)

**UNITED STATES HISTORY TO 1877***
Light Cummins and Arnold M. Rice
ISBN 978-0-06-088159-7 (paperback)

**WESTERN CIVILIZATION TO 1500**
John Chuchiak and Walter Kirchner
ISBN 978-0-06-088162-7 (paperback)

**ABNORMAL PSYCHOLOGY**
Sarah Sifers
ISBN 978-0-06-088145-0 (paperback)

**UNITED STATES HISTORY FROM 1865***
John Baick and Arnold M. Rice
ISBN 978-0-06-088158-0 (paperback)

**ELEMENTARY ALGEBRA**
Joan Van Glabek
ISBN 978-0-06-088148-1 (paperback)

**SPANISH GRAMMAR**
Ana Fairchild and Juan Mendez
ISBN 978-0-06-088157-3 (paperback)

***PERFECT FOR AP REVIEW**

Available wherever books are sold, or call 1-800-331-3761 to order.